Evidence-based Management of

LIPID DISORDERS

Maud N. Vissers
John J. P. Kastelein
Erik S. Stroes

i

tfm Publishing Limited, Castle Hill Barns, Harley, Nr Shrewsbury, SY5 6LX, UK.
Tel: +44 (0)1952 510061; Fax: +44 (0)1952 510192
E-mail: nikki@tfmpublishing.com; Web site: www.tfmpublishing.com

Design & Typesetting: Nikki Bramhill BSc Hons Dip Law
First Edition: © August 2010
ISBN: 978 1 903378 71 7

Cover image: © 2010 3d4medical, www.3d4medical.com

Printed by Gutenberg Press Ltd., Gudja Road, Tarxien, PLA 19, Malta.
Tel: +356 21897037; Fax: +356 21800069.

Contents

Foreword

Worldwide, cardiovascular diseases are among the leading causes of death, and atherosclerosis is by far their most common cause. A century has passed since the term 'atherosclerosis' was first introduced by F. Marchand in 1904, who suggested that atherosclerosis was responsible for almost all obstructive processes in the arteries. A few years later, the relationship between cholesterol and atherosclerotic plaques was discovered, first by A. Windaus, who detected cholesterol in human atheromatous lesions in 1910, and shortly thereafter, in 1914, by N. Anichkov and S. Chalatow, who discovered the significance and role of cholesterol in atherosclerosis pathogenesis based on their landmark experiments in rabbits. These discoveries heralded a spectacular research effort in the relation between cholesterol and atherosclerosis.

A century of studies on atherosclerosis later, we not only acknowledge the crucial role of LDL-cholesterol in the development of cardiovascular diseases, but we also recognize other players in the field. These risk factors include, but are not restricted to, low HDL-cholesterol levels, high triglyceride levels and the size of the lipoproteins, as well as lifestyle and diseases that impair a healthy lipoprotein balance, such as diabetes, metabolic syndrome, inflammatory diseases, renal insufficiency, and – although not related to lipids – hypertension. Along with these discoveries, several therapeutic strategies have been developed during the last decades. Some of them have been proven to improve lipid levels and to reduce cardiovascular risk, whereas others are still in the investigational phase.

The authors were asked to look systematically at the literature and to evaluate and interpret the available evidence on the selected topics in order to provide the reader with a reliable summary of the current knowledge on the management of lipid disorders. Each chapter concludes with a series of key points that present a summary of evidence-based recommendations for best practice, graded according to the quality of the evidence. For certain topics, however, there are no data from well-designed randomized controlled trials (RCTs), just because it is too early or RCTs are not feasible. As outlined in the first chapter by Dr. Steinberg, RCTs provide by far the most valuable evidence guiding decisions regarding medical intervention, but other relevant evidence must be considered as well. In such cases we have to rely on case reports, descriptive studies or opinions and/or clinical experience of respected authorities.

We are grateful to all the authors for their phenomenal task in putting all the available evidence-based information together. We hope that readers will enjoy all the chapters as much as we did.

Maud N. Vissers PhD
John J.P. Kastelein MD PhD
Erik S. Stroes MD PhD
Amsterdam, May 2010

Contributors

Rob E. Aarnoutse PharmD PhD Hospital Pharmacist, Department of Clinical Pharmacy, Radboud University Nijmegen Medical Centre, Nijmegen, The Netherlands

Evertine J. Abbink MD PhD Research Physician, Department of General Internal Medicine, Radboud University Nijmegen Medical Centre, Nijmegen, the Netherlands

Martin Adiels MSc PhD Assistant Researcher, Sahlgrenska Center for Metabolism and Cardiovascular Research, Wallenberg Laboratory for Cardiovascular Research and the Department of Molecular and Clinical Medicine, The Sahlgrenska Academy, University of Gothenburg, Gothenburg, Sweden

Jane Armitage FFPH FRCP Professor of Clinical Trials and Epidemiology, Clinical Trial Service Unit & Epidemiological Studies Unit (CTSU), University of Oxford, Oxford, UK

Benoit J. Arsenault PhD Researcher, Centre de Recherche de l'Institut Universitaire de Cardiologie et de Pneumologie de Québec, Canada

Vincent W. Bloks Research Officer, Center for Liver, Digestive and Metabolic Diseases, Beatrix Children's Hospital – University Medical Center Groningen, University of Groningen, The Netherlands

Jan Borén MD PhD Professor of Cardiovascular Medicine, Sahlgrenska Center for Metabolism and Cardiovascular Research, Wallenberg Laboratory for Cardiovascular Research and the Department of Molecular and Clinical Medicine, The Sahlgrenska Academy, University of Gothenburg, Gothenburg, Sweden

Louise Bowman MD MRCP Clinical Research Fellow, Clinical Trial Service Unit & Epidemiological Studies Unit (CTSU), University of Oxford, Oxford, UK

David M. Burger PharmD PhD Hospital Pharmacist - Clinical Pharmacologist, Department of Clinical Pharmacy, Radboud University Nijmegen Medical Centre, Nijmegen, The Netherlands

Jacqueline de Graaf MD PhD Vascular Specialist, Department of General Internal Medicine, Radboud University Nijmegen Medical Centre, Nijmegen, the Netherlands

Jean-Pierre Després PhD FAHA Director of Research, Cardiology, Centre de Recherche de l'Institut Universitaire de Cardiologie et de Pneumologie de Québec, Canada

Christiane Drechsler MD Fellow, Nephrology and Clinical Research, Department of Nephrology, Leiden University Medical Center, Leiden, The Netherlands

Henk-Jan Guchelaar PhD Professor of Clinical Pharmacy and Hospital Pharmacist, Department of Clinical Pharmacy & Toxicology, Leiden University Medical Center, Leiden, The Netherlands

Robert A. Hegele MD FRCPC FACP Director, Blackburn Cardiovascular Genetics Laboratory; Scientist, Vascular Biology Research Group, Robarts Research Institute, London, Ontario, Canada

G. Kees Hovingh MD PhD Resident, Internal Medicine and Vascular Medicine, Department of Vascular Medicine, Academic Medical Center, Amsterdam, The Netherlands

Tisha R. Joy MD FRCPC Assistant Professor, Department of Medicine, Schulich School of Medicine and Dentistry, University of Western Ontario, London, Ontario, Canada

John J.P. Kastelein MD PhD Professor of Medicine, Department of Vascular Medicine, Academic Medical Centre, University of Amsterdam, Amsterdam, The Netherlands

Folkert Kuipers PhD Professor, Dean of Faculty of Medical Sciences, Center for Liver, Digestive and Metabolic Diseases, Beatrix Children's Hospital – University Medical Center Groningen, University of Groningen, The Netherlands

Peter J. Lansberg MD PhD Co-ordinator, Durrer Center for Cardiogenetic Research, Department of Vascular Medicine, Academic Medical Center, Amsterdam, The Netherlands

Sarah Lewington MSc DPhil Senior Research Fellow, Clinical Trial Service Unit & Epidemiological Studies Unit (CTSU), University of Oxford, Oxford, UK

Ronald P. Mensink PhD MSc Professor of Molecular Nutrition, Department of Human Biology, Maastricht University, Maastricht, The Netherlands

Michael T. Nurmohamed MD PhD Consultant Rheumatologist, Departments of Internal Medicine & Rheumatology, VU University Medical Centre; Department of Rheumatology, Jan van Breemen Institute, Amsterdam, The Netherlands

Sven-Olof Olofsson MD PhD Professor of Medical Biochemistry, Sahlgrenska Center for Metabolism and Cardiovascular Research, Wallenberg Laboratory for Cardiovascular Research and the Department of Molecular and Clinical Medicine, The Sahlgrenska Academy, University of Gothenburg, Gothenburg, Sweden

Frans L. Opdam MD Fellow, Vascular Medicine, Section of Vascular Medicine, Department of Endocrinology and Internal Medicine, Leiden University Medical Center, Leiden, The Netherlands

Shailendra B. Patel BM ChB DPhil FRCP Professor of Medicine, Medical College of Wisconsin, and the Clement J. Zablocki Veterans Affairs Medical Center, Milwaukee, Wisconsin, USA

Jogchum Plat PhD Associate Professor, Human Biology, Department of Human Biology, Maastricht University, Maastricht, The Netherlands

Ton Rabelink MD PhD Professor of Nephrology, Department of Nephrology, Leiden University Medical Center, Leiden, The Netherlands

Gerald Salen MD Professor of Medicine, University of Medicine and Dentistry of New Jersey, New Jersey Medical School, Newark, New Jersey, USA

Anton F. Stalenhoef MD PhD FRCP Professor of Medicine, Department of General Internal Medicine, Radboud University Nijmegen Medical Centre, Nijmegen, the Netherlands

Daniel Steinberg MD PhD Professor of Medicine Emeritus, University of California San Diego, La Jolla, California, USA

Erik S. Stroes MD PhD Professor of Medicine, Department of Vascular Medicine, Academic Medical Centre, University of Amsterdam, Amsterdam, The Netherlands

Jouke T. Tamsma MD PhD Consultant, Vascular Medicine, Section of Vascular Medicine, Department of Endocrinology and Internal Medicine, Leiden University Medical Center, Leiden, The Netherlands

Marja-Riitta Taskinen MD PhD Professor of Medicine, Division of Cardiology, University of Helsinki, Biomedicum, Helsinki, Finland

Serena Tonstad MD PhD Head Physician, Department of Preventive Cardiology, Oslo University Hospital Ullevål, Oslo, Norway; Professor, Clinical Nutrition, Department of Nutrition, University of Oslo, Oslo, Norway

Sotirios Tsimikas MD FACC FAHA FSCAI Professor of Medicine, Division of Cardiology, Vascular Medicine Program, University of California San Diego, La Jolla, California

Hester van Meer MD Paediatrician, Fellow Paediatric Gastroenterology, Center for Liver, Digestive and Metabolic Diseases, Beatrix Children's Hospital – University Medical Center Groningen, University of Groningen, The Netherlands

Menno Vergeer MD Resident, Internal Medicine and Vascular Medicine, Department of Vascular Medicine, Academic Medical Center, Amsterdam, The Netherlands

Henkjan J. Verkade MD Professor, Paediatric Gastroenterologist and Chair, Department of Paediatrics, Center for Liver, Digestive and Metabolic Diseases, Beatrix Children's Hospital – University Medical Center Groningen, University of Groningen, The Netherlands

Adie Viljoen MBBS FRCPath Consultant Chemical Pathologist, Lister Hospital, Stevenage, Hertfordshire, UK

Maud N. Vissers PhD Researcher, Department of Vascular Medicine, Academic Medical Centre, University of Amsterdam, Amsterdam, The Netherlands

Christoph Wanner MD PhD Professor of Nephrology, Department of Medicine, Division of Nephrology, University Hospital Würzburg, Germany

Anthony S. Wierzbicki DM DPhil FRCPath FAHA Consultant Metabolic Physician & Chemical Pathologist, Guy's & St Thomas' Hospitals, London, UK

Acknowledgements

We are grateful to all of the contributors for taking on this important task and hope they will be proud to be part of a book which attempts to set out the evidence-based management of lipid disorders.

We would also like to thank Nikki Bramhill and Jonathan Gregory from tfm Publishing Limited for their invaluable assistance.

Using evidence-based medicine

The process of gathering evidence is a time-consuming task. One of the main reasons for supporting the use of evidence-based medicine, is the rate of change of new practices, and the increasing tendency for specialisation. Medical information is widely available from a variety of sources for clinicians but keeping up-to-date with current literature remains an almost impossible task for many with a busy clinical workload. *Evidence-based Management of Lipid Disorders* has been written to aid this process. The chapters in this book have been written by internationally renowned experts who have applied the principles of evidence-based medicine and taken relevant clinical questions and examined the current evidence for the answers. The authors were asked to quote levels and grades of evidence for each major point, and to provide a summary of key points and their respective evidence levels at the end of each chapter. The levels of evidence and grades of evidence used in this book are shown in Tables 1 and 2 and are widely used in evidence-based medicine.

Table 1. Levels of evidence.

Level	Type of evidence
Ia	Evidence obtained from systematic review or meta-analysis of randomised controlled trials
Ib	Evidence obtained from at least one randomised controlled trial
IIa	Evidence obtained from at least one well-designed controlled study without randomisation
IIb	Evidence obtained from at least one other type of well-designed quasi-experimental study
III	Evidence obtained from well-designed non-experimental descriptive studies, such as comparative studies, correlation studies and case studies
IV	Evidence obtained from expert committee reports or opinions and/or clinical experience of respected authorities

Table 2. Grades of evidence.

Grade of evidence	Evidence
A	At least one randomised controlled trial as part of a body of literature of overall good quality and consistency addressing the specific recommendation (evidence levels Ia and Ib)
B	Well-conducted clinical studies but no randomised clinical trials on the topic of recommendation (evidence levels IIa, IIb, III)
C	Expert committee reports or opinions and/or clinical experience of respected authorities. This grading indicates that directly applicable clinical studies of good quality are absent (evidence level IV)

Chapter 1

How much evidence is enough?

Daniel Steinberg MD PhD, Professor of Medicine Emeritus
University of California San Diego, La Jolla, California, USA

Introduction

The title is deliberately vague. One needs to know more. "Enough for what?" If, for example, the issue is whether or not to approve clinical use of a promising new cancer drug even though it may have potentially lethal side effects, the evidence for efficacy had better be all but overwhelming. If, at the other extreme, the only issue is whether or not to pursue further animal research on a promising drug, a few preliminary *in vitro* studies might be sufficient evidence. Obviously, the bar has to be set at the level appropriate to the specific question under consideration. This chapter discusses the criteria we use in deciding whether or not to accept a given hypothesis as proven and, most important, whether or not to go ahead and recommend its incorporation into medical practice.

Evidence-based medicine

The large-scale, randomized, double-blinded, placebo-controlled clinical trial (RCT) continues to be the gold standard for evaluation of a new medical or surgical intervention. This is as it should be. Everyone will agree that the best way to find out if an intervention really works is to do an RCT, a single-variable experiment that tests the new intervention against a placebo or against an alternative intervention already in use. However, in the minds of many clinicians and investigators, this is the *only kind of evidence* that counts. The 'evidence' in evidence-based medicine has come to be almost synonymous with results from RCTs. Yet evidence-based medicine was originally meant to call for integrating clinical expertise and the best external evidence [1]. There was never an intention to confine the relevant evidence to the results of RCTs. For example, if there is already evidence from animal model studies that a certain inborn error of metabolism responds favourably to a simple dietary intervention, that should be taken into account. If that dietary intervention is totally harmless, and especially if the disease is so rare that a large-scale trial is out of the question, few would argue against testing the treatment in a few selected cases. Over 200 years ago Thomas Bayes formally proposed using what he called a "prior probability", based on previous trials and/or other relevant lines of evidence, in evaluating the truth of a hypothesis. In the present context the Bayesian view is that you should consider the likelihood of a hypothesis based on all the relevant evidence available to you before you enter into a clinical trial and weight the significance of the results of the current trial accordingly. Now, pooling the results of previous clinical trials with the results of a new clinical trial can and should be done using the Bayesian approach [2]. Unfortunately, there is no easy way to quantify and weigh other kinds of evidence so that they can be taken account of in a mathematically rigorous fashion. For example, let's assume you have a new antibiotic that has cured septicemia due to a penicillin-resistant *S. aureus* in 90% of 100 rats treated with it. You carry out a clinical trial in 100 cases of septicemia due to this same organism and find a cure rate of 70%. However, the p value is 0.07. Should the FDA give approval even though the p value is >0.05? Most of us would probably vote for approval, taking into account the remarkable results of the prior animal studies. But what if the cure rate in the clinical trial were only 1.5% with a p value of 0.04? With such a numerically small (even though statistically significant) cure rate, we would probably defer judgment until additional evidence became available.

How much of what we do is based exclusively on RCT data?

Many, perhaps most, of the things we do in clinical medicine do not have the imprimatur of an RCT to back them up. For example, the hypothesis that cigarette smoking causes lung cancer has never been proved by an RCT… and almost certainly never will be. However, the strikingly high morbidity and mortality in cigarette smokers, together with the facts that risk decreases when they quit and that cigarette smoke contains carcinogens, was more than sufficient to justify the current vigorous public health programs to help people stop smoking [3]. Unfortunately, most of the major chronic disease problems that face us have multiple rather than single etiologies and their prevention is not nearly so straightforward. Still, here is an example of a major public health problem in which prevention and treatment is based not on RCT data but ancillary evidence of several different kinds.

When a clinician today prescribes statins or other cholesterol-lowering drugs for hypercholesterolemia, he has strong RCT data to back him up. Yet his confidence that he is doing the right thing is importantly based also – directly or indirectly, knowingly or unknowingly, – on the many additional lines of evidence that have supported the lipid hypothesis over the years. The first large-scale RCT to critically test the lipid hypothesis was the National Institutes of Health Coronary Primary Prevention Trial (CPPT) published in 1984 [4]. However, for many years before that some physicians were already recommending dietary and drug regimens for lowering blood cholesterol. They felt justified in doing so because of the lines of evidence coming from several different biomedical disciplines (Table 1).

Table 1. The multiple different kinds of evidence supporting the lipid hypothesis available prior to the large-scale randomized clinical trials.

Source of the evidence	Nature of the evidence	References
Human pathology	Cholesterol derived from plasma lipoproteins is a consistent and striking feature of atherosclerotic lesions	(5)
Experimental pathology	Lesions similar to those of human atherosclerosis can be produced in many different animal species by raising the level of cholesterol in their blood to a high enough level and maintaining it for a long enough time	(6)
Genetic studies	People with dramatically high blood cholesterol levels, as in familial hypercholesterolemia, have dramatically premature coronary heart disease	(7)
Epidemiology	People with even relatively modest elevations of blood cholesterol levels are at significantly higher risk. This is true across a wide spectrum of blood cholesterol levels and holds on comparison of populations from different countries and also within populations	(8, 9)
Clinical investigation	Blood cholesterol level is increased when dietary saturated fat intake is increased, as shown by carefully controlled metabolic ward studies	(10, 11)
Epidemiology	Populations with dietary habits that include a high saturated fat intake have higher blood cholesterol levels and a higher coronary heart disease incidence than populations with lower saturated fat intake	(12)
Geographic epidemiology	The wide differences in blood cholesterol levels and coronary heart disease risk between populations of different countries is largely due to environmental factors (probably diet) rather than genetic factors, as shown, for example, by the Japanese migration studies	(13)
Pilot clinical trials	Dietary intervention to lower blood cholesterol decreased the risk of coronary heart disease in several studies, small and flawed in some ways, but offering support to the lipid hypothesis	(14-17)

All of these findings were already in hand by the early '70s but there was no truly definitive RCT until the 1984 CPPT [4]. Still most research workers in the relevant fields were already convinced of the causal relationship between blood cholesterol and coronary heart disease. In 1978, Norum surveyed 211 scientists involved in one or another way in atherosclerosis research – epidemiologists, nutritionists, geneticists, clinical investigators [18]. The response rate was a remarkable 90% so the results are representative. He asked: "Do you think there is a connection between plasma cholesterol level and the development of coronary heart disease?" Almost 98% said "Yes". To the question, "Do you think that our knowledge about diet and coronary heart disease is sufficient to recommend a moderate change in the diet for the population in an affluent society?", 91% said "Yes". In other words for years prior to the publication of a large definitive RCT almost 90% of experts in the field already believed that blood cholesterol levels were causally linked to heart attacks.

Nevertheless, most clinicians were unwilling to take hypercholesterolemia seriously and most authorities were unwilling to extrapolate from the lines of evidence listed above and get on with developing intervention guidelines and treatment programs. In retrospect they were too conservative and cholesterol levels below 300mg/dL continued to be considered 'in the normal range'. How many myocardial infarctions could have been prevented had measures to reduce hypercholesterolemia been actively pursued in the 1970s? But policy makers were unwilling to take action without RCT evidence, the gold standard.

The history of how we have approached the management of hypercholesterolemia over the years is marked by extraordinary conservatism. In fact even after the 1984 Coronary Primary Prevention Trial had provided the RCT data that should have convinced even the skeptics about the causative linkage between hypercholesterolemia and coronary heart disease, there was continuing resistance to implementing appropriate interventions. It was argued that the CPPT study was done in men only and therefore did not justify treatment in women. It was argued that the study was done using a drug (cholestyramine) and therefore did not justify recommendations for diet treatment. It was argued that the study was done in middle-aged men with very high cholesterol levels and therefore did not justify treatment in the very old or in the very young. While the CPPT showed a statistically significant reduction in coronary heart disease morbidity and mortality, all-cause mortality was not reduced. It was argued then that lowering cholesterol levels might be increasing deaths due to other causes. Well, as we all know now, each and every one of these objections to extrapolation from the CPPT was laid to rest by subsequent clinical trials using statins because blood cholesterol was lowered more effectively and therefore the decrease in hard endpoints was greater. There is little doubt that the foot dragging that held back full implementation of cholesterol-lowering programs for years was responsible for many thousands of preventable coronary events.

Today we are being asked to consider another extrapolation: should we consider initiating cholesterol-lowering treatment at an earlier age, say age 30, in patients at only moderately high risk?

The case for earlier intervention

The war against coronary heart disease is going well: statins reduce events by about one third. Yet many are asking: what about the two thirds that go on and have their infarction despite statin treatment? Some have concluded that this 30% salvage rate is the best that can be done with current methods of treatment... that better results will require alternative interventions such as the use of anti-inflammatory agents. But if treatment were started at an earlier age, say 30 rather than 50 or 60, the salvage rate could be considerably higher, possibly as high as 80-90%. The evidence to support this point of view is extensive and persuasive, as reviewed by Steinberg, Glass and Witztum [19]. Why do we think we can do better?

Human pathology

The Japanese in 1952 had a mortality rate from coronary heart disease that was about 10% that in the United States [20, 21] and this large difference was not genetically based. Epidemiologic studies have shown that the Japanese who migrate to Hawaii or to San Francisco have higher blood cholesterol levels and a higher incidence of coronary heart disease [13, 22]. This occurs within a few generations so the gene pool has not had time to change significantly. There is good reason to believe that the major change in the new environment is diet. Keys reported that the fat content of the diet rose from 10-15% of total calories in Japanese on the home island to about 30% in Japanese migrants to Hawaii and to almost 40% in migrants to Los Angeles [12].

Now the Japanese follow the dietary patterns of their country for their entire lifetime and thus they have their lower cholesterol levels over that lifetime. In contrast, most of our clinical trials only last for 5 years. Even if the drop in blood cholesterol during that 5-year trial is profound enough to bring it down to Japanese levels, the event rate is unlikely to drop to the Japanese event rates. The canonical 5-year trials give us a minimum estimate of the impact of preventive management.

Fatty streak lesions

Fatty streak lesions begin in childhood and are extensive by age 30 [23, 24]. These fatty streaks themselves are clinically benign. However, they are the precursors of the fibrous plaque and, ultimately, the vulnerable plaque that is the site of fatal thrombosis. We know that the risk factors correlating with the extent of fatty streaks in the young, including hypercholesterolemia, hypertension and obesity, also correlate with coronary heart disease risk in adults [25, 26]. So we are dealing with a single disease entity that evolves slowly over many decades. The PDAY study [27] showed that the arterial sites susceptible to fatty streak formation are anatomically the same as those susceptible to plaque formation. It follows that if we intervened early and were able to limit fatty streak formation we would prevent or at least defer the later evolution to the fibrous plaque and the vulnerable plaque. Instead of deferring treatment until middle age, as most clinicians do with patients at only moderate short-term risk, why not nip the fatty streak in the bud? *Reductio ad absurdum*, no one would seriously advocate deferring treatment of diabetes until microvascular disease became clinically evident. We should not be waiting until an age when clinical coronary heart disease is just around the corner.

Early statin treatment

There are no serious untoward effects of early statin treatment, even in children. We already treat very high-risk patients in childhood (e.g. patients with familial hypercholesterolemia). It has been shown that it works and that it is safe. In children ages 8 to 18, pravastatin treatment for 2 years did not impair growth or maturation [28]. Starting treatment at an earlier age would entail a longer exposure to drug so both risk/benefit and cost/benefit would have to be taken into account. New guidelines would have to balance the anticipated improvement in prognosis against the risk and cost of treatment.

A low LDL level from birth

Having a low LDL level from birth confers much greater protection from coronary heart disease than does a comparable degree of cholesterol-lowering over the 5 years of a clinical trial. This is dramatically demonstrated by recent studies by Cohen, Hobbs and colleagues on a new gene importantly involved in regulation of the LDL receptor [28, 29]. This gene (*PCSK9*) codes for a protein that plays a major role in regulating cell surface expression of the LDL receptor. Adults with a nonsense mutation in *PCSK9* have plasma LDL levels that are 28% lower than that found in those with the normal gene. Now, in the 5-year statin trials a 28% drop in LDL would be associated with a 25-35% drop in risk. In contrast, risk in these subjects with the mutations was reduced by fully 88% [30, 31]. As nicely pointed out by Brown and Goldstein [32], the implication is that having a low LDL from birth almost triples the magnitude of the effect on risk compared to that seen in a 5-year trial starting in middle age. The findings of Cohen and Hobbs have been confirmed by two groups [33, 34]. They strongly support a mandate to treat earlier. Drugs that regulate the expression and function of PCSK9 are probably in the pipeline. Since PCSK9 works by a different mechanism, such inhibitors would probably have effects additive to those of other drugs.

Levels of LDL currently considered 'normal' or 'acceptable'

The levels of LDL currently considered 'normal' or 'acceptable' are not benign with regard to atherogenesis. The results of the recent JUPITER Trial make that clear [35]. This trial randomized 17,802 apparently healthy men (age 50 or older) and women (age 60 or older) to placebo or to 20mg rosuvastatin daily. An entry hsCRP level of 2.0mg/L was required but other major risk factors were a basis for exclusion. The combined primary endpoint was myocardial infarction, stroke, arterial revascularisation, hospitalisation for unstable angina or cardiovascular death. Initial LDL had to be less than 130mg/dL and the median value for the cohort was 108mg/dL. The study was interrupted after only a little less than 2 years because of a striking 44% reduction in endpoints in the treated group (hazard ratio 0.56, p<0.00001). LDL was reduced to a median of 50mg/dL. Because subjects with high-risk factors (other than CRP) were excluded, the absolute incidence of endpoints was very low – 0.77 and 1.36 per 100 person-years in the treated and untreated groups, respectively, but the relative risk reduction was as great as that in the groups at much higher risk in other statin trials. The JUPITER results further underscore the need to treat more aggressively and to widen the net both in terms of LDL level and age.

So what should be recommended?

It is already best practice to treat those at very highest risk, e.g. patients with familial hypercholesterolemia, from childhood. Patients with established clinical coronary heart disease or diabetes are also treated aggressively on discovery, at whatever age. On the other hand, according to current guidelines [36], a 40-year-old man with a cholesterol level of 229mg/dL would not qualify for aggressive treatment because his 10-year Framingham risk might be only 5%. However, even though he develops no additional risk factors, over the years his calculated Framingham risk rises progressively and his life-time risk, the probability of his having a major cardiovascular event sooner or later, is 43% [37, 38]. At age 40 the extent of atherosclerosis is already quite significant and gets progressively worse over the ensuing decades. It would seem reasonable to recommend that this man and others with a similarly high life-time risk should be treated more aggressively beginning no later than age 30. A recent analysis by the Heart Protection Study Collaborative Group concludes that life-time treatment with 40mg/d of simvastatin at current generic prices would be cost effective in people age 35-85, even in those with risk of a major cardiovascular event as low as 1% per year [39].

However, because there are no RCTs in 30-year-olds, those responsible for developing guidelines are unlikely to make such a proposal. They will more likely tend to be conservative and only make recommendations that bear the imprimitur "evidence-based medicine". They are more likely to say "Let's wait for the clinical trial". But in this instance a clinical trial is not feasible. A clinical trial of drug treatment initiated at age 30 would have to span 25 years or more and would be forbiddingly expensive. It surely isn't going to happen soon, if ever. If, as we believe, treatment started at 30 would double current salvage rates with statin therapy, each year we delay the 'treat early' strategy may be costing thousands of lives. Doing nothing is *de facto* making a decision. Do we sit on our hands? Or do we invoke the power of the lipid hypothesis and urge those who write the guidelines to think outside the box and consider departing from current practice. There are so many lines of evidence justifying the extrapolation that Bayes himself would no doubt concur and so would most clinicians.

Conclusions

In this chapter we have chosen for analysis the particular case of the management of hypercholesterolemia but similar dilemmas are bound to arise in other areas of medicine. We should not be rigidly wedded to the RCT as the only arbiter of what is best medical practice. This is obviously the case when an RCT trial is not feasible or is many decades down the road. Even when RCT data are available, decisions about intervention should take into consideration all of the relevant evidence, not just the RCT data.

Key points	Evidence level
◆ While the results of a randomized, double-blind clinical trial (RCT) provide by far the most valuable evidence guiding decisions regarding medical intervention, other relevant evidence must be considered as well.	Not applicable
◆ Evidence from clinical observations, basic studies of pathogenesis, animal model studies, epidemiologic correlations, genetic studies, and any other relevant sources should be considered along with the RCT results in deciding whether or not to recommend a new intervention.	Not applicable
◆ In some instances an RCT may not even be feasible and yet a recommendation for intervention may be warranted on the basis of other lines of evidence. This was the case with respect to cigarette smoking and lung cancer. With appropriate attention to risk/benefit ratio, the same may be true of earlier intervention to correct hypercholesterolemia and other risk factors for coronary heart disease.	Not applicable

References

1.   Sackett DL, Rosenberg WM, Gray JA, Haynes RB, Richardson WS. Evidence based medicine: what it is and what it isn't. *BMJ* 1996; 312(7023): 71-2.
2.   Diamond GA, Kaul S. Prior convictions: Bayesian approaches to the analysis and interpretation of clinical megatrials. *J Am Coll Cardiol* 2004; 43(11):1929-39.
3.   Doll R. An epidemiological perspective of the biology of cancer. *Cancer Res* 1978; 38(11 Pt 1): 3573-83.
4.   The Lipid Research Clinics Coronary Primary Prevention Trial results. I. Reduction in incidence of coronary heart disease. *JAMA* 1984; 251(3): 351-64.
5.   Windaus A. Uber den Gehalt normaler und atheromatoser Aorten an Cholsterin und Cholesterinestern. *Hoppe-Seyler Z Physiol Chemie* 1910; 67: 174-6.
6.   Anitschkow N. Experimental atherosclerosis in animals. In: *Arteriosclerosis*. Cowdry EV, Ed. New York: Macmillan, 1933: 271-322.
7.   Muller C. Angina pectoris in hereditary xanthomatosis. *Arch Int Med* 1939; 64: 675-700.
8.   Keys A. Coronary disease in seven countries. *Circulation* 1970; 41 Suppl. 1): 1-211.
9.   Kannel WB, Dawber TR, Kagan A, Revotskie N, Stokes J, III. Factors of risk in the development of coronary heart disease - six year follow-up experience. The Framingham Study. *Ann Intern Med* 1961; 55: 33-50.
10.   Kinsell LW, Partridge J, Boling L, Margen S, Michael G. Dietary modification of serum cholesterol and phospholipid levels. *J Clin Endocrinol Metab* 1952; 12(7): 909-13.

11. Ahrens EH, Jr., Blankenhorn DH, Tsaltas TT. Effect on human serum lipids of substituting plant for animal fat in diet. *Proc Soc Exp Biol Med* 1954; 86(4): 872-8.

12. Keys A. Diet and the epidemiology of coronary heart disease. *J Am Med Assoc* 1957; 164(17): 1912-9.

13. Robertson TL, Kato H, Rhoads GG, *et al*. Epidemiologic studies of coronary heart disease and stroke in Japanese men living in Japan, Hawaii and California. Incidence of myocardial infarction and death from coronary heart disease. *Am J Cardiol* 1977; 39(2): 239-43.

14. Leren P. The effect of plasma cholesterol lowering diet in male survivors of myocardial infarction. A controlled clinical trial. *Acta Med Scand Suppl* 1966; 466: 1-92.

15. Leren P. The Oslo diet-heart study. Eleven-year report. *Circulation* 1970; 42(5): 935-42.

16. Dayton S, Pearce ML, Goldman H, Harnish A, Plotkin D, Shickman M, *et al*. Controlled trial of a diet high in unsaturated fat for prevention of atherosclerotic complications. *Lancet* 1968; 2(7577): 1060-2.

17. Miettinen M, Turpeinen O, Karvonen MJ, Elosuo R, Paavilainen E. Effect of cholesterol-lowering diet on mortality from coronary heart-disease and other causes. A twelve-year clinical trial in men and women. *Lancet* 1972; 2(7782): 835-8.

18. Norum KR. Some present concepts concerning diet and prevention of coronary heart disease. *Nutr Metab* 1978; 22(1): 1-7.

19. Steinberg D, Glass CK, Witztum JL. Evidence mandating earlier and more aggressive treatment of hypercholesterolemia. *Circulation* 2008; 118(6): 672-7.

20. Kimura N. Analysis of 10,000 postmortem examinations in Japan. In: *World trends in cardiology; selected papers from Second World Congress of Cardiology*. Keys A, White PD, Eds. New York: Hoeber-Harper, 1956: 22-33.

21. Gore I, Nakashima T, Imai T, White PD. Coronary atherosclerosis and myocardial infarction in Kyushu, Japan, and Boston, Massachusetts. *Am J Cardiol* 1962; 10: 400-6.

22. Marmot MG, Syme SL, Kagan A, Kato H, Cohen JB, Belsky J. Epidemiologic studies of coronary heart disease and stroke in Japanese men living in Japan, Hawaii and California: prevalence of coronary and hypertensive heart disease and associated risk factors. *Am J Epidemiol* 1975; 102(6): 514-25.

23. Enos WF, Holmes RH, Beyer J. Coronary disease among United States soldiers killed in action in Korea; preliminary report. *J Am Med Assoc* 1953; 152(12): 1090-3.

24. Tuzcu EM, Kapadia SR, Tutar E, *et al*. High prevalence of coronary atherosclerosis in asymptomatic teenagers and young adults: evidence from intravascular ultrasound. *Circulation* 2001; 103(22): 2705-10.

25. Berenson GS, Srinivasan SR, Bao W, Newman WP, III, Tracy RE, Wattigney WA. Association between multiple cardiovascular risk factors and atherosclerosis in children and young adults. The Bogalusa Heart Study. *N Engl J Med* 1998; 338(23): 1650-6.

26. Malcom GT, Oalmann MC, Strong JP. Risk factors for atherosclerosis in young subjects: the PDAY Study. Pathobiological Determinants of Atherosclerosis in Youth. *Ann N Y Acad Sci* 1997; 817: 179-88.

27. McMahan CA, McGill HC, Gidding SS, *et al*. PDAY risk score predicts advanced coronary artery atherosclerosis in middle-aged persons as well as youth. *Atherosclerosis* 2007; 190: 370-7.

28. Abifadel M, Varret M, Rabes JP, *et al*. Mutations in *PCSK9* cause autosomal dominant hypercholesterolemia. *Nat Genet* 2003; 34(2): 154-6.

29. Maxwell KN, Soccio RE, Duncan EM, Sehayek E, Breslow JL. Novel putative SREBP and LXR target genes identified by microarray analysis in liver of cholesterol-fed mice. *J Lipid Res* 2003; 44(11): 2109-19.

30. Cohen J, Pertsemlidis A, Kotowski IK, Graham R, Garcia CK, Hobbs HH. Low LDL cholesterol in individuals of African descent resulting from frequent nonsense mutations in *PCSK9*. *Nat Genet* 2005; 37(2): 161-5.

31. Cohen JC, Boerwinkle E, Mosley TH, Jr., Hobbs HH. Sequence variations in *PCSK9*, low LDL, and protection against coronary heart disease. *N Engl J Med* 2006; 354(12): 1264-72.

32. Brown MS, Goldstein JL. Biomedicine. Lowering LDL - not only how low, but how long? *Science* 2006; 311(5768): 1721-3.

33. McPherson R, Kavaslar N. Statins for primary prevention of coronary artery disease. *Lancet* 2007; 369: 1078.

34. Myocardial Infarction Genetics Consortium. Proprotein convertase subtilisin/kexin type 9 (PCSK9) missense variant is reproducibly associated with early-onset myocardial infarction in >1500 cases and 1500 controls. *Circulation* 2007; 116: II, 806.

35. Ridker PM, Danielson E, Fonseco FAH, *et al*. Rosuvastatin to prevent vascular events in men and women with elevated C-reactive protein. *N Engl J Med* 2008; 359: 2195-207.

36. Executive Summary of The Third Report of The National Cholesterol Education Program (NCEP) Expert Panel on Detection, Evaluation, And Treatment of High Blood Cholesterol In Adults (Adult Treatment Panel III). *JAMA* 2001; 285(19): 2486-97.

37. Lloyd-Jones DM, Wilson PW, Larson MG, *et al.* Framingham risk score and prediction of lifetime risk for coronary heart disease. *Am J Cardiol* 2004; 94(1): 20-4.

38. Lloyd-Jones DM. Short-term versus long-term risk for coronary artery disease: implications for lipid guidelines. *Curr Opin Lipidol* 2006; 17(6): 619-25.

39. Mihaylova B, Briggs A, Armitage J, Parish S, Gray A, Collins R. Lifetime cost effectiveness of simvastatin in a range of risk groups and age groups derived from a randomised trial of 20,536 people. *BMJ* 2006; 333(7579): 1145.

Chapter 2

A brief review of lipoprotein metabolism

Martin Adiels [1] MSc PhD, Assistant Researcher
Sven-Olof Olofsson [1] MD PhD, Professor of Medical Biochemistry
Marja-Riitta Taskinen [2] MD PhD, Professor of Medicine
Jan Borén [1] MD PhD, Professor of Cardiovascular Medicine
1 Sahlgrenska Center for Metabolism and Cardiovascular Research
Wallenberg Laboratory for Cardiovascular Research and the
Department of Molecular and Clinical Medicine, The Sahlgrenska Academy
University of Gothenburg, Gothenburg, Sweden
2 Division of Cardiology, University of Helsinki, Biomedicum, Helsinki, Finland

Introduction

Neutral lipids, such as cholesterol and triglycerides, are insoluble in plasma. As a result, circulating lipid is bound to lipoproteins that transport the lipid to various tissues for energy utilization, lipid deposition, steroid hormone production, and bile acid formation. The lipoprotein consists of lipid (esterified and unesterified cholesterol, triglycerides, and phospholipids), and protein. The protein components of the lipoprotein are known as apolipoproteins or apoproteins. The different apolipoproteins serve as cofactors for enzymes and ligands for receptors.

The handling of lipoproteins in the body is referred to as lipoprotein metabolism. This is divided into two pathways, exogenous and endogenous, depending mainly on whether the lipoproteins in question are composed chiefly of dietary (exogenous) lipids or whether they originated in the liver (endogenous). There are five major classes of lipoproteins, each of which has a different function. These are chylomicrons (CM), very-low-density lipoproteins (VLDL), intermediate-density lipoproteins (IDL), low-density lipoproteins (LDL) and high-density lipoproteins (HDL)(Figure 1). The metabolism of the different lipoprotein classes are not separated but are closely interrelated. Here we give a brief review of lipoprotein metabolism, which is important for the understanding of the pathophysiology of coronary vascular disease, and for understanding mechanisms of drug actions.

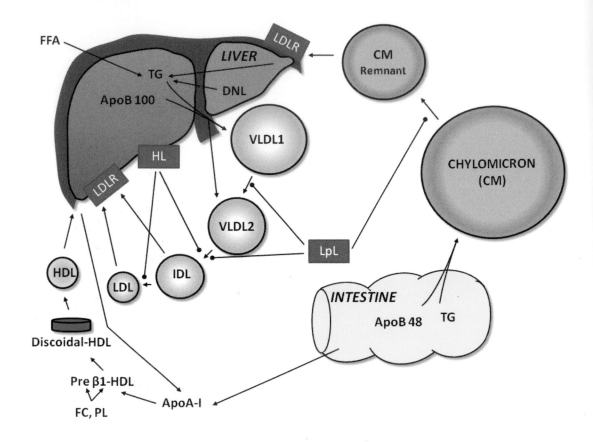

Figure 1. Dietary lipids enter the circulation as cargo on the apolipoprotein (apo) B48 containing chylomicrons (CM), synthesised in the intestine. Using lipids from the circulation (free fatty acids [FFA]), *de novo* lipogenesis (DNL), or diet (as chylomicron remnants), the liver synthesizes very-low-density lipoprotein (VLDL)1 and VLDL2 particles around the major protein apoB100. Chylomicrons, VLDL1 and VLDL2 are delipidated by the lipoprotein lipase (LPL), which liberates fatty acids which are taken up by skeletal muscle and adipose tissue. As VLDL1 loses lipids, it becomes VLDL2, while VLDL2 becomes intermediate-density lipoprotein (IDL) particles. IDL can be further delipidated by hepatic lipase (HL) and becomes a low-density lipoprotein (LDL). CM remnants, IDL and LDL can be taken up by the liver through the LDL receptor (LDLR). In contrast, high-density lipoprotein (HDL) is formed in the extracellular space, where apoAI is associated with phospholipids (PL) and free cholesterol (FC), and forms a discoidal HDL particle. The HDL particle is further matured by lecithin:cholesterol acyltransferase (LCAT) which produces cholesterol esters which form the core of the HDL particle. Ultimately the cholesterol is taken up by the liver and the apoAI can be recycled. Both the intestine and the liver secrete apoAI.

Metabolism of triglyceride-rich lipoproteins

Assembly and secretion

The assembly of VLDL occurs in the hepatocytes and starts with the lipidation of the structural protein apolipoprotein B100 (apoB100) [1]. The apoB100 is cotranslationally lipidated by microsomal triglyceride transfer protein (MTP) as it enters the rough endoplasmic reticulum (ER). The resulting primordial particle, pre-VLDL [1-3], is further lipidated and is converted to a VLDL2 particle [4], which can be secreted from the hepatocyte. A second step in the assembly of VLDL can occur in the Golgi apparatus where VLDL2 can be converted to VLDL1 by the addition of a major amount of lipids [4, 5]. This second step is not dependent on MTP, but requires the small GTP binding protein, ADP ribosylation factor 1 (ARF-1) [6], which is involved in trafficking between the ER and the Golgi apparatus [7].

Some regulation of apoB100 secretion occurs within the secretory pathway as apoB100 can be sorted to degradation both cotranslationally and post-translationally. In the cotranslational degradation, apoB100 is retracted from the lumen of the ER to the cytosol, where it conjugates with ubiquitin and is thus targeted to proteosomal degradation [8-11]. When the MTP activity or lipid availability is low the apoB100 remains associated with the translocon and is sorted to degradation through cotranslational degradation [12]. Post-translational degradation seems to occur later in the secretory pathway. The mechanisms are not yet known, but it has been shown to be promoted by polyunsaturated fatty acids in cell cultures [11].

Chylomicrons are assembled in a similar process as VLDL, except that apoB48 is the major structural protein. ApoB48 consists of the first 48% of the amino acids of apoB100 and is the product of an apobec-I edited apoB100 mRNA. The dietary lipids form micelles in the gut lumen and lipases secreted from the pancreas into the gut lipolyse the lipids to cholesterol, fatty acids, and monoacylglycerols. These forms of lipids are taken up by the enterocytes, are re-esterified and secreted as chylomicrons [13].

Metabolism of VLDL in the plasma

Circulating VLDL is exposed to several possible modifications. Newly synthesised VLDL interacts with circulating HDL and becomes enriched in apoC and apoE by transfer from the HDL. The enriched VLDL is now fully functional and is primarily modified by lipoprotein lipase (LPL) in the vascular surface of the capillary endothelium of skeletal muscle and adipose tissue. LPL is activated by apoCII [14, 15], but is inhibited by apoCIII [16]. LPL hydrolyses the 1(3)-ester bonds of the triglycerides in both chylomicrons and VLDL. The liberated fatty acids and 2-monoacylglycerols are taken up by the tissues. Skeletal muscle mainly uses the fatty acid as an energy source through beta-oxidation. Adipose tissue re-esterifies the fatty acids for storage as triglycerides, which are released into the circulation during fasting through the action of adipose triglyceride lipase (ATGL) [17] and hormone-sensitive lipase (HSL) [18].

When triglycerides are removed from the VLDL, the particle shrinks and lowers the proportion of lipids and consequently the density increases. As the density increases, VLDL1 becomes VLDL2 and VLDL2 is further transformed to IDL. Some IDL is cleared directly by the liver through receptor-mediated uptake via the LDL receptor [19]. However, the majority of IDL (50-70%) is transferred to LDL in a process where IDL is modified by hepatic lipase (HL) and cholesteryl ester transfer protein (CETP). The activity of LPL determines the residence time of the circulating VLDL1 and VLDL2 particles. Thus, the plasma level of triglycerides is determined by the production rate and the residence time of VLDL1 and VLDL2 particles.

In vivo studies of triglyceride-rich lipoprotein (TRL) metabolism

While traditional measurements of blood lipids are important as diagnostic tools, they do not give any insight into the underlying mechanisms. Similarly, in vitro studies can reveal a basic understanding of VLDL assembly, but cannot provide any insight into dysregulation and therapies of lipoprotein disorders. Abnormal concentrations of lipids and apolipoproteins can result from changes in the production, conversion, or catabolism of lipoprotein particles. Thus, although static measurements are important, they do not reveal the underlying mechanisms involved in the dysregulation of lipid disorders. To infer this information, it is necessary to perform in vivo tracer/tracee studies in which the rates of synthesis or catabolism of a particular lipoprotein or apolipoprotein can be determined [20].

Using stable isotope tracers, gas chromatography-mass spectroscopy (GC-MS) techniques and mathematical modelling, it has been possible to study and quantify production and clearance of lipoproteins in humans. These techniques have been employed to study the kinetics of the protein content of the particles: apoB100 in the VLDL-IDL-LDL cascade, VLDL1-VLDL2 separately or VLDL1-VLDL2-IDL-LDL. Chylomicron metabolism has been investigated by studying the apoB48 protein and HDL metabolism has been characterised by studying the apoAI and apoAII proteins. Since VLDL consists mostly of triglycerides it is possible to study the metabolism of these lipoproteins by labelling the core lipid content with labelled glycerol or a labelled fatty acid.

Regulators of VLDL synthesis

The synthesis and secretion of VLDL is dependent on substrate availability. Stable isotope studies have shown that circulating free fatty acids are the main source of lipids for VLDL triglycerides, contributing 66-80% [21, 22] in healthy subjects and 43-56% in subjects with non-alcoholic fatty liver disease [22, 23] (III/B). Increasing free fatty acid availability increases VLDL secretion both in vivo and in vitro [24-26]. De novo lipogenesis and dietary lipids are additional sources of lipids for VLDL secretion.

Recent kinetic studies show a correlation between liver fat content and VLDL secretion rate [22, 27, 28] (III/B). This is probably a reflection of an overall increased lipid flux through the liver and when the influx of lipids exceeds the efflux of lipids, lipids start to accumulate. Insulin lowers plasma free fatty acid concentration by inhibiting the hormone-sensitive lipase (HSL), an enzyme that releases free fatty acids from adipose tissue. This reduces substrate availability for VLDL-triglyceride synthesis which in turn lowers the VLDL secretion. Furthermore, studies have shown that insulin also has direct effects on VLDL assembly and secretion [24, 27, 29, 30].

Disturbances in lipoprotein metabolism in metabolic diseases

Kinetic studies have revealed that dyslipidemia seen in subjects with type 2 diabetes and insulin resistance is associated with increased secretion of VLDL [31-34] **(III/B)**. In particular, secretion of the large triglyceride-rich VLDL1 is increased, with VLDL2 production being relatively constant [35, 36]. The dyslipidemia is further augmented by decreased hepatic clearance of VLDL, IDL and LDL.

Likewise, central obesity in men is associated with increased VLDL production [37, 38] **(III/B)** and slower clearance of IDL and LDL [38]. In contrast, obese women only have a reduced clearance [39]. In more detailed studies it has been shown that visceral fat depot [40], insulin resistance [41] and liver fat [22, 27, 28] have been linked to oversecretion of large VLDL particles.

Familial combined hypercholesterolemia (FCH) can be caused by several different mutations and therefore kinetic studies show inconsistent results. However, most results point to a decreased clearance of LDL (and most often VLDL), while VLDL, IDL and LDL production is increased [42].

The effect of interventions on lipoprotein metabolism

Weight loss improves lipoprotein metabolism by decreasing VLDL secretion [43, 44] **(IIa/B)**. The improvement is mostly achieved by the reduction of intraperitoneal adipose tissue mass. Weight loss also upregulates LDL catabolism. Omega-3 fatty acids are known to regulate lipoprotein metabolism, and have been shown to decrease VLDL apoB secretion in normal subjects [45] and subjects with metabolic syndrome [46] **(IIa/B)**.

Metabolism of LDL

LDL is the major carrier of cholesterol in human plasma and is thus intimately involved in the process of atherosclerosis [47]. LDL is cleared from the circulation by the LDL receptor which is primarily expressed by the liver [48]. As LDL is the end product of VLDL, its particle count is dependent on the rate of production of VLDL and the LDL receptor-mediated uptake of IDL and LDL. The lipoprotein class comprises a number of distinct subfractions, and can be divided into large, intermediate and small sized particles [49]. Examination of the properties of LDL subfractions has led to the belief that small, dense LDL is a particularly atherogenic form of the lipoprotein. Small, dense LDL is generated by intravascular lipoprotein remodelling as a result of disturbances such as type 2 diabetes, metabolic syndrome and renal disease. Studies from several laboratories indicate that LDL will lose cholesteryl ester (via the cholesteryl ester transfer protein [CETP] mechanism) and gain triglycerides in the presence of elevated VLDL1 levels. It is postulated that exposure of the resulting triglyceride-enriched LDL to hepatic lipase (HL) will lead to the removal of sufficient core lipid (triglycerides) and surface lipid (as HL also acts on phospholids) to promote a shift in particle size into the small, dense range. The key regulatory factors in this model of small dense LDL formation are, therefore, the concentration of VLDL1 [50] and the activities of HL and CETP.

Small dense LDL is slowly metabolized (approximate residence time of 5 days) compared with LDL derived from smaller VLDL or IDL precursors (which has a residence time of approximately 2 days) [49]. One explanation for this slow metabolism is that small, dense LDL binds less well to the LDL receptor compared with its larger counterparts, which has the consequence of prolonging its lifetime in the circulation. Furthermore, the particle appears to interact more strongly with arterial wall proteoglycans [51]. In the 'response to retention' hypothesis of atherosclerosis, this property will increase the time that lipoprotein spends trapped in the subendothelial space of the artery wall and, hence, increase the opportunity to promote atherogenic changes [51]. Indeed, epidemiological studies have demonstrated a correlation between small, dense LDL and an increased risk of coronary heart disease (CHD) [52]. However, LDL size has not been shown to be fully independent of related factors such as elevated plasma triglyceride concentrations [52]. Thus, small, dense LDL may indicate a metabolic condition associated with increased CHD risk more than a direct promotion of atherosclerosis by the small, dense LDL particles *per se* [52].

Metabolism of HDL

Mature HDL consists of a core of cholesterol esters, some triglycerides and an outer shell of phospholipids and cholesterol. The major protein classes on the surface are apoAI and apoAII. ApoAI is secreted by the liver and intestine, and combines with phospholipids to form small, discoidal HDL particles that can bind cholesterol and some phospholipids from peripheral cells. The further maturation of HDL is catalysed by lecithin:cholesterol acyltransferase (LCAT), which esterifies a free cholesterol with a fatty acid from a phosphatidylcholine and forms a cholesterol ester and a lysophosphatidylcholine. The movement of cholesteryl ester to the core of the HDL particle converts the small HDL into larger HDL particles. Lipoprotein lipase hydrolyses the triglyceride carried on triglyceride-rich lipoproteins to provide surface components (phospholipids, free cholesterol and apolipoproteins) to the HDL particle.

Triglycerides from triglyceride-rich lipoproteins are exchanged for cholesterol ester on the maturating HDL particle through CETP. The plasma enzymes, hepatic lipase, endothelial lipase and secretory phospholipase A2 (sPLA2), hydrolyse and remove phospholipids from the newly formed HDL. In the final step of cholesterol transport the scavenger receptor class

B1 (SR-B1) is critical for the uptake of cholesterol into the liver [53, 54]. SR-B1 mediates the uptake of cholesteryl esters via binding to primarily large HDL particles. The selective uptake of cholesterol is an obligatory step for the removal of cholesterol into the bile and its subsequent excretion in faeces. This process generates lipid-poor small HDL particles. Recognition of the dynamic nature and heterogeneity of HDL particles is essential to understand the metabolic fate of HDL and its regulation.

The efflux of cholesterol from the cells is a highly regulated process where specific transport proteins including ATP-binding cassette transporters, ABCA1 and ABCG1, play a crucial role [55-57]. Cholesterol efflux from macrophages via both ABCA1 and ABCG1 is considered to be critical for the anti-atherogenic action of HDL. Recent evidence indicates that large HDL particles may be the preferential acceptor for cholesterol efflux via ABCG1 action [54, 58]. Like apoB100, apoAI and apoAII kinetics can be studied using stable isotope techniques [59]. Collectively, several studies indicate that the main reason for the low HDL and apoAI levels in the metabolic syndrome and related disorders is an increased clearance rate [59-63]. As a balancing factor, apoAI production is often increased [59, 63]. The HDL clearance rate itself is correlated with the plasma triglyceride levels [61, 63].

Results from kinetic studies of HDL metabolism have recently been reviewed [20, 59] and updated [64]. Interestingly, recent findings from both weight loss studies and omega-3 supplement studies show that both apoAI clearance and production rate are decreased and therefore no change in HDL concentrations were detected [65, 66].

Lipoprotein metabolism is closely linked

It is now recognized that the different components of diabetic dyslipidemia are not isolated abnormalities but are closely linked to each other metabolically [47, 67, 68], and are mainly initiated by the hepatic overproduction of large triglyceride-rich VLDL1 [47, 68]. Kinetic studies have shown that the LDL fractional catabolic rate is inversely correlated with plasma triglyceride concentration which is largely determined by VLDL1 concentration. In subjects with triglyceride concentrations between 150-200mg/dL (1.36-2.26mmol/L), the prevailing small dense LDL is mainly derived from VLDL precursors, and catabolized more slowly than the large buoyant LDL prevailing in subjects with lower triglyceride levels. These studies show that triglyceride-rich VLDL is the precursor of slowly catabolized LDL particles. Increased levels of VLDL1 also alter the composition of HDL through the actions of CETP and hepatic lipase, leading to the formation of small, dense HDL and increased catabolism of these particles [69] (Figure 2).

The intestinally derived apoB48-containing chylomicrons and chylomicron-remnants are cleared from the circulation by the same pathway as hepatically derived apoB100-containing lipoproteins, and therefore compete for clearance [70]. Thus, increased production of VLDL1 is linked to high levels of plasma triglycerides, low levels of HDL cholesterol, the appearance of small, dense LDL and excessive post-prandial lipemia [47, 49, 67, 68, 71].

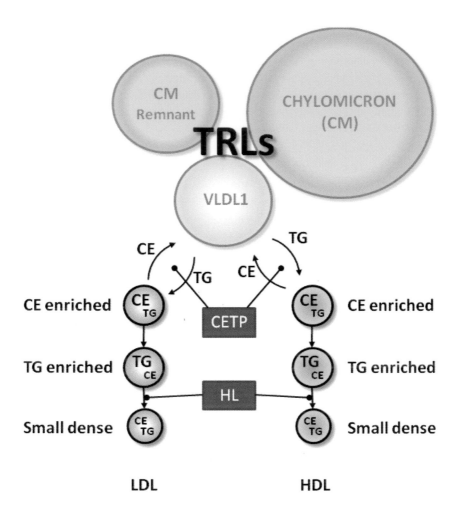

Figure 2. Both the low-density lipoproteins (LDL) and high-density lipoproteins (HDL) can interact with the triglyceride-rich lipoproteins (TRLs). In this process, the cholesterol ester (CE)-rich particles lose CE which is replaced by triglycerides (TG), through the action of cholesteryl ester transfer protein (CETP). The resulting products are TG enriched, and are good substrates for hepatic lipase (HL), which removes the TG and produces small dense particles.

The effects of drugs on lipoprotein metabolism

The possibility of examining lipoprotein kinetics using stable isotopes and mathematical models has provided tools to study *in vivo* the effects of drugs targeting the lipid metabolism. In particular it is possible to discriminate between the effects on lipoprotein synthesis and catabolism. HMG-CoA reductase inhibitors, commonly known as statins, primarily lower LDL cholesterol but also lower plasma triglyceride levels. Several kinetic studies on statins show an increased clearance rate across VLDL, IDL and LDL as the primary factor of LDL cholesterol lowering [33, 72-75] **(Ib/A)**, whereas decreased production rates, in particular of VLDL, are observed in some studies [33, 75, 76]. However, most studies have shown little or no effects on HDL metabolism [20].

Fenofibrates also increase the clearance of apoB **(Ib/A)**, while also increasing apoAI production [60, 75]. Nicotinic acid lowers LDL cholesterol, triglycerides and apoB, while increasing the levels of HDL cholesterol and apoAI **(IIa/B)**. New formulations of nicotinic acid, with extended or intermediate release have fewer side effects (such as flushing) [77]. Recent studies have shown that a major effect on lipoprotein metabolism of nicotinic acid is an increase in the fractional catabolic rate (FCR) of triglyceride-rich lipoproteins (both apoB100 and apoB48), while HDL is raised by an increased production rate of apoAI [78]. However, the results are inconclusive as earlier studies have shown a decreased production of apoB100 [79, 80]. As of today the exact mechanisms of how nicotinic acid lowers LDL cholesterol are not known.

Conclusions

In conclusion, the metabolic pathways of lipids and lipoproteins are closely interrelated and even though there are several potent lipid-lowering drugs available on the market, their exact functions still remain unknown to some extent. Hopefully, clarification of these molecular mechanisms will be translated into further improved treatment for dyslipidemia, which is of key importance given the high risk for cardiovascular disease in patients with dyslipidemia.

Due to the methodological complexity and high costs of kinetic studies, these are often small and underpowered and it will not be until the results from several studies are combined that some general conclusions can be made. Therefore, the grades of evidence are generally low when it comes to kinetic intervention studies.

Key points	Evidence level
◆ Statins increase clearance rates of VLDL, IDL, and LDL, and decrease production rates of, in particular VLDL, thereby improving the lipoprotein profile.	Ib/A
◆ Fibrates increase the clearance rate of apoB particles and the production of apoAI particles.	Ib/A
◆ Nicotinic acid lowers LDL cholesterol and triglycerides and increases HDL.	IIa/B
◆ Weight loss decreases VLDL secretion, thereby improving lipoprotein metabolism.	IIa/B
◆ Omega-3 fatty acids decrease VLDL secretion thereby regulating lipoprotein metabolism.	IIa/B

References

1. Olofsson SO, Boren J. Apolipoprotein B: a clinically important apolipoprotein which assembles atherogenic lipoproteins and promotes the development of atherosclerosis. *J Intern Med* 2005; 258: 395-410.
2. Olofsson SO, Asp L, Boren J. The assembly and secretion of apolipoprotein B-containing lipoproteins. *Curr Opin Lipidol* 1999; 10: 341-6.
3. Boren J, Graham L, Wettesten M, Scott J, White A, Olofsson SO. The assembly and secretion of ApoB 100-containing lipoproteins in Hep G2 cells. ApoB 100 is cotranslationally integrated into lipoproteins. *J Biol Chem* 1992; 267: 9858-67.
4. Stillemark-Billton P, Beck C, Boren J, Olofsson SO. Relation of the size and intracellular sorting of apoB to the formation of VLDL 1 and VLDL 2. *J Lipid Res* 2005; 46: 104-14.
5. Stillemark P, Boren J, Andersson M, Larsson T, Rustaeus S, Karlsson KA, Olofsson SO. The assembly and secretion of apolipoprotein B-48-containing very low density lipoproteins in McA-RH7777 cells. *J Biol Chem* 2000; 275: 10506-13.
6. Asp L, Claesson C, Boren J, Olofsson SO. ADP-ribosylation factor 1 and its activation of phospholipase D are important for the assembly of very low density lipoproteins. *J Biol Chem* 2000; 275: 26285-92.
7. Asp L, Magnusson B, Rutberg M, Li L, Boren J, Olofsson SO. Role of ADP ribosylation factor 1 in the assembly and secretion of ApoB-100-containing lipoproteins. *Arterioscler Thromb Vasc Biol* 2005; 25: 566-70.
8. Mitchell DM, Zhou M, Pariyarath R, Wang H, Aitchison JD, Ginsberg HN, Fisher EA. Apoprotein B100 has a prolonged interaction with the translocon during which its lipidation and translocation change from dependence on the microsomal triglyceride transfer protein to independence. *Proc Natl Acad Sci USA* 1998; 95: 14733-8.
9. Liang S, Wu X, Fisher EA, Ginsberg HN. The amino-terminal domain of apolipoprotein B does not undergo retrograde translocation from the endoplasmic reticulum to the cytosol. Proteasomal degradation of nascent apolipoprotein B begins at the carboxyl terminus of the protein, while apolipoprotein B is still in its original translocon. *J Biol Chem* 2000; 275: 32003-10.
10. Pariyarath R, Wang H, Aitchison JD, Ginsberg HN, Welch WJ, Johnson AE, Fisher EA. Co-translational interactions of apoprotein B with the ribosome and translocon during lipoprotein assembly or targeting to the proteasome. *J Biol Chem* 2001; 276: 541-50.
11. Fisher EA, Pan M, Chen X, Wu X, Wang H, Jamil H, Sparks JD, Williams KJ. The triple threat to nascent apolipoprotein B. Evidence for multiple, distinct degradative pathways. *J Biol Chem* 2001; 276: 27855-63.
12. Fisher EA, Ginsberg HN. Complexity in the secretory pathway: the assembly and secretion of apolipoprotein B-containing lipoproteins. *J Biol Chem* 2002; 277: 17377-80.
13. Williams KJ. Molecular processes that handle - and mishandle - dietary lipids. *J Clin Invest* 2008; 118: 3247-59.
14. Havel RJ, Shore VG, Shore B, Bier DM. Role of specific glycopeptides of human serum lipoproteins in the activation of lipoprotein lipase. *Circ Res* 1970; 27: 595-600.
15. LaRosa JC, Levy RI, Herbert P, Lux SE, Fredrickson DS. A specific apoprotein activator for lipoprotein lipase. *Biochem Biophys Res Commun* 1970; 41: 57-62.
16. Ginsberg HN, Le NA, Goldberg IJ, Gibson JC, Rubinstein A, Wang-Iverson P, Norum R, Brown WV. Apolipoprotein B metabolism in subjects with deficiency of apolipoproteins CIII and AI. Evidence that apolipoprotein CIII inhibits catabolism of triglyceride-rich lipoproteins by lipoprotein lipase *in vivo*. *J Clin Invest* 1986; 78: 1287-95.
17. Zimmermann R, Strauss JG, Haemmerle G, Schoiswohl G, Birner-Gruenberger R, Riederer M, Lass A, Neuberger G, Eisenhaber F, Hermetter A, et al. Fat mobilization in adipose tissue is promoted by adipose triglyceride lipase. *Science* 2004; 306: 1383-6.
18. Vaughan M, Berger JE, Steinberg D. Hormone-sensitive lipase and monoglyceride lipase activities in adipose tissue. *J Biol Chem* 1964; 239: 401-9.
19. Brown MS, Goldstein JL. A receptor-mediated pathway for cholesterol homeostasis. *Science* 1986; 232: 34-47.
20. Chan DC, Barrett PH, Watts GF. Recent studies of lipoprotein kinetics in the metabolic syndrome and related disorders. *Curr Opin Lipidol* 2006; 17: 28-36.

21. Barrows BR, Parks EJ. Contributions of different fatty acid sources to very low-density lipoprotein-triacylglycerol in the fasted and fed states. *J Clin Endocrinol Metab* 2006; 91: 1446-52.

22. Fabbrini E, Mohammed BS, Magkos F, Korenblat KM, Patterson BW, Klein S. Alterations in adipose tissue and hepatic lipid kinetics in obese men and women with nonalcoholic fatty liver disease. *Gastroenterology* 2008; 134: 424-31.

23. Donnelly KL, Smith CI, Schwarzenberg SJ, Jessurun J, Boldt MD, Parks EJ. Sources of fatty acids stored in liver and secreted via lipoproteins in patients with nonalcoholic fatty liver disease. *J Clin Invest* 2005; 115: 1343-51.

24. Lewis GF, Uffelman KD, Szeto LW, Weller B, Steiner G. Interaction between free fatty acids and insulin in the acute control of very low density lipoprotein production in humans. *J Clin Invest* 1995; 95:158-66.

25. Lewis GF. Fatty acid regulation of very low density lipoprotein production. *Curr Opin Lipidol* 1997; 8: 146-53.

26. Duez H, Lamarche B, Valero R, Pavlic M, Proctor S, Xiao C, Szeto L, Patterson BW, Lewis GF. Both intestinal and hepatic lipoprotein production are stimulated by an acute elevation of plasma free fatty acids in humans. *Circulation* 2008; 117: 2369-76.

27. Adiels M, Taskinen MR, Packard C, Caslake MJ, Soro-Paavonen A, Westerbacka J, Vehkavaara S, Hakkinen A, Olofsson SO, Yki-Jarvinen H, *et al.* Overproduction of large VLDL particles is driven by increased liver fat content in man. *Diabetologia* 2006; 49: 755-65.

28. Tsekouras YE, Magkos F, Kavouras SA, Panagiotakos DB, Sidossis LS. Estimated liver weight is directly related to hepatic very low-density lipoprotein-triglyceride secretion rate in men. *Eur J Clin Invest* 2008; 38: 656-62.

29. Malmstrom R, Packard CJ, Caslake M, Bedford D, Stewart P, Yki-Jarvinen H, Shepherd J, Taskinen MR. Effects of insulin and acipimox on VLDL1 and VLDL2 apolipoprotein B production in normal subjects. *Diabetes* 1998; 47: 779-87.

30. Malmstrom R, Packard CJ, Watson TD, Rannikko S, Caslake M, Bedford D, Stewart P, Yki-Jarvinen H, Shepherd J, Taskinen MR. Metabolic basis of hypotriglyceridemic effects of insulin in normal men. *Arterioscler Thromb Vasc Biol* 1997; 17: 1454-64.

31. Kissebah AH, Alfarsi S, Evans DJ, Adams PW. Integrated regulation of very low density lipoprotein triglyceride and apolipoprotein-B kinetics in non-insulin-dependent diabetes mellitus. *Diabetes* 1982; 31: 217-25.

32. Duvillard L, Pont F, Florentin E, Galland-Jos C, Gambert P, Verges B. Metabolic abnormalities of apolipoprotein B-containing lipoproteins in non-insulin-dependent diabetes: a stable isotope kinetic study. *Eur J Clin Invest* 2000; 30: 685-94.

33. Ouguerram K, Magot T, Zair Y, Marchini JS, Charbonnel B, Laouenan H, Krempf M. Effect of atorvastatin on apolipoprotein B100 containing lipoprotein metabolism in type-2 diabetes. *J Pharmacol Exp Ther* 2003; 306: 332-7.

34. Cummings MH, Watts GF, Umpleby AM, Hennessy TR, Naoumova R, Slavin BM, Thompson GR, Sonksen PH. Increased hepatic secretion of very-low-density lipoprotein apolipoprotein B-100 in NIDDM. *Diabetologia* 1995; 38: 959-67.

35. Adiels M, Boren J, Caslake MJ, Stewart P, Soro A, Westerbacka J, Wennberg B, Olofsson SO, Packard C, Taskinen MR. Overproduction of VLDL1 driven by hyperglycemia is a dominant feature of diabetic dyslipidemia. *Arterioscler Thromb Vasc Biol* 2005; 25: 1697-703.

36. Taskinen MR, Packard CJ, Shepherd J. Effect of insulin therapy on metabolic fate of apolipoprotein B-containing lipoproteins in NIDDM. *Diabetes* 1990; 39: 1017-27.

37. Riches FM, Watts GF, Naoumova RP, Kelly JM, Croft KD, Thompson GR. Hepatic secretion of very-low-density lipoprotein apolipoprotein B-100 studied with a stable isotope technique in men with visceral obesity. *Int J Obes Relat Metab Disord* 1998; 22: 414-23.

38. Chan DC, Watts GF, Redgrave TG, Mori TA, Barrett PH. Apolipoprotein B-100 kinetics in visceral obesity: associations with plasma apolipoprotein C-III concentration. *Metabolism* 2002; 51: 1041-6.

39. Mittendorfer B, Patterson BW, Klein S, Sidossis LS. VLDL-triglyceride kinetics during hyperglycemia-hyperinsulinemia: effects of sex and obesity. *Am J Physiol Endocrinol Metab* 2003; 284: E708-15.

40. Watts GF, Chan DC, Barrett PH, Susekov AV, Hua J, Song, S. Fat compartments and apolipoprotein B-100 kinetics in overweight-obese men. *Obes Res* 2003; 11:152-9.

41. Ginsberg HN, Huang LS. The insulin resistance syndrome: impact on lipoprotein metabolism and atherothrombosis. *J Cardiovasc Risk* 2000; 7: 325-31.

42. Parhofer KG, Barrett PH. Thematic review series: patient-oriented research. What we have learned about VLDL and LDL metabolism from human kinetics studies. *J Lipid Res* 2006; 47: 1620-30.

43. Riches FM, Watts GF, Hua J, Stewart GR, Naoumova RP, Barrett PH. Reduction in visceral adipose tissue is associated with improvement in apolipoprotein B-100 metabolism in obese men. *J Clin Endocrinol Metab* 1999; 84: 2854-61.

44. James AP, Watts GF, Barrett PH, Smith D, Pal S, Chan DC, Mamo JC. Effect of weight loss on postprandial lipemia and low-density lipoprotein receptor binding in overweight men. *Metabolism* 2003; 52: 136-41.

45. Bordin P, Bodamer OA, Venkatesan S, Gray RM, Bannister PA, Halliday D. Effects of fish oil supplementation on apolipoprotein B100 production and lipoprotein metabolism in normolipidaemic males. *Eur J Clin Nutr* 1998; 52: 104-9.

46. Chan DC, Watts GF, Barrett PH, Beilin LJ, Redgrave TG, Mori TA. Regulatory effects of HMG CoA reductase inhibitor and fish oils on apolipoprotein B-100 kinetics in insulin-resistant obese male subjects with dyslipidemia. *Diabetes* 2002; 51: 2377-86.

47. Taskinen MR. Diabetic dyslipidaemia: from basic research to clinical practice. *Diabetologia* 2003; 46: 733-49.

48. Goldstein JL, Brown MS. The LDL receptor. *Arterioscler Thromb Vasc Biol* 2009; 29: 431-8.

49. Packard CJ. Triacylglycerol-rich lipoproteins and the generation of small, dense low-density lipoprotein. *Biochem Soc Trans* 2003; 31: 1066-9.

50. Adiels M, Olofsson SO, Taskinen MR, Boren J. Overproduction of very low-density lipoproteins is the hallmark of the dyslipidemia in the metabolic syndrome. *Arterioscler Thromb Vasc Biol* 2008; 28: 1225-36.

51. Tabas I, Williams KJ, Boren J. Subendothelial lipoprotein retention as the initiating process in atherosclerosis: update and therapeutic implications. *Circulation* 2007; 116: 1832-44.

52. Lada AT, Rudel LL. Associations of low density lipoprotein particle composition with atherogenicity. *Curr Opin Lipidol* 2004; 15: 19-24.

53. Rader DJ. Molecular regulation of HDL metabolism and function: implications for novel therapies. *J Clin Invest* 2006; 116: 3090-100.

54. Tall AR, Yvan-Charvet L, Terasaka N, Pagler T, Wang N. HDL, ABC transporters, and cholesterol efflux: implications for the treatment of atherosclerosis. *Cell Metab* 2008; 7: 365-75.

55. Rye KA, Bursill CA, Lambert G, Tabet F, Barter PJ. The metabolism and anti-atherogenic properties of HDL. *J Lipid Res* 2009; 50 Suppl: S195-200.

56. Kontush A, Chapman MJ. Functionally defective high-density lipoprotein: a new therapeutic target at the crossroads of dyslipidemia, inflammation, and atherosclerosis. *Pharmacol Rev* 2006; 58: 342-74.

57. Linsel-Nitschke P, Tall AR. HDL as a target in the treatment of atherosclerotic cardiovascular disease. *Nat Rev Drug Discov* 2005; 4: 193-205.

58. Sankaranarayanan S, Oram JF, Asztalos BF, Vaughan AM, Lund-Katz S, Adorni MP, Phillips MC, Rothblat GH. Effects of acceptor composition and mechanism of ABCG1-mediated cellular free cholesterol efflux. *J Lipid Res* 2009; 50: 275-84.

59. Rashid S, Patterson BW, Lewis GF. Thematic review series: patient-oriented research. What have we learned about HDL metabolism from kinetics studies in humans? *J Lipid Res* 2006; 47: 1631-42.

60. Watts GF, Barrett PH, Ji J, Serone AP, Chan DC, Croft KD, Loehrer F, Johnson AG. Differential regulation of lipoprotein kinetics by atorvastatin and fenofibrate in subjects with the metabolic syndrome. *Diabetes* 2003. 52: 803-11.

61. Verges B, Petit JM, Duvillard L, Dautin G, Florentin E, Galland F, Gambert P. Adiponectin is an important determinant of apoA-I catabolism. *Arterioscler Thromb Vasc Biol* 2006; 26: 1364-9.

62. Frenais R, Ouguerram K, Maugeais C, Mahot P, Maugere P, Krempf M, Magot T. High density lipoprotein apolipoprotein AI kinetics in NIDDM: a stable isotope study. *Diabetologia* 1997; 40: 578-83.

63. Ji J, Watts GF, Johnson AG, Chan DC, Ooi EM, Rye KA, Serone AP, Barrett PH. High-density lipoprotein (HDL) transport in the metabolic syndrome: application of a new model for HDL particle kinetics. *J Clin Endocrinol Metab* 2005; 91: 973-9.

64. Watts GF, Barrett PH, Chan DC. HDL metabolism in context: looking on the bright side. *Curr Opin Lipidol* 2008; 19: 395-404.

65. Ng TW, Watts GF, Barrett PH, Rye KA, Chan DC. Effect of weight loss on LDL and HDL kinetics in the metabolic syndrome: associations with changes in plasma retinol-binding protein-4 and adiponectin levels. *Diabetes Care* 2007; 30: 2945-50.

66. Chan DC, Watts GF, Nguyen MN, Barrett PH. Factorial study of the effect of n-3 fatty acid supplementation and atorvastatin on the kinetics of HDL apolipoproteins A-I and A-II in men with abdominal obesity. *Am J Clin Nutr* 2006; 84: 37-43.

67. Ginsberg HN, Zhang YL, Hernandez-Ono A. Metabolic syndrome: focus on dyslipidemia. *Obesity* (Silver Spring) 2006; 14 Suppl 1: 41S-49S.

68. Adiels M, Olofsson SO, Taskinen MR, Boren J. Diabetic dyslipidaemia. *Curr Opin Lipidol* 2006; 17: 238-46.

69. Rashid S, Watanabe T, Sakaue T, Lewis GF. Mechanisms of HDL lowering in insulin resistant, hypertriglyceridemic states: the combined effect of HDL triglyceride enrichment and elevated hepatic lipase activity. *Clin Biochem* 2003; 36: 421-9.

70. Brunzell JD, Hazzard WR, Porte D, Jr., Bierman EL. Evidence for a common, saturable, triglyceride removal mechanism for chylomicrons and very low density lipoproteins in man. *J Clin Invest* 1973; 52: 1578-85.

71. Verges B. New insight into the pathophysiology of lipid abnormalities in type 2 diabetes. *Diabetes Metab* 2005; 31: 429-39.

72. Forster LF, Stewart G, Bedford D, Stewart JP, Rogers E, Shepherd J, Packard CJ, Caslake MJ. Influence of atorvastatin and simvastatin on apolipoprotein B metabolism in moderate combined hyperlipidemic subjects with low VLDL and LDL fractional clearance rates. *Atherosclerosis* 2002; 164: 129-45.

73. Verges B, Florentin E, Baillot-Rudoni S, Monier S, Petit JM, Rageot D, Gambert P, Duvillard L. Effects of 20mg rosuvastatin on VLDL1-, VLDL2-, IDL- and LDL-ApoB kinetics in type 2 diabetes. *Diabetologia* 2008; 51: 1382-90.

74. Ooi EM, Barrett PH, Chan DC, Nestel PJ, Watts GF. Dose-dependent effect of rosuvastatin on apolipoprotein B-100 kinetics in the metabolic syndrome. *Atherosclerosis* 2008; 197: 139-46.

75. Bilz S, Wagner S, Schmitz M, Bedynek A, Keller U, Demant T. Effects of atorvastatin versus fenofibrate on apoB-100 and apoA-I kinetics in mixed hyperlipidemia. *J Lipid Res* 2004; 45: 174-85.

76. Myerson M, Ngai C, Jones J, Holleran S, Ramakrishnan R, Berglund L, Ginsberg HN. Treatment with high-dose simvastatin reduces secretion of apolipoprotein B-lipoproteins in patients with diabetic dyslipidemia. *J Lipid Res* 2005; 46: 2735-44.

77. McKenney JM, Proctor JD, Harris S, Chinchili VM. A comparison of the efficacy and toxic effects of sustained- vs immediate-release niacin in hypercholesterolemic patients. *JAMA* 1994; 271: 672-7.

78. Lamon-Fava S, Diffenderfer MR, Barrett PH, Buchsbaum A, Nyaku M, Horvath KV, Asztalos BF, Otokozawa S, Ai M, Matthan NR, *et al.* Extended-release niacin alters the metabolism of plasma apolipoprotein (Apo) A-I and ApoB-containing lipoproteins. *Arterioscler Thromb Vasc Biol* 2008; 28: 1672-8.

79. Grundy SM, Mok HY, Zech L, Berman M. Influence of nicotinic acid on metabolism of cholesterol and triglycerides in man. *J Lipid Res* 1981; 22: 24-36.

80. Wang W, Basinger A, Neese RA, Shane B, Myong SA, Christiansen M, Hellerstein MK. Effect of nicotinic acid administration on hepatic very low density lipoprotein-triglyceride production. *Am J Physiol Endocrinol Metab* 2001; 280: E540-7.

Chapter 3

Epidemiological aspects of lipid and lipoprotein levels in relation to cardiovascular diseases

Jane Armitage FFPH FRCP, Professor of Clinical Trials and Epidemiology
Louise Bowman MD MRCP, Clinical Research Fellow
Sarah Lewington MSc DPhil, Senior Research Fellow
Clinical Trial Service Unit & Epidemiological Studies Unit (CTSU)
University of Oxford, Oxford, UK

Introduction

Worldwide, half of all adult mortality (and extensive severe disability) is caused by vascular diseases, and most of those deaths involve coronary heart disease or stroke. Many of those killed by these conditions are still in middle age (i.e. aged 35-69) when they die, losing about 20 years of life expectancy. About 3 million such deaths occur among people under 60 years of age, and over 3 million among people aged 60-69[1]. In both developing and developed regions, blood lipids, blood pressure, tobacco, and excessive alcohol consumption are major causes of the vascular disease burden. This chapter concentrates on the effects of blood lipids which represent one of the most important modifiable risk factors and account for about half the population attributable risk of myocardial infarction[2].

The principal determinants of blood lipid levels are dietary intake of saturated fat, polyunsaturated fat and cholesterol[3-5], although cholesterol concentrations are also affected by reduced energy intakes resulting in weight loss, genetic and other factors[6, 7]. Much of the international variation in cardiovascular disease rates is therefore dietary in origin. Metabolic ward studies suggest that, in a typical western diet, replacing 60% of saturated fat intake by mono- or polyunsaturates and avoiding 60% of dietary cholesterol would reduce blood total cholesterol (mainly LDL cholesterol) by about 10-15% (typically about 0.8mmol/L)[5] **(Ia/A)**. At a population level this difference would be associated with about 40% less coronary disease in middle age[8]. Individualised intensive dietary advice has a more modest effect in free-living subjects with typical reductions of about 6% in blood cholesterol which tend to decrease over time[9]. Failure to comply fully with dietary recommendations is the likely explanation for the limited efficacy seen of dietary advice. However, if such dietary changes can be sustained, then the cardiovascular benefits are, as with other treatment strategies, dependent on the degree of LDL-lowering achieved [10].

Blood lipids and coronary heart disease risk

The association of blood cholesterol with the risk of coronary heart disease (CHD) has been assessed in a number of prospective observational studies and brought together in two large collaborative individual-patient-data meta-analyses which have published relevant data: the Prospective Studies Collaboration (PSC), which contains data on 1 million participants from 61 studies mainly from Europe (70% of participants) and North America or Australia (20%), with 10% of participants from studies conducted in China or Japan [11]; and the Asia Pacific Cohort Studies Collaboration (APCSC), which contains data on over 650,000 participants from 44 separate cohort studies in mainland China, Hong Kong, Taiwan, Japan, South Korea, Singapore, Thailand, New Zealand and Australia [12, 13].

These observational studies show a continuous positive association between usual levels of total cholesterol (a surrogate for LDL cholesterol – see below) and the risk of CHD, with a prolonged difference of 1mmol/L lower total cholesterol being associated in both men and women with about a halving in CHD mortality in early middle age (i.e. 40-49 years), about a third lower CHD mortality in later middle age (i.e. 50-69) and about a sixth lower in old age (i.e. 70-89 years)(Figure 1) [8] **(III/B)**. However, although the proportional differences in risk decrease with age, the absolute effects of cholesterol on annual CHD mortality rates are much greater at older than younger ages so that the absolute difference in the annual risk of CHD death per 1mmol/L difference in total cholesterol is about ten times greater at age 80 than at age 40. Although the positive association between total cholesterol and CHD has been known for some time, the effects of other vascular risk factors – particularly blood pressure and smoking – on this association remained uncertain. Recent evidence suggests that the proportional effects at a specific age are similar for smokers and non-smokers, and for obese and non-obese individuals [8], so that the absolute increase in risk associated with a given increase in cholesterol is greater among smokers and those who are obese. At a specific age, however, blood pressure somewhat attenuates the proportional effects of blood cholesterol on CHD risk (Figure 2), so the absolute effects of cholesterol and of blood pressure on CHD risk are approximately independent of each other (i.e. the absolute effects of cholesterol and blood pressure are roughly additive rather than multiplicative) [8, 12] **(III/B)**.

Many, but not all of the prospective studies in these meta-analyses also measured HDL cholesterol, but most did not have fasting triglyceride levels and so calculation of LDL cholesterol was not possible. Nevertheless, from the studies where it is available, HDL cholesterol adds greatly to the predictive ability of total cholesterol and higher HDL cholesterol and lower non-HDL cholesterol levels are approximately independently associated with lower CHD risk (Figure 3) **(III/B)**. Consequently, the ratio of total/HDL cholesterol is substantially more informative about CHD risk than either alone, and is more than twice as informative as total cholesterol [8]. Because higher non-HDL cholesterol levels predict similar relative risks regardless of the level of HDL cholesterol, the absolute relevance of non-HDL cholesterol is likely to be greater if HDL cholesterol levels are low.

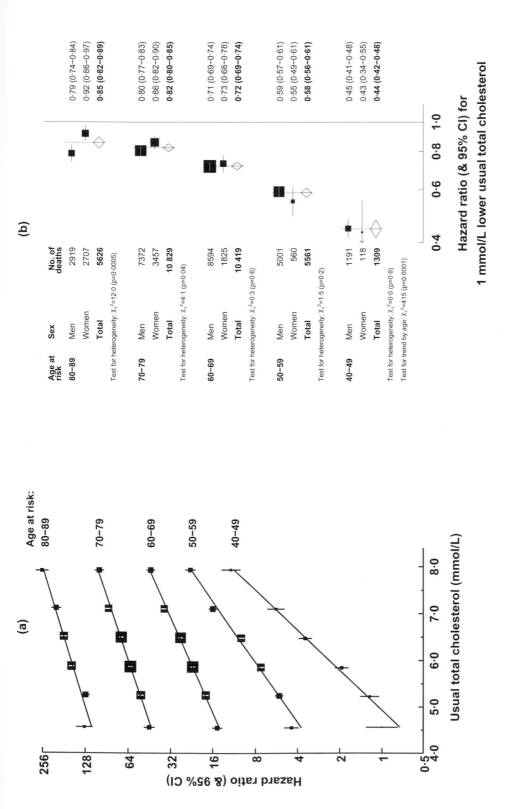

Figure 1. CHD mortality (33,744 deaths) versus usual total cholesterol by age and sex [8]: (a) age-specific associations; and (b) age- and sex-specific hazard ratios for 1mmol/L lower usual total cholesterol.

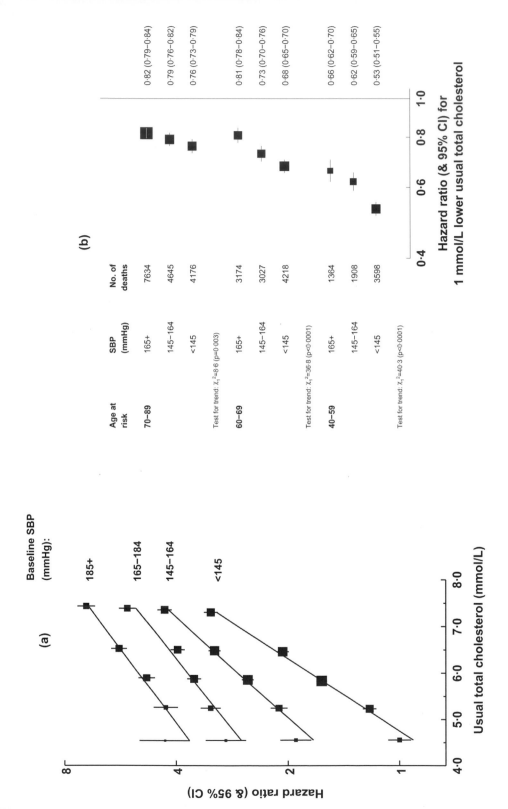

Figure 2. CHD mortality (33,744 deaths) versus usual total cholesterol by baseline blood pressure [8]: (a) systolic blood pressure-specific associations; and (b) systolic blood pressure-specific hazard ratios for 1mmol/L lower usual total cholesterol.

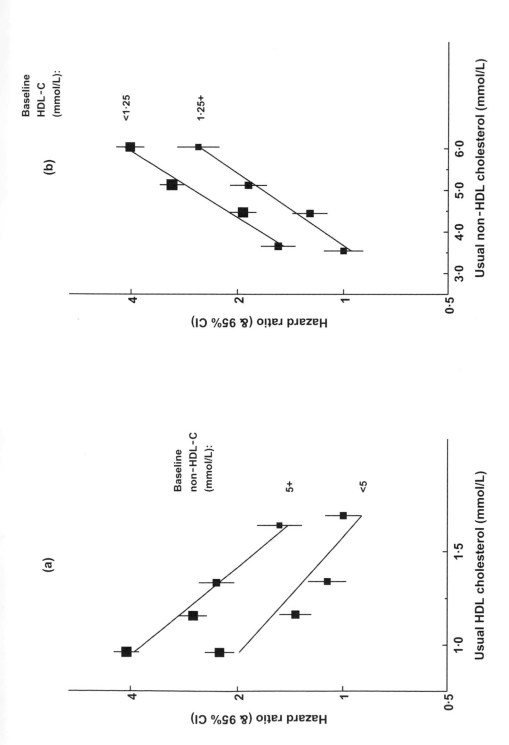

Figure 3. CHD mortality (3020 deaths) versus HDL and non-HDL cholesterol [8]: (a) usual HDL cholesterol by baseline measurement of non-HDL cholesterol; and (b) usual non-HDL cholesterol by baseline measurement of HDL cholesterol.

A meta-analysis of 14 large randomized clinical trials involving 90,000 participants which looked at the effects of cholesterol-lowering using statins on coronary events (fatal or non-fatal) is largely in keeping with these observational findings [14]. On average in these trials there was a 19% (95% CI: 15%-24%) reduction in coronary mortality per 1mmol/L reduction in LDL cholesterol and a 23% (20%-26%) reduction in the combined endpoint of non-fatal myocardial infarction (MI) or coronary death **(Ia/A)**. Hence, about half the risk associated with a life-long higher blood cholesterol appears to be reversed over about 5 years in these clinical trials. To illustrate this: among 40-59-year-olds with systolic blood pressure of 145-164mm Hg, the CHD mortality risk associated with a long-term difference in blood cholesterol of 1mmol/L was 38% (Figure 2) and in the trials (also mainly in middle-aged people) reducing LDL cholesterol by 1mmol/L for about 5 years reduced CHD mortality risk by 19%. Again in line with the observational evidence, the proportional benefits in the trials were slightly lower among those aged over 65 years compared with those aged 65 years or less (19% vs 26%; p for interaction=0.01) but, there was no difference between those treated or untreated for hypertension or between those whose diastolic blood pressure was above or below 90mm Hg at randomization. It seems plausible that longer term or earlier statin treatment may produce larger proportional benefits, i.e. reversing more of the epidemiologically expected risk, but this remains speculative.

Blood lipids and stroke risk

Stroke is the third most common cause of death and a leading cause of severe disability worldwide [15, 16]. Moreover, the burden of stroke will increase as the population ages. But, unlike CHD, stroke is a much more heterogeneous disease consisting of two major subdivisions (hemorrhagic and ischemic) and within these subdivisions different types (e.g. intracerebral and subarachnoid hemorrhage for hemorrhagic and embolic, lacunar and large artery ischemic strokes), may each have different associations with blood lipids. During the twentieth century, ischaemic stroke showed a rise and fall – mirroring that for CHD – while hemorrhagic stroke declined consistently. These different secular trends are in keeping with the risk factors for the two main stroke subtypes being different, and that ischemic stroke shares at least some risk factors with CHD. The role of blood cholesterol as a cause of stroke mortality remains uncertain [8, 12] but there is now no doubt that lowering LDL cholesterol with statins reduces the risk of an ischemic stroke [14, 17] **(Ia/A)**.

In the 1990s, a meta-analysis of observational studies predominantly in western populations showed no association between total cholesterol and total stroke at older ages, but a suggestion of a positive association in early middle age [18] **(III/B)**. However, some limitations of these older observational data need to be understood:

- it is all based only on mortality and hemorrhagic strokes (although substantially less common than non-hemorrhagic) are more likely to be fatal than non-hemorrhagic;
- many of the strokes are of unknown type since CT or MRI scanning was not routinely available at the time these studies were performed and, even when a subtype is attributed, there may be substantial misclassification [19]; and

* most studies had only baseline total cholesterol and no information on lipid subfractions.

A more recent meta-analysis of prospective studies conducted in China and Japan reported that lower total cholesterol was associated with non-significantly lower risk of non-hemorrhagic stroke and non-significantly higher risk of hemorrhagic stroke [20]. In the most recent meta-analysis of 11,663 stroke deaths from the Prospective Studies Collaboration, total stroke mortality and ischemic stroke mortality were weakly positively associated with total cholesterol only in middle age (aged less than 70) and only in those with lower blood pressure (baseline measurement of systolic blood pressure less than about 145mm Hg) [8] (III/B). Moreover, even in middle age, the weak positive association can approximately be accounted for by the association of each 1mmol/L usual total cholesterol with about 2mm Hg usual systolic blood pressure. Even before allowance for blood pressure, total cholesterol was not positively associated with ischemic stroke mortality at older ages or at higher levels of blood pressure, and was negatively associated with hemorrhagic and total stroke mortality in these subgroups. Other observational studies have also suggested that total cholesterol is negatively associated with hemorrhagic stroke in people with high blood pressure [21-23]. In the Korean Medical Insurance Corporation (KMIC) study of 13,445 fatal and non-fatal strokes (6328 ischemic strokes, 3947 hemorrhagic strokes, 3170 undefined strokes), increased risk of hemorrhagic stroke with low concentrations of total cholesterol (<4.14mmol/L) was restricted to heavy drinkers and the authors suggest that low blood cholesterol may be acting as a marker of the health damaging effects of alcohol, rather than be a cause of hemorrhagic stroke [23] (III/B). Recent information from the AMORIS cohort including information on about 6000 fatal and non-fatal strokes does indicate a positive association between blood total cholesterol and ischemic but not hemorrhagic stroke [24] (III/B).

Nonetheless, the large-scale randomized trials of cholesterol-lowering with statins show unequivocally that reducing LDL cholesterol by 1mmol/L reduces total stroke risk by about 17% (95% CI: 12%-22%), due to a 19% (11%-26%) reduction in ischemic stroke with no apparent adverse impact on hemorrhagic stroke [14] (Ia/A). In these trials there was a non-significant 9% reduction in stroke death per mmol/L LDL cholesterol reduction. The contrast between these statistically reliable results from randomized trials and the statistically reliable observational epidemiological results of no association between total cholesterol and stroke mortality is substantial and puzzling. Further investigation of exactly how lipoprotein particles affect stroke risks or of how cholesterol may affect different stroke subtypes may help to explain this discrepancy.

The role of cholesterol fractions – namely, HDL cholesterol and LDL cholesterol – as a cause of stroke is even more uncertain, with quite limited data available from either observational studies or randomized controlled trials. In the Asia Pacific Studies Collaboration, there was no association between HDL cholesterol and stroke risk of any type based on 845 fatal or non-fatal stroke events (271 ischemic, 222 hemorrhagic, remainder unknown etiology) [25] (III/B). Comparing risks of people in the top third of the distribution of HDL cholesterol with those in the bottom third (i.e. HDL cholesterol ≥1.5mmol/L vs

≤1.1mmol/L), the hazard ratio (95% confidence interval) was 0.89 (0.70-1.12) for ischemic stroke, 0.81 (0.62-1.07) for hemorrhagic stroke, 1.06 (0.94-1.20) for unclassified strokes giving 0.95 (0.86-1.06) for all stroke events. The PSC was also unable to show any statistically significant association with total stroke mortality for either HDL or non-HDL cholesterol. However, there was a weak positive association of stroke mortality with the ratio of total/HDL cholesterol in middle age (hazard ratio [95% confidence interval]: 0.86 [0.74-0.99]), but no association at older ages [8].

Lipoprotein particle number may be more relevant

Although there is clear and consistent epidemiological and trial data demonstrating that blood levels of LDL and HDL cholesterol are associated, positively and negatively respectively, with CHD risk, it is being increasingly recognized that the number of atherogenic particles may be a more important determinant of the risk of vascular disease than these conventional lipid measures.

The theory is that the number of lipoprotein particles of a particular type may better determine the likelihood of their entering and lodging within an arterial wall rather than the amount of cholesterol held in the particles. The lipid composition of the principal atherogenic lipoproteins differs substantially between individuals and it has been accepted that small dense LDL particles are relatively more atherogenic than larger ones [26]. Therefore, although they are highly correlated, levels of LDL cholesterol do not necessarily reflect LDL particle number. Each of the atherogenic lipoprotein particles (LDL, IDL, VLDL and Lp(a)) contains a single molecule of apolipoprotein (apo) B, and therefore the concentration of apoB provides a direct measure of the number of circulating atherogenic lipoproteins.

By contrast, HDL particles may have between one and four molecules of apoAI per particle and account for virtually all plasma apoAI. HDL particles vary considerably in size, cholesterol content and probably in biological activity. Small HDL particles, which are more numerous, typically carry only two molecules of apoAI and a few dozen cholesterol molecules, while large ones might carry three molecules of apoAI and over 100 cholesterol molecules. Thus, apoAI does not directly reflect the HDL particle concentration. Despite this, HDL cholesterol concentration and levels of apoAI are highly correlated and both measures are negatively associated with vascular risk.

Apolipoproteins and coronary heart disease risk

Consistent with the hypothesis that particle number is an important factor in the development of atherosclerosis, apolipoproteins have been shown in several studies to be superior to plasma lipid levels in predicting the risk of coronary heart disease. Over 30 years ago, a case control study of 218 MI survivors and 160 controls demonstrated significant differences in measures of total cholesterol, HDL cholesterol, apoB and apoAI between the two groups [27] (III/B).

In the last decade, similar results have begun to emerge from large-scale prospective epidemiological studies. The AMORIS study had measures of apolipoproteins and total cholesterol in 175,000 subjects who were followed up for a mean of 5.5 years, during which time 1200 patients suffered a fatal myocardial infarction [28]. Baseline levels of apoB, apoAI and, particularly apoB/apoAI were strongly related to risk of fatal MI, after adjustment for age, total cholesterol and triglycerides **(III/B)**. In multivariate analyses apoB was a stronger predictor of risk than LDL cholesterol in both sexes. In INTERHEART, a much larger case control study of acute myocardial infarction involving about 12,000 cases of acute MI and 15,000 controls, the apoB/apoAI ratio had the highest odds ratio (OR) for each 1 SD difference in all ethnic groups, in men and women, and at all ages [29] **(III/B)** (overall OR per 1 SD change was: apoB/apoAI 1.59 [95% CI 1.52-1.64]; apoB 1.32 [1.28-1.36]; non-HDL cholesterol 1.21 [1.17-1.24]; total/HDL cholesterol 1.17 [1.13-1.20]; apoAI 0.67 [0.65-0.70]; HDL cholesterol 0.85 [0.83-0.88]). Nuclear magnetic resonance can also be used to assess particle number and in a small number of studies similar results showing LDL and HDL particle number to be important predictors of risk have been published [30, 31].

Most recently, analyses from the ISIS resource have allowed these relationships to be studied in more detail [32]. Levels of apoB, apoAI, LDL cholesterol, HDL cholesterol and total cholesterol were assayed in 3500 MI patients without prior vascular disease and 9800 controls. Repeat assays of blood samples taken 2-3 years later from about 1000 controls importantly allowed correction for regression dilution bias. Myocardial infarction risk was found to be more strongly related to apoB than to LDL cholesterol and, given apoB, was more strongly negatively related to apoAI than to HDL cholesterol **(III/B)**. ApoB and apoAI were largely uncorrelated and were both strongly predictive of risk. The apoB/apoAI ratio encapsulated almost all the predictive power of these four measurements. As in the INTERHEART study [29], the association of MI risk with the apoB/apoAI ratio was continuous, substantial (relative risk for top vs bottom decile of 7.3 with a 95% CI 5.8-9.2) and varied little with age. The apoB/apoAI ratio was substantially more informative about risk (χ^2_1=550) than commonly used measures such as LDL-C/HDL-C, total/HDL cholesterol, non-HDL cholesterol and total cholesterol (χ^2_1=407, 334, 204 and 105, respectively, Figure 4 [32]).

Several of the major statin clinical trials have also measured baseline apolipoprotein levels. Data from the placebo groups of these trials show weaker associations (as would be expected given their prior disease) than observational studies in people who are healthy at baseline, but again apoB is generally found to be more informative than LDL cholesterol as an index of the risk of future coronary events with the ratio of apoB/apoAI remaining the most informative measure [33-36].

Apolipoproteins and stroke disease risk

As described above, the observed associations of conventional lipid measures with risk of stroke are less clear than those for coronary heart disease and the heterogeneous nature of stroke make interpretation of the data difficult. However, in general, it seems that the associations of stroke risk with apolipoprotein measures are stronger and rather more

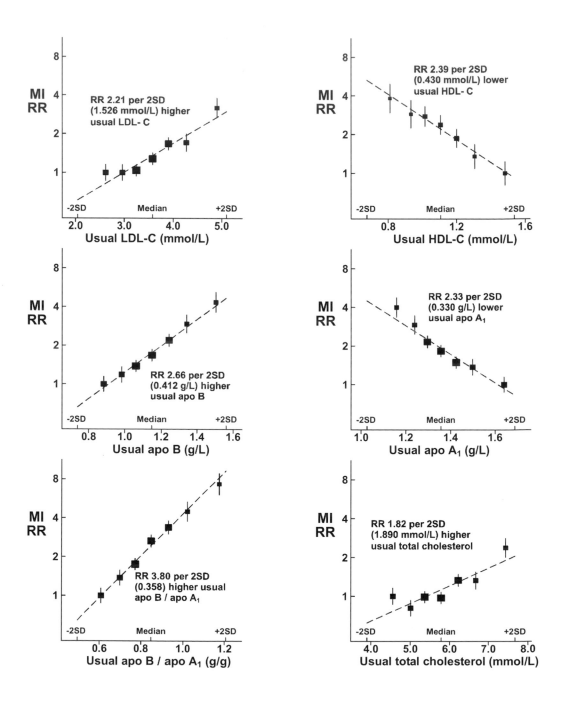

Figure 4. Relative risk of myocardial infarction at different usual levels of LDL, HDL and total cholesterol, apoB, apoAI, and their ratio [32]. Relative risks (RR) and 95% confidence intervals, adjusted for age, sex, smoking and BMI, are plotted against the mean usual value. The seven groups are based on deciles or, for the middle three groups, quintiles of the values among cases.

consistent than those seen with standard lipid measures. Most notably, a recent analysis from the AMORIS cohort, in which it was possible to exclude patients with prior stroke, included 148,600 participants with follow-up ranging from 7 to 17 years [24] and provided information regarding etiology (ischemic vs hemorrhagic) of the stroke. All lipoprotein components were associated with ischemic stroke, although the apoB/apoAI ratio gave the strongest predictive information in multivariate analyses **(III/B)**. The risk of hemorrhagic stroke was found to be unrelated to apolipoproteins in line with the lack of association with conventional lipid measures. Other smaller studies support the association of stroke with apolipoproteins and, as with CHD, the ratio of apoB/apoAI is generally found to be the most predictive of risk [37-40].

Practical advantages of apolipoprotein versus conventional lipid measures

In addition to improved predictive value, apolipoproteins have methodological advantages over conventional lipid measures in clinical practice. The measurement of apoB and apoAI is standardised, simple and inexpensive. In contrast to the estimation of blood LDL cholesterol levels (which, in most laboratories is calculated based on total cholesterol and triglyceride levels, and therefore potentially affected by degree of fasting) apolipoproteins may be reliably measured on non-fasting samples.

Conclusions

As is clear from the above, lipids and lipoproteins are fundamental and causal in the pathogenesis of ischemic cardiovascular disease. It is now clear that reducing the number of atherogenic particles (as measured by either LDL cholesterol or apolipoprotein B) reduces the risk of subsequent cardiovascular events (heart attacks and strokes). Typically, about half of the risk seen in observational studies in association with a given long-term higher blood lipid level can be reversed by cholesterol-lowering treatment. It may be possible to reverse a higher proportion if treatment were initiated earlier [41]. Recent evidence showing no effect in randomized studies of lipid lowering in people with end-stage vascular disease (e.g. heart failure [42, 43] or on renal dialysis [44]) suggests that waiting until there is significant structural damage may be too late. Again this argues the case for treatment to be initiated in time to minimise the damage caused by acute non-fatal events and before there is accumulated damage.

The observational studies all indicate that measures of HDL cholesterol or apolipoprotein AI are inversely associated with cardiovascular risk. However, as explained in Chapter 6 it is currently uncertain whether raising HDL cholesterol with drugs will also reduce cardiovascular risk. But, if HDL-raising is found to successfully reduce risk, it offers substantial further opportunities for preventing disease. Newer measures of lipoproteins in large well characterised cohorts may help us understand better where we need to target new treatments. In the meantime, wider use of the safe and readily available lipid-lowering drugs – statins – could prevent millions more disabling cardiovascular events and deaths.

Key points	Evidence level
◆ Lipids and lipoproteins are causal in the pathogenesis of ischemic cardiovascular disease.	Ia/A
◆ Reducing the number of atherogenic particles (as measured by either LDL cholesterol or apoB) reduces the risk of subsequent cardiovascular events.	Ia/A
◆ Measures of HDL cholesterol or apolipoprotein AI are inversely associated with cardiovascular risk.	III/B
◆ It is currently uncertain whether raising HDL cholesterol with drugs will also reduce cardiovascular risk.	Ib/A
◆ Newer measures of lipoproteins may help us understand better where we need to target new treatments.	III/B

References

1. Murray CJ, Lopez AD. Mortality by cause for eight regions of the world: Global Burden of Disease Study. *Lancet* 1997; 349: 1269-76.
2. Yusuf PS, Hawken S, Ounpuu S, *et al.* Effect of potentially modifiable risk factors associated with myocardial infarction in 52 countries (the INTERHEART study): case-control study. *Lancet* 2004; 364: 937-52.
3. Hegsted DM, Ausman LM, Johnson JA, Dallal GE. Dietary fat and serum lipids: an evaluation of the experimental data. *Am J Clin Nutr* 1993; 57: 875-83.
4. Keys A, Anderson JT, Grande F. Prediction of serum-cholesterol responses of man to changes in fats in the diet. *Lancet* 1957; 273: 959-66.
5. Clarke R, Frost C, Collins R, Appleby P, Peto R. Dietary lipids and blood cholesterol: quantitative meta-analysis of metabolic ward studies. *BMJ* 1997; 314: 112-7.
6. Dattilo AM, Kris-Etherton PM. Effects of weight reduction on blood lipids and lipoproteins: a meta-analysis. *Am J Clin Nutr* 1992; 56: 320-8.
7. Goldstein JL, Brown MS. The low-density lipoprotein pathway and its relation to atherosclerosis. *Annu Rev Biochem* 1977; 46: 897-930.
8. Lewington S, Whitlock G, Clarke R, *et al.* Blood cholesterol and vascular mortality by age, sex, and blood pressure: a meta-analysis of individual data from 61 prospective studies with 55,000 vascular deaths. *Lancet* 2007; 370: 1829-39.
9. Tang JL, Armitage JM, Lancaster T, Silagy CA, Fowler GH, Neil HA. Systematic review of dietary intervention trials to lower blood total cholesterol in free-living subjects. *BMJ* 1998; 316: 1213-20.
10. Hooper L, Summerbell CD, Higgins JP, *et al.* Dietary fat intake and prevention of cardiovascular disease: systematic review. *BMJ* 2001; 322: 757-63.
11. Collaborative overview ('meta-analysis') of prospective observational studies of the associations of usual blood pressure and usual cholesterol levels with common causes of death: protocol for the second cycle of the Prospective Studies Collaboration. *J Cardiovasc Risk* 1999; 6: 315-20.
12. Zhang X, Patel A, Horibe H, *et al.* Cholesterol, coronary heart disease, and stroke in the Asia Pacific region. *Int J Epidemiol* 2003; 32: 563-72.
13. Woodward M, Barzi F, Martiniuk A, *et al.* Cohort profile: the Asia Pacific Cohort Studies Collaboration. *Int J Epidemiol* 2006; 35: 1412-6.
14. Cholesterol Treatment Trialists' Collaboration. Efficacy and safety of cholesterol-lowering treatment: prospective meta-analysis of data from 90,056 participants in 14 randomised trials of statins. *Lancet* 2005; 366: 1267-78.

15. Yusuf S, Reddy S, Ounpuu S, Anand S. Global burden of cardiovascular diseases: part I: general considerations, the epidemiologic transition, risk factors, and impact of urbanization. *Circulation* 2001; 104: 2746-53.

16. Yusuf S, Reddy S, Ounpuu S, Anand S. Global burden of cardiovascular diseases: Part II: variations in cardiovascular disease by specific ethnic groups and geographic regions and prevention strategies. *Circulation* 2001; 104: 2855-64.

17. Heart Protection Study Collaborative Group. Effects of cholesterol-lowering with simvastatin on stroke and other major vascular events in 20,536 people with cerebrovascular disease or other high-risk conditions. *Lancet* 2004; 363: 757-67.

18. Cholesterol, diastolic blood pressure, and stroke: 13,000 strokes in 450,000 people in 45 prospective cohorts. Prospective Studies Collaboration. *Lancet* 1995; 346: 1647-53.

19. Wardlaw JM, Keir SL, Dennis MS. The impact of delays in computed tomography of the brain on the accuracy of diagnosis and subsequent management in patients with minor stroke. *J Neurol Neurosurg Psychiatry* 2003; 74: 77-81.

20. Blood pressure, cholesterol, and stroke in eastern Asia. Eastern Stroke and Coronary Heart Disease Collaborative Research Group. *Lancet* 1998; 352: 1801-7.

21. Noda H, Iso H, Irie F, et al. Low-density lipoprotein cholesterol concentrations and death due to intraparenchymal hemorrhage: the Ibaraki Prefectural Health Study. *Circulation* 2009; 119: 2136-45.

22. Iso H, Jacobs DRJ, Wentworth D, Neaton JD, Cohen JD. Serum cholesterol levels and six-year mortality from stroke in 350,977 men screened for the multiple risk factor intervention trial. *N Engl J Med* 1989; 320: 904-10.

23. Ebrahim S, Sung J, Song YM, Ferrer RL, Lawlor DA, Davey Smith G. Serum cholesterol, haemorrhagic stroke, ischaemic stroke, and myocardial infarction: Korean National Health System Prospective Cohort Study. *BMJ* 2006; 333: 22.

24. Holme I, Aastveit AH, Hammar N, Jungner I, Walldius G. Relationships between lipoprotein components and risk of ischaemic and haemorrhagic stroke in the Apolipoprotein MOrtality RISk study (AMORIS). *J Intern Med* 2009; 265: 275-87.

25. Woodward M, Barzi F, Feigin V, et al. Associations between high-density lipoprotein cholesterol and both stroke and coronary heart disease in the Asia Pacific region. *Eur Heart J* 2007; 28: 2653-60.

26. Austin MA, Edwards KL. Small, dense low density lipoproteins, the insulin resistance syndrome and noninsulin-dependent diabetes. *Curr Opin Lipidol* 1996; 7: 167-71.

27. Avogaro P, Bon GB, Cazzolato G, Quinci GB. Are apolipoproteins better discriminators than lipids for atherosclerosis? *Lancet* 1979; 1: 901-3.

28. Walldius G, Jungner I, Holme I, Aastveit AH, Kolar W, Steiner E. High apolipoprotein B, low apolipoprotein A-I, and improvement in the prediction of fatal myocardial infarction (AMORIS study): a prospective study. *Lancet* 2001; 358: 2026-33.

29. McQueen MJ, Hawken S, Wang X, et al. Lipids, lipoproteins, and apolipoproteins as risk markers of myocardial infarction in 52 countries (the INTERHEART study): a case-control study. *Lancet* 2008; 372: 224-33.

30. Otvos JD, Collins D, Freedman DS, et al. Low-density lipoprotein and high-density lipoprotein particle subclasses predict coronary events and are favorably changed by gemfibrozil therapy in the Veterans Affairs High-Density Lipoprotein Intervention Trial. *Circulation* 2006; 113: 1556-63.

31. Mora S, Otvos JD, Rifai N, Rosenson RS, Buring JE, Ridker PM. Lipoprotein particle profiles by nuclear magnetic resonance compared with standard lipids and apolipoproteins in predicting incident cardiovascular disease in women. *Circulation* 2009; 119: 931-9.

32. Parish S, Peto R, Palmer A, et al. The joint effects of Apo B, Apo A1, LDL cholesterol and HDL cholesterol on risk: 3510 cases of acute myocardial infarction and 9805 controls. *Eur Heart J* 2009; 30: 2137-46.

33. Charlton-Menys V, Betteridge DJ, Colhoun H, et al. Apolipoproteins, cardiovascular risk and statin response in type 2 diabetes: the Collaborative Atorvastatin Diabetes Study (CARDS). *Diabetologia* 2009; 52: 218-25.

34. Simes RJ, Marschner IC, Hunt D, et al. Relationship between lipid levels and clinical outcomes in the Long-term Intervention with Pravastatin in Ischemic Disease (LIPID) Trial: to what extent is the reduction in coronary events with pravastatin explained by on-study lipid levels? *Circulation* 2002; 105: 1162-9.

35. Pedersen TR, Olsson AG, Faergeman O, *et al*. Lipoprotein changes and reduction in the incidence of major coronary heart disease events in the Scandinavian Simvastatin Survival Study (4S). *Circulation* 1998; 97: 1453-60.

36. Gotto AM, Jr., Whitney E, Stein EA, *et al*. Relation between baseline and on-treatment lipid parameters and first acute major coronary events in the Air Force/Texas Coronary Atherosclerosis Prevention Study (AFCAPS/TexCAPS). *Circulation* 2000; 101: 477-84.

37. Chien KL, Sung FC, Hsu HC, Su TC, Lin RS, Lee YT. Apolipoprotein A-I and B and stroke events in a community-based cohort in Taiwan: report of the Chin-Shan Community Cardiovascular Study. *Stroke* 2002; 33: 39-44.

38. Koren-Morag N, Goldbourt U, Graff E, Tanne D. Apolipoproteins B and AI and the risk of ischemic cerebrovascular events in patients with pre-existing atherothrombotic disease. *J Neurol Sci* 2008; 270: 82-7.

39. Qureshi AI, Giles WH, Croft JB, Guterman LR, Hopkins LN. Apolipoproteins A-1 and B and the likelihood of non-fatal stroke and myocardial infarction - data from The Third National Health and Nutrition Examination Survey. *Med Sci Monit* 2002; 8: CR311-6.

40. Sharobeem KM, Patel JV, Ritch AE, Lip GY, Gill PS, Hughes EA. Elevated lipoprotein (a) and apolipoprotein B to AI ratio in South Asian patients with ischaemic stroke. *Int J Clin Pract* 2007; 61: 1824-8.

41. Ridker PM, Danielson E, Fonseca FA, *et al*. Rosuvastatin to prevent vascular events in men and women with elevated C-reactive protein. *N Engl J Med* 2008; 359: 2195-207.

42. Kjekshus J, Apetrei E, Barrios V, *et al*. Rosuvastatin in older patients with systolic heart failure. *N Engl J Med* 2007; 357: 2248-61.

43. Tavazzi L, Maggioni AP, Marchioli R, *et al*. Effect of rosuvastatin in patients with chronic heart failure (the GISSI-HF trial): a randomised, double-blind, placebo-controlled trial. *Lancet* 2008; 372: 1231-9.

44. Wanner C, Krane V, Marz W, *et al*. Atorvastatin in patients with type 2 diabetes mellitus undergoing hemodialysis. *N Engl J Med* 2005; 353: 238-48.

Chapter 4

Are LDL cholesterol-lowering functional food ingredients successful in the long term?

Jogchum Plat PhD, Associate Professor, Human Biology
Ronald P. Mensink PhD MSc, Professor of Molecular Nutrition
Department of Human Biology, Maastricht University
Maastricht, The Netherlands

Introduction

Despite huge improvements in treating and preventing cardiovascular diseases (CVD), it remains a leading cause of mortality and disability worldwide. Atherosclerosis is the process underlying CVD in which elevated (oxidized) low-density lipoprotein (LDL) cholesterol is recognized as a causal factor [1, 2]. The first indication, that increased circulating serum total cholesterol concentrations are related to lesion formation, already originates from the beginning of the previous century. Since then, a long and winding road has resulted at least four decades ago in the current situation, i.e. recognition that lowering serum total and particularly LDL cholesterol concentrations is a major target to reduce cardiovascular risk. Dietary guidelines recommended by many different health agencies particularly focus on reducing saturated and trans-fatty acid intake, as this effectively lowers serum total and LDL cholesterol concentrations. For saturated fatty acids, this could already be unequivocally concluded from the prediction equations, as formulated by Keys *et al* [3] several decades ago. It further appeared that reductions in serum total cholesterol that could be achieved by reducing dietary cholesterol intake, were less strong than those achieved by decreasing saturated-fat intake, though still present [4].

Further, numerous epidemiological studies have shown that elevated serum LDL cholesterol concentrations raise the risk for CVD. Also, genetic studies show the causal role of elevated LDL cholesterol in CVD. For example, subjects that are carriers of a specific variation (*PCSK9*[142X] or *PCSK9*[679X]) in the gene encoding proprotein convertase subtilisin-like / kexin type 9 (PCSK9) had 28% lower serum LDL cholesterol concentrations [5]. PCSK9 is a secreted protease that is responsible for degradation of the LDL receptor after binding to its extracellular domain. Individuals with the above-mentioned loss of function mutations have, therefore, a lower serum LDL cholesterol concentration. Interestingly, the carriers characterised by a life-long 28% lower serum LDL cholesterol had an approximate 88% lower CVD risk over a period of 15 years. Carriers of another mutation (*PCSK9*[46L]), resulting in a 15% lower serum LDL cholesterol concentration, were characterised by a 47% reduced CHD risk [5]. This illustrates not only that lower LDL cholesterol concentrations are protective, but also that effects are particularly evident if LDL cholesterol concentrations are low from childhood onwards. Fully in line with the *PCSK9* data, LDL cholesterol-lowering drugs also reduce cardiovascular mortality. The first drugs showing these effects were the statins. One of the confirmative statin studies carried out in the 1990s was the 4S study, performed in 4444 patients in Scandinavia [6]. Since then, there has been a constant attempt to further lower the targets set as optimal LDL cholesterol concentrations. Behind this drive to further lower LDL cholesterol, a continuous and progressive relationship was suggested between serum LDL cholesterol concentrations and CVD risk.

Although statins have become more effective over the years, patients on statin treatment often still do not reach the goal for LDL cholesterol concentrations as set by the National Cholesterol Education Program (NCEP) [7]. Moreover, even doubling the dose of statins, may not be helpful, since it was found to provide an additional LDL cholesterol reduction of only 3-7% [8]. However, it can be argued that doubling the dose is more beneficial than can be concluded solely based on observed changes in LDL cholesterol, because of the suggested pleiotropic effects of statins. On the other hand, doubling the dose of statins might also increase the risk for adverse effects, especially in older people who often use a lot of co-medication as well. Besides doubling the dose of a statin, an alternative approach for further lowering elevated LDL cholesterol concentrations is the use of functional foods – such as products enriched with plant sterol or stanol esters – on top of statin treatment [9]. In fact, combining plant sterol / stanol-enriched products with statins is more effective in further lowering LDL cholesterol than doubling the statin dose. This may be due to the fact that plant sterols and stanols inhibit the absorption of dietary and biliary cholesterol in the intestine, whereas statins lower endogenous cholesterol synthesis. Thus, these two differing mechanisms apparently complement each other. Consuming around 2.5g of plant sterols or stanols / day lowers serum LDL cholesterol concentrations by approximately 10%, not only as solo intervention but also as an add-on treatment to statins.

Besides plant sterol or stanol-enriched foods, there are other functional ingredients with a potential effect on serum LDL cholesterol concentrations. Although not confirmed by the same number of studies as available for plant sterols and stanols, viscous fibers, such as β-glucans, pectins, and gums, have been shown to be effective in lowering serum LDL cholesterol concentrations. For all these FDA approved ingredients the question is whether this will be a successful means for controlling serum lipid levels in the long term. An additional question is whether long-term reductions in LDL cholesterol induced by these dietary components do translate into healthier vessels.

Plant sterols and stanols

Plant sterols (β-sitosterol, campesterol, and stigmasterol) are the natural occurring equivalents of the mammalian cholesterol. Although in much lower quantities plant stanols (sitostanol and campestanol) – being the saturated derivatives of plant sterols – are also present in nature. Due to the structural similarity of these so-called 4-desmethylsterols with cholesterol (Figure 1), plant sterols and stanols can replace cholesterol in membranes, mixed micelles, and lipoproteins. The replacement of cholesterol from mixed micelles in the intestinal lumen lowers the supply of intestinal cholesterol available for absorption. It is thought that this is the mechanism underlying the known decrease in intestinal cholesterol absorption. The decrease in intestinal cholesterol absorption ultimately results in decreased serum LDL cholesterol concentrations, possibly through increases in hepatic LDL-receptor expression. This was suggested by the results from a well-controlled placebo-controlled intervention study, in which plant stanol ester consumption reduced cholesterol absorption and increased expression of the LDL receptor in human peripheral mononuclear blood cells (PBMCs). Since the expression of the LDL receptor in PBMCs highly correlated with the expression in the liver [10], this data can be interpreted in that hepatic expression of the LDL receptor increased due to plant stanol ester consumption. In addition, there was a highly significant correlation between the changes in serum LDL cholesterol concentrations and protein expressions of the LDL receptor on the cell surface (Figure 2) [11]. This clearly explains the observed reductions in serum LDL cholesterol concentrations in human intervention studies after plant sterol and stanol consumption (Figure 3).

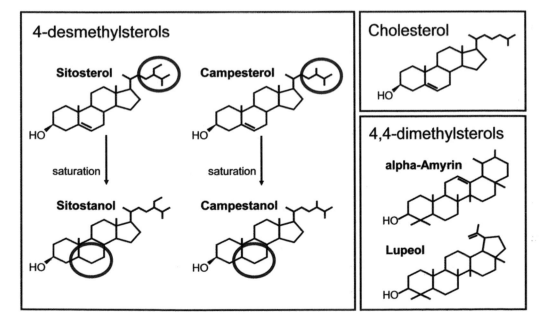

Figure 1. Structures of different plant sterols as compared to cholesterol. On the left the structures of two 4-desmethylsterols (sitosterol and campesterol) are shown, while it is also indicated how plant stanols can be made out of sterols by saturation of the double bond. Examples of 4,4 dimethylsterols, such as alpha-amyrin and lupeol, are depicted on the right side.

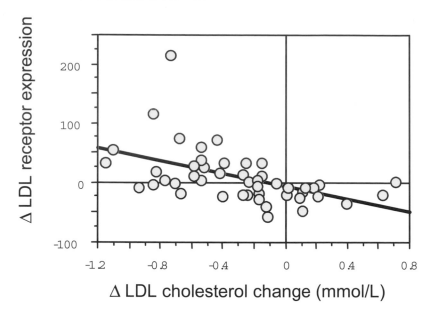

Figure 2. The relationship between changes in LDL receptor cell-surface protein of monocytes and changes in serum LDL cholesterol concentrations [11].

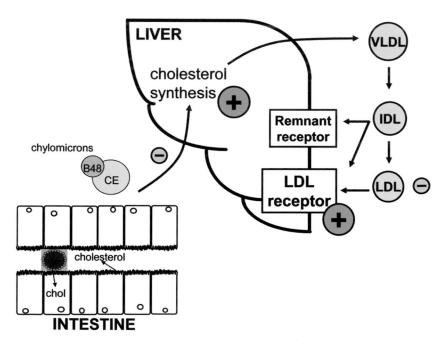

Figure 3. Plant stanol esters lower intestinal cholesterol absorption. Since less cholesterol enters the circulation this induces a compensatory increase in the endogenous cholesterol synthesis. Despite this increased synthesis, the net effect is a reduction in serum LDL cholesterol concentrations. From the literature it is known that LDL production from VLDL and IDL is reduced in male NIDDM patients. We have now shown that LDL receptor expression increases. This might not only enhance LDL clearance from the circulation, but IDL clearance as well and therefore also explains the reduced LDL formation.

A meta-analysis including all randomized, double-blind, dietary intervention trials concluded that plant sterols and stanols lowered serum LDL cholesterol by an average 6.7% (range 4.9-8.6%), 8.5% (7.0-10.1%), 8.9% (7.4-10.5%) and 11.3% (10.3-12.3%) at daily intakes of 0.7-1.1, 1.5-1.9, 2.0-2.4, or ≥2.5g, respectively **(Ia/A)**, with no effects on HDL-cholesterol or triacylglycerol [9]. In line with the comparable effects on serum LDL cholesterol concentrations, it was found that plant sterol and stanol esters lowered cholesterol absorption to the same extent [12]. In ileostomy patients, small bowel cholesterol absorption decreased from 56% to 38-39%, irrespective of the fact that the diet was enriched for 3 days with 1.5g plant sterol or stanol esters. However, not all plant sterols lower plasma LDL cholesterol. In contrast to spreads enriched with free 4-desmethylsterols (sitosterol and campesterol) from soybean oil, spreads enriched with 4,4-dimethylsterols from sheanut oil, such as lupeol and α-amyrin (Figure 1), did not decrease serum LDL cholesterol [13]. It may be that 4,4-dimethylsterols, of which the molecular structures show less overlap with cholesterol than 4-desmethylsterols, cannot replace intestinal cholesterol from the mixed micelles. However, cholesterol absorption was not measured, and it is therefore also possible that other effects of 4,4-dimethylsterols have counteracted cholesterol absorption.

In addition to the effects on serum LDL cholesterol concentrations, we have recently suggested that plant stanols not only lower serum LDL cholesterol but also triacylglycerol concentrations [14]. Effects were only evident in subjects with increased serum triacylglycerol concentrations before the start of the study. This suggestion was confirmed in a placebo controlled intervention study in metabolic syndrome subjects showing a reduction of 29% in serum triacylglycerol concentrations after consuming 2g plant stanols as their fatty acid esters for 9 weeks [15], an effect comparable to that described for fish oils [16]. Regarding long-term functional effects of these compounds on cardiovascular risk, this of course offers additional possibilities.

Although most placebo-controlled studies had a relatively short duration, the longer-term efficacy of plant sterols and stanols has also been demonstrated. Both plant sterol esters as well as plant stanol esters were still effective in maintaining the lowered serum LDL cholesterol values after 1 year of follow-up [17, 18]. Our own group recently showed in patients who were already on statin treatment for several years, that both plant sterol and plant stanol esters were effective as add-on treatment to further lowering serum LDL cholesterol concentrations during an 18-month intervention period [19]. In brief, in the plant sterol group, the average changes in serum total and LDL cholesterol concentrations were 0.38mmol/L (or 6.8%) and 0.33mmol/L (or 9.7%), respectively, whereas plant stanol esters lowered serum total and LDL cholesterol concentrations by 0.48mmol/L (or 8.8%) and 0.38mmol/L (or 11.2%), respectively (Figure 4) **(Ib/A)**.

Although promising, the ultimate question is whether these lipid-lowering effects translate into a reduced cardiovascular risk. In this respect, animal studies are supportive. In both apoE*3-Leiden mice and in heterozygous LDL receptor-deficient mice, plant sterol and stanol esters not only lowered serum cholesterol concentrations, but also attenuated atherosclerotic lesion development [20, 21]. In humans, this question is more difficult to answer. Instead, studies have been carried out with functional effects on vessel wall characteristics as endpoints.

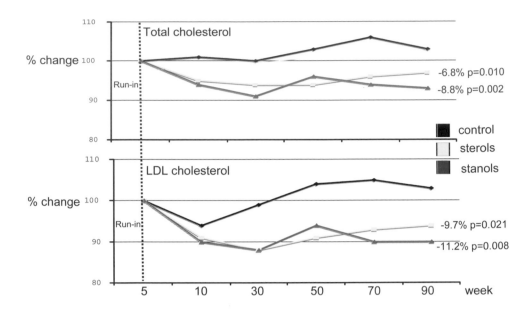

Figure 4. Relative concentrations of serum total and LDL cholesterol during the study [19]. Average concentrations of lipids and lipoproteins in weeks 4 and 5 were set at 100%.

Moreover, using outcome data from studies using pharmaceutical cholesterol absorption inhibitors can be supportive in drawing conclusions about the usefulness of this approach. For this purpose, ezetimibe, a Niemann-Pick C1 like 1 protein (NPC1L1) inhibitor, is a good drug candidate. Ezetimibe has been shown to be a highly effective inhibitor of intestinal cholesterol absorption [22]. With respect to the efficacy in terms of risk reduction by lowering intestinal cholesterol absorption, it needs to be emphasized that the recent ENHANCE trial has clearly indicated that an additional reduction in serum LDL cholesterol concentration does not always translate into improved intima media thickness (IMT). The ENHANCE trial demonstrated that adding ezetimibe (10mg/day) – a powerful cholesterol absorption inhibitor – on top of treatment with simvastatin (80mg/day) did indeed further lower serum LDL cholesterol concentrations in familial hypercholesterolemia (FH) as a priori hypothesized [23]. After 2 years of follow-up, serum LDL cholesterol concentrations were lowered by 55.6% in the ezetimibe + simvastatin group versus 39.1% in the group only receiving simvastatin. However, despite the additional 16.5% reduction in LDL cholesterol there was no further improvement in IMT of the carotid artery. However, there is a very good explanation for this. The baseline IMT was already very low because of highly effective treatment of the heterozygous FH patients before inclusion, that further improvement by the addition of ezetimibe to simvastatin treatment was hardly possible. Therefore, the question is whether the effects of plant sterol or stanol esters will be beneficial in the end for all consumers are more than justified. In humans, the effects of plant sterol or stanol ester consumption on vessel wall characteristics have been evaluated as well. So far, only a few studies have analyzed the effects of plant sterols or stanols on arterial wall properties in humans. These studies showed no effects of plant sterol or stanol ester consumption on flow-mediated dilation (FMD) in children [24, 25] and adults [26]. Also, on carotid artery elasticity, no effect of plant sterol or stanol ester consumption was found in healthy volunteers [27] or in hypercholesterolemic patients already on statin treatment [28] **(Ib/A)**. However, both studies in which arterial elasticity parameters were calculated found that subjects at risk, i.e. with a disturbed compliance of the carotid artery [27] or elevated matrix metalloproteinase (MMP9) concentrations [28] at baseline, did show improvements in arterial compliance **(Ib/A)**. This illustrates that the reduction in serum LDL cholesterol concentrations are not by definition translated into functional improvements of the vessel wall, at least not in subjects with relatively healthy vessels. Since the effects seem promising in subjects at risk, there is a need for a study specifically designed to answer the question of whether the effects are indeed beneficial in these patients in terms of slowing down progression of (validated markers for) cardiovascular disease.

Viscous fibers

Dietary fibers are plant compounds that are resistant to digestion by enzymes in the small intestine, although some fermentation into short chain fatty acids in the colon is possible. A simple classification is based on their capacity to bind water or not. Insoluble fibers are structural fibers such as cellulose and lignins, as present in plants. Soluble or viscous gel-forming fibers are, for example, β-glucans, psyllium, pectins, and gums, as present in oats, barley, rye, vegetables and fruits.

β-glucans are carbohydrates consisting of linked glucose molecules, and as such form major structural components of the cell walls of yeast and fungi, but are also found in cell walls of cereals such as barley and oats. Depending on the source, there are substantial differences in macromolecular structure between β-glucans. The oat and barley cell walls contain unbranched β-glucans with β-(1→3) and β-(1→4)-linked glycopyranosyl residues (Figure 5) [29]. These oat and barley derived β-glucans, which are basically the most important sources for cereal glucans, are known for their serum cholesterol-lowering effects **(Ia/A)**. Besides cereals, β-glucans – with a slightly different molecular structure – can also be found in fungi and yeast. However, their effects on cholesterol metabolism have hardly been evaluated in well-controlled human intervention studies. Therefore, making firm conclusions about their efficacy in lowering serum LDL cholesterol concentrations is too early. As well as β-glucans there is also another viscous fiber called psyllium, which is recognised by the FDA for its effects on serum cholesterol concentration. A meta-analysis containing several well-controlled studies showed that four major viscous fiber types (β-glucan [from cereals], psyllium, pectin and guar gum) effectively lowered serum LDL cholesterol concentrations [30]. Despite the fact that there are large differences in molecular structure between the different fiber types, there appeared to be hardly any differences in the efficacy of the individual fibers. This may suggest that there is a common underlying mechanism. This mechanism is unfortunately not fully delineated, but there are clear indications that the enterohepatic circulation of bile acids is hindered by the fact that viscous fibers can bind the bile acids or otherwise interfere with the enterohepatic circulation within the intestinal lumen.

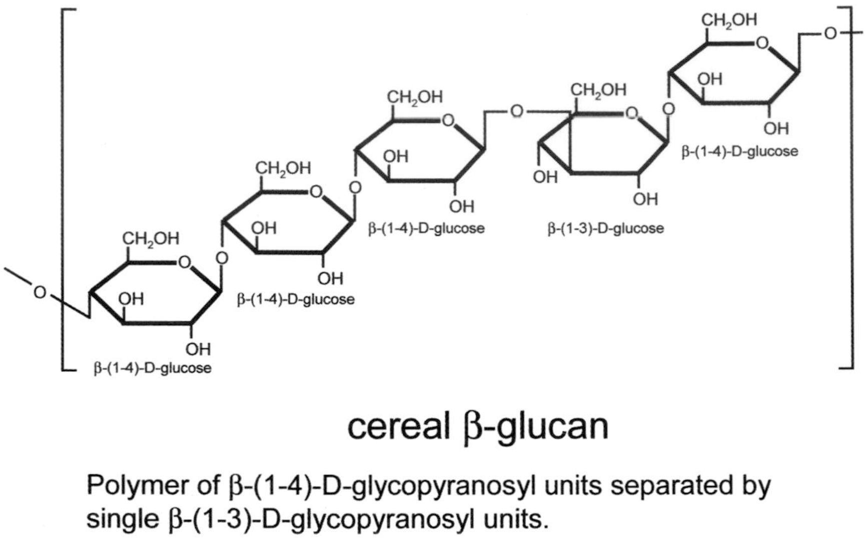

cereal β-glucan

Polymer of β-(1-4)-D-glycopyranosyl units separated by single β-(1-3)-D-glycopyranosyl units.

Figure 5. General structure of a β-glucan molecule.

Consequently, bile acids are secreted with the faeces and the conversion of cholesterol into newly formed bile acids in the liver is increased. This enhanced bile acid production demands a higher uptake of LDL particles from the circulation explaining reductions in serum LDL cholesterol. On the other hand, the absorption of dietary cholesterol itself from the intestine also seems to be lowered [31].

On a gram-to-gram basis, the effects of β-glucans on serum LDL cholesterol concentration are not as large as those of plant sterols and stanols. Estimations are that for each gram of oat-derived β-glucans, serum LDL cholesterol is lowered by 0.032mmol/L. At a daily intake of 5g which can actually only be reached by enriched products, the effect is a reduction of 0.16mmol/L[30], or approximately 5-6% at a baseline LDL cholesterol concentration of around 3mmol/L. Whether effects remain after long-term consumption of these viscous fibers is not known, since such studies have not been performed. Also, studies describing effects on arterial wall properties are missing. However, epidemiological prospective cohort studies suggest that an increased intake of soluble fibers (such as β-glucans) is associated with a reduction in CVD risk [32].

Combining products enriched with plant sterols or stanols and β-glucans

Pharmacologically, it is common to combine two drugs with different working mechanisms to achieve additional benefits. Therefore, it is not to be unexpected that nutritionists have also started thinking in this direction. In theory, products enriched with plant sterols or stanols should be effective on top of the effects of one of the viscous fibers. Indeed, Yoshida *et al* have shown that adding glucomannan (10g/day), another viscous fiber derived from konjac root, to 1.8g plant sterols as their fatty acid esters, further lowered serum LDL cholesterol concentrations [33]. It was found that plant sterol esters lowered serum LDL cholesterol by 5.4%, glucomannan by 13.8% and the combination by 21.7% **(Ia/A)**. However, Theuwissen *et al* have suggested that combining plant stanols with β-glucans did have a smaller effect on serum LDL cholesterol concentrations than the sum of the effects for both individual interventions [34]. A likely explanation for this latter finding can be found in the possible effect of β-glucans on intestinal absorption of cholesterol. This explanation was based on the observation that circulating plant sterol concentrations were lowered when β-glucan-enriched products were consumed. It is generally accepted that serum plant sterol concentrations relate positively to intestinal cholesterol absorption [35]. This can be explained by the current knowledge that cholesterol and plant sterols share the same transporter molecules responsible for absorption and secretion within the enterocytes. For example, the NPC1L1 protein seems crucial in the uptake of cholesterol from the intestine, as shown by studies using the cholesterol absorption inhibitor, ezetimibe. However, studies with NPC1L1-deficient mice also suggested that NPC1L1 plays a crucial role in the absorption of plant sterols [36]. Therefore, ezetimibe is nowadays also prescribed for patients with sitosterolemia – a rare inheritable disease caused by mutations in the ATP binding cassette transporters G5 or G8 and characterized by elevated intestinal plant sterol absorption together with a reduced capacity to secrete plant sterols in bile – and as such responsible for lowering intestinal plant sterol absorption.

However, we have earlier hypothesized on the mechanisms of plant sterols and stanols explaining that the reduced intestinal cholesterol absorption involves changes in regulatory processes within the enterocytes [37]. This assumption also means that plant sterols or stanols need to be absorbed from the intestinal lumen into the enterocytes to become effective, i.e activate for example a sterol efflux pump. If this assumption is true, combining plant sterols or stanols with another compound that lowers cholesterol absorption (and therefore most likely plant sterols or stanol absorption) may interfere with the efficacy of plant sterols and stanols. In other words, if less plant sterols and stanols can enter the enterocytes, the effect of the sterols or stanols is diminished. Therefore, in our view, since β-glucans may also lower intestinal absorption of cholesterol, the effects of plant sterols or stanols and β-glucans on serum LDL cholesterol concentrations are not *per se* additive. In line with this explanation, combining plant stanols with ezetimibe showed the same result, i.e. the effects were not additive [38]. Again, we assume that the reduced absorption of plant stanols into the enterocytes due to ezetimibe treatment has possibly blocked stanols interfering with intracellular cholesterol metabolism.

Over the coming years the number of functional foods and drugs that interfere with intestinal cholesterol absorption will expand. Therefore, predicting the long-term efficacy of functional foods aiming to improve serum lipid levels will become more speculative. It will all depend on the use of other functional food ingredients and co-medication that are used. In that respect, understanding the underlying mechanisms will be helpful.

Conclusions

The evidence suggests that functional foods enriched with plant sterol or stanol esters effectively lower serum LDL cholesterol concentrations in short- and long-term placebo-controlled intervention studies. Reductions in serum LDL cholesterol concentrations are not translated into functional improvements in subjects with relatively healthy vessels. Since the effects seem promising in subjects at risk, there is a need for a study specifically designed to answer the question on whether the effects are indeed beneficial in these patients in terms of slowing down progression of cardiovascular disease. Also, functional foods enriched with the viscous fiber, β-glucans, effectively lower serum LDL cholesterol concentrations, although the effects are less pronounced. Whether the effects of these viscous fibers remain after long-term consumption or even if they affect arterial wall properties is not known, since those studies have not been performed. The combination of different functional food ingredients might even be counteractive. This will make the prediction of long-term efficacy of functional foods aiming to improve serum lipid levels even more speculative.

Key points	Evidence level
◆ Plant sterols and stanols lower serum LDL cholesterol in studies with a short duration.	Ia/A
◆ Plant sterols and stanols lower serum LDL cholesterol in studies with a longer duration up to 18 months.	Ib/A
◆ Plant sterols and stanols have no effect on arterial wall properties in healthy subjects.	Ib/A
◆ Plant sterols and stanols may improve arterial wall properties in subjects with disturbed endothelial function.	Ib/A
◆ β-glucans from oats lower serum LDL cholesterol in studies with a short duration.	Ia/A
◆ Combining different functional food ingredients aiming at lowering serum LDL cholesterol concentrations can be more or less effective in lowering serum LDL cholesterol.	Ia/A

References

1. Davidson MH. Overview of prevention and treatment of atherosclerosis with lipid-altering therapy for pharmacy directors. *Am J Manag Care* 2007; 13 Suppl 10: S260-9.
2. Ross R. Atherosclerosis - an inflammatory disease. *N Engl J Med* 1999; 340: 115-26.
3. Keys A, Parlin RW. Serum cholesterol response to changes in dietary lipids. *Am J Clin Nutr* 1966; 19: 175-81.
4. Howell WH, McNamara DJ, Tosca MA, Smith BT, Gaines JA. Plasma lipid and lipoprotein responses to dietary fat and cholesterol: a meta-analysis. *Am J Clin Nutr* 1997; 65: 1747-64.
5. Cohen JC, Boerwinkle E, Mosley TH, Hobbs HH. Sequence variations in PCSK9, low LDL, and protection against coronary heart disease. *N Engl J Med* 2006; 354; 1264-72.

6. Randomised trial of cholesterol lowering in 4444 patients with coronary heart disease: the Scandinavian Simvastatin Survival Study (4S). *Lancet* 1994; 344: 1383-89.

7. Expert panel on detection evaluation, and treatment of high blood cholesterol in adults. Executive summary of the third report of the National Cholesterol Education Program (NCEP) Expert Panel on Detection, Evaluation, and Treatment of High Blood Cholesterol in Aduls (Adult Treatment Panel III). *J Am Med Assoc* 2003; 285: 2486-97.

8. Jones PH, Davidson MH, Stein EA, Bays HE, McKenney JM, Miller E, Cain VA, Blasetto JW. Comparison of the efficacy and safety of rosuvastatin versus atorvastatin, simvastatin, and pravastatin across doses (STELLAR* Trial). *Am J Cardiol* 2003; 92: 152-60.

9. Katan MB, Grundy SM, Jones P, Law M, Miettinen T, Paoletti R. Efficacy and safety of plant stanols and sterols in the management of blood cholesterol levels. *Mayo Clin Proc* 2003; 78: 965-78.

10. Powell EE, Kroon PA. Low density lipoprotein receptor and 3-hydroxy-3 methylglutaryl coenzyme A reductase gene expression in human mononuclear leukocytes is regulated coordinately and parallels gene expression in human liver. *J Clin Invest* 1994; 93: 2168-74.

11. Plat J, Mensink RP. Hypocholesterolemic mechanisms of plant stanol esters; effects on LDL receptor mRNA and cell surface protein expression, and HMG-CoA reductase mRNA expression in non-hypercholesterolemic subjects. *FASEB J* 2002; 16: 258-60.

12. Normén L, Dutta P, Lia A, Andersson H. Soy sterol esters and b-sitostanol ester as inhibitors of cholesterol absorption in human small bowel. *Am J Clin Nutr* 2000; 71: 908-13.

13. Weststrate, JA, Meijer GW. Plant sterol-enriched margarines and reduction of plasma total- and LDL-cholesterol concentrations in normocholesterolaemic and mildly hypercholesterolaemic subjects. *Eur J Clin Nutr* 1998; 52: 334-43.

14. Naumann E, Plat J, Kester ADM, Mensink RP. The baseline serum lipoprotein profile is related to plant stanol induced changes in serum lipids and lipoproteins. *J Am Coll Nutr* 2008; 27: 117-26.

15. Plat J, Brufau G, Dallinga-ThiE GM, Dasselaar M, Mensink RP. A plant stanol yogurt drink alone or combined with a low-dose OTC statin lowers triacylglycerol and non-HDL cholesterol concentrations in metabolic syndrome patients. *J Nutr* 2009; 139: 1143-9.

16. Harris WS. N-3 fatty acids and serum lipoproteins: human studies. *Am J Clin Nutr* 1997; 65: 1645S-54.

17. Hendriks HF, Brink EJ, Meijer GW, Princen HM, Ntanios FY. Safety of long-term consumption of plant sterol esters-enriched spread. *Eur J Clin Nutr* 2003; 57: 681-92.

18. Miettinen TA, Puska P, Gylling H, Vanhanen H, Vartiainen E. Reduction of serum cholesterol with sitostanol-ester margarine in a mildly hypercholesterolemic population. *N Engl J Med* 1995; 333: 1308-12.

19. Jong NA, Plat J, Lutjohann D, Mensink RP. Effects of long-term plant sterol or stanol consumption on lipid and lipoprotein metabolism in subjects on statin treatment. *Br J Nutr* 2008; 100: 937-41.

20. Volger OL, Mensink RP, Plat J, Hornstra G, Havekes LM, Princen HM. Dietary vegetable oil and wood derived plant stanol esters reduce atherosclerotic lesion size and severity in apoE*3-Leiden transgenic mice. *Atherosclerosis* 2001; 157: 375-81.

21. Plat J, Beugels I, Gijbels MJ, de Winther MP, Mensink RP. Plant sterol or stanol esters retard lesion formation in LDL receptor-deficient mice independent of changes in serum plant sterols. *J Lipid Res* 2006; 47: 2762-71.

22. Altmann SW, Davis HR Jr, Zhu L, Yao X, Hoos LM, Tetzloff G, Lyer SPN, Maguire M, Golovko A, Zeng M, *et al*. Niemann-Pick C1 like 1 protein is critical for intestinal cholesterol absorption. *Science* 2005; 303: 1201-4.

23. Kastelein JJ, Akdim F, Stroes ESG, Zwinderman AH, Bots ML, Stalenhoef AFH, Visseren FLJ, Sijbrands EJG, Trip MD, Stein EA, Gaudet D, Duivenvoorden R, Veltri EP, Marais D, de Groot E. Simvastatin with or without ezetimibe in familial hypercholesterolemia. *N Engl J Med* 2008; 358: 1431-3.

24. de Jongh S, Vissers MN, Rol P, Bakker HD, Kastelein JJ, Stroes ES. Plant sterols lower LDL cholesterol without improving endothelial function in prepubertal children with familial hypercholesterolaemia. *J Inherit Metab Dis* 2003; 26: 343-51.

25. Jakulj L, Vissers MN, Rodenburg J, Wiegman A, Trip MD, Kastelein JJ. Plant stanols do not restore endothelial function in pre-pubertal children with familial hypercholesterolemia despite reduction of low-density lipoprotein cholesterol levels. *J Pediatr* 2006; 148: 495-500.

26. Hallikainen M, Lyyra-Laitinen T, Laitinen T, Agren JJ, Pihlajamaki J, Rauramaa R, Miettinen TA, Gylling H. Endothelial function in hypercholesterolemic subjects: Effects of plant stanol and sterol esters. *Atherosclerosis* 2006; 188: 425-32.

27. Raitakari OT, Salo P, Gylling H, Miettinen TA. Plant stanol ester consumption and arterial elasticity and endothelial function. *Br J Nutr* 2008; 100: 603-8.

28. Jong NA, Plat J, Hoeks A, Mensink RP. Effects of long-term consumption of plant sterol or plant stanol esters on endothelial function and arterial stiffness in patients on stable statin treatment. *Atherosclerosis* 2007; 8: 1.

29. Estrada A, Yun CH, Van Kessel A, Li B, Hauta S, Laarveld B. Immunomodulatory activities of oat beta-glucan *in vitro* and *in vivo*. *Microbiol Immunol* 1997; 41: 991-8.

30. Brown L, Rosner B, Willett WW, Sacks FM. Cholesterol-lowering effects of dietary fiber: a meta-analysis. *Am J Clin Nutr* 1999; 69: 30-42.

31. Naumann E, van Rees AB, Onnig G, Oste R, Wydra M, Mensink RP. Beta-glucan incoporated into a fruit drink effectively lowers serum LDL cholesterol concentrations. *Am J Clin Nutr* 2006; 83: 601-5.

32. Pereira MA, O'Reilly E, Augustsson K. Dietary fiber and risk of coronary heart disease: a pooled analysis of cohort studies. *Arch Intern Med* 2004;1 64: 370-6.

33. Yoshida M, Vanstone CA, Parsons WD, Zawistowski J, Jones PJ. Effect of plant sterols and glucomannan on lipids in individuals with and without type II diabetes. *Eur J Clin Nutr* 2006; 60: 529-37.

34. Theuwissen E, Mensink RP. Simultaneous intake of β-glucan and plant stanol esters affects lipid metabolism in slightly hypercholesterolemic subjects. *J Nutr* 2007; 137: 583-8.

35. Miettinen TA, Tilvis RS, Kesäniemi YA. Serum plant sterols and cholesterol precursors reflect cholesterol absorption and synthesis in volunteers of a randomly selected male population. *Am J Epidemiol* 1990; 131: 20-31.

36. Davis HR Jr, Zhu LJ, Hoos LM, Tetzloff G, Maguire M, Liu J, Yao X, Iyer SPN, Lam MH, Lund EG, Detmers PA, Graziano MP, Altmann SW. Niemann-Pick C1 like 1 (NPC1L1) is the intestinal phytosterol and cholesterol transporter and a key modulator of whole-body cholesterol homeostasis. *J Biol Chem* 2004; 279: 33586-92.

37. Plat J, Onselen van ENM, Heugten van MMA, Mensink RP. Effects on serum lipids, lipoproteins and fat-soluble antioxidant concentrations of consumption frequency of margarines and shortenings enriched with plant stanol esters. *Eur J Clin Nutr* 2000; 54: 671-7.

38. Jakulj L, Trip MD, Sudhop T, von Bergmann K, Kastelein JJ, Vissers MN. Inhibition of cholesterol absorption by the combination of dietary plant sterols and ezetimibe: effects on plasma lipid levels. *J Lipid Res* 2005; 46: 2692-8.

Chapter 5

Evidence-based treatment of primary hypo-
and hypercholesterolemic disorders

Tisha R. Joy MD FRCPC, Assistant Professor
Department of Medicine, Schulich School of Medicine and Dentistry
University of Western Ontario, London, Ontario, Canada

Robert A. Hegele MD FRCPC FACP
Director, Blackburn Cardiovascular Genetics Laboratory
Scientist, Vascular Biology Research Group
Robarts Research Institute, London, Ontario, Canada

Introduction

Dyslipidemia affects up to 47% of US adults [1]. The most prevalent dyslipidemias in the general population include elevated low-density lipoprotein cholesterol (LDL-C), elevated triglyceride (TG), and/or depressed high-density lipoprotein cholesterol (HDL-C) levels. Both high LDL-C and low HDL-C levels have been independently linked to cardiovascular disease (CVD), while elevated TG levels are often associated with pancreatitis. Although the vast majority of patients have dyslipidemia due to secondary causes such as diabetes, obesity or medications often on a polygenic background of susceptibility, a small proportion has primary dyslipidemia such as familial hypercholesterolemia (FH), abetalipoproteinemia (ABL), familial hypertriglyceridemia, and familial hypoalphalipoproteinemia. Insights from the pathogenesis and treatment of these monogenic lipid disorders has had important implications for the more common dyslipidemias. In fact, therapeutic strategies such as statins, proprotein convertase subtilisin/kexin 9 (PCSK9) inhibitors, and apolipoprotein (apo) AI-based strategies (apoAI Milano) have been developed for the more common secondary dyslipidemias based on an understanding of primary dyslipidemias. This chapter will discuss the evidence-based management of FH and ABL as well as primary hypertriglyceridemia and hypoalphalipoproteinemia (see Table 1).

Table 1. Recommendations for management for selected primary lipid disorders.

Disorder	Therapeutic option	Level of evidence
Familial hypercholesterolemia		
	Lifestyle intervention	Level Ia, Grade A
Heterozygotes	*Pharmacologic intervention in adults*	
	Statins	Level Ib, Grade A
	Ezetimibe	
	• If statin intolerant or contraindications to statin therapy	Level IV, Grade C
	• As add-on therapy	Level Ib, Grade A
	Fibrates	
	• If statin intolerant or contraindications to statin therapy	Level IV, Grade C
	• As add-on therapy	Level IIb, Grade B
	Bile acid sequestrants	
	• If statin intolerant or contraindications to statin therapy	Level IV, Grade C
	• As add-on therapy	Level Ib, Grade A
	Niacin	
	• If statin intolerant or contraindications to statin therapy	Level IV, Grade C
	• As add-on therapy	Level III, Grade B
	Pharmacologic intervention in children	
	Statins	Level Ia, Grade A
	Bile acid sequestrants	Level Ib, Grade A
Homozygotes	LDL apheresis	Level IIa, Grade B
	Liver transplantation	Level IV, Grade C
Primary hypertriglyceridemia		
	Lifestyle intervention	Level IV, Grade C
	Pharmacologic intervention	
	Fibrates	Level Ib, Grade A
	Statins	Level IIb, Grade B
	Niacin	Level Ib, Grade A
	Omega-3 fatty acids	Level III, Grade B
	Ezetimibe	Level IV, Grade C
Abetalipoproteinemia		
	Dietary modification	Level III, Grade B
	Pharmacologic intervention	
	High-dose oral vitamin A and E replacement	Level III, Grade B
	Vitamin D replacement	Level IV, Grade C
	Vitamin K replacement	Level IV, Grade C
Hypoalphalipoproteinemia		
	Lifestyle intervention	Level IV, Grade C
	Pharmacologic intervention	
	Niacin	Level IIb, Grade B
	Fibrates	Level IIb, Grade B

Familial hypercholesterolemia

FH (*OMIM* 143890), is an autosomal co-dominant disorder, with a frequency of ~1:500 people for heterozygous FH (HeFH) and $1:10^6$ for homozygous (or compound heterozygous) FH (HoFH) [2]. Importantly, a higher prevalence is found in certain populations such as Quebecois, Lebanese, and South Afrikaners [3]. FH is genetically characterized by loss-of-function mutations in the LDL receptor gene (*LDLR*). The LDL receptor binds to apolipoprotein (apo) B, and clears LDL particles from the plasma. In FH, the impaired hepatic catabolism of LDL increases plasma LDL-C levels by six- to ten-fold in individuals with HoFH and by two-fold in HeFH [2]. The increased LDL-C levels accelerate atherogenesis, with CVD presenting sometimes in the third to fourth decades of life [2]. There is a 25-fold increased incidence of early myocardial infarction (<60 years) among those with HeFH compared to the general population [2]. Furthermore, cholesterol can also be deposited in ectopic locations such as eyelids, cornea, and extensor tendons, leading to classic clinical manifestations such as xanthelasmas, corneal arcus, and tendon xanthomas, respectively. Two other less common monogenic disorders, heterozygous familial defective apoB resulting from loss-of-function mutations in the *APOB* gene and hypercholesterolemia secondary to gain-of-function mutations in *PCSK9*, can present clinically and biochemically similar to HeFH. These disorders each result in significant elevations in LDL-C and thus the treatment strategies are similar. Interestingly, certain heterozygous loss-of-function mutations in both *APOB* and *PCSK9* (but not *LDLR*) can cause low LDL-C levels.

Therapeutic strategies for HeFH

Non-pharmacologic management

Adequate exercise, smoking cessation, and maintenance of a healthy weight are important lifestyle interventions in guidelines for FH treatment [4]. A diet with ≤100mg/day of cholesterol, 20% of calories from fat and 6% from saturated fatty acids will decrease LDL-C levels by 18-30% among FH-affected adults and children [5]. In a randomized cross-over study of 19 HeFH patients already treated with simvastatin, a low-fat diet decreased LDL-C levels by 6% while a randomized controlled trial (RCT) examining low-fat diet with or without pravastatin in 20 HeFH patients demonstrated a 15% decrease in LDL-C levels attributed to diet alone [6, 7]. A meta-analysis of four RCTs revealed a 10-15% LDL-C decrease with the addition of fat spreads enriched with 2.3 ± 0.5g of phytosterols/stanols per day in the diet of HeFH patients treated for 6.5 ± 1.9 weeks, without any adverse effects [8]. Consequently, a low-fat diet supplemented with phytosterols/stanols has been recommended by the International Panel on Management of Familial Hypercholesterolemia [4] as initial therapy for FH patients including children >3 years old **(Ia/A)**.

Pharmacologic management

Pharmacologic lowering of LDL-C levels in FH patients includes statins or 3-hydroxy-3-methyl-glutaryl-coenzyme (HMG-CoA) reductase inhibitors. HMG-CoA reductase is the rate-limiting step in *de novo* cholesterol synthesis, and its pharmacologic inhibition upregulates hepatic LDLRs and enhances removal of LDL from plasma. Statins can lower LDL-C levels by up to 60%, supporting their role as first-line therapy in FH [7, 9-17] **(Ib/A)**. The introduction of statins has been associated with decreased mortality in FH [18]. Importantly, only atorvastatin has thus far been documented to cause carotid intima-media thickness regression in HeFH [17]. No RCT with statins in FH has reported decreased CVD, although this would be expected based on extrapolation from RCTs in non-FH populations [19] as well as from cohort studies [20] (Figure 1).

The use of statins as first-line therapy in FH is often not sufficient to attain LDL-C goals. Furthermore, statins may not be well tolerated in some patients. Thus, second-line lipid-lowering agents are required, including ezetimibe, bile acid sequestrants (BAS), fibrates, and extended-release niacin. Ezetimibe inhibits intestinal cholesterol absorption by blocking the

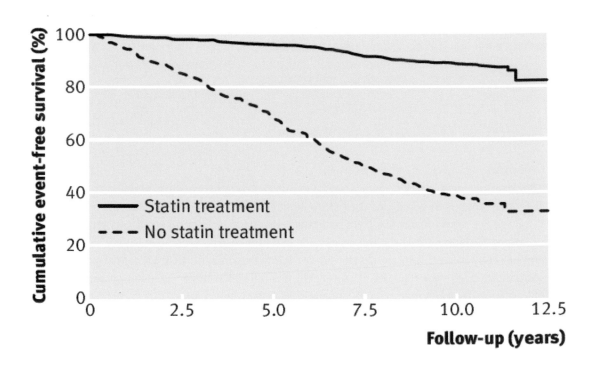

Figure 1. Kaplan-Meier curve estimates of cumulative coronary heart disease-free survival among patients with familial hypercholesterolemia according to statin treatment (p<0.001 for difference). *Reproduced with permission from the BMJ Publishing Group Ltd, © 2008. From Versmissen J, et al [20],*

Niemann-Pick C1 like 1 (NPC1L1) transporter. It reduces LDL-C by ~18% as monotherapy and by ~25% as an add-on to existing statin therapy [21-23]. Among FH patients, the addition of ezetimibe to existing statin therapy resulted in a further 13-23% reduction in LDL-C, with a greater percentage achieving their LDL-C targets [11, 24]. Importantly, no trial evidence yet supports improved CVD or surrogate outcomes with ezetimibe as either monotherapy or add-on therapy [11] in FH and non-FH populations. Because ezetimibe tends to be well-tolerated, it has been recommended by the National Institute for Health and Clinical Excellence (NICE) [25] as a therapeutic option in those who either are statin-intolerant or have contraindications to statin therapy **(IV/C)**, or as add-on therapy in those unable to achieve their LDL-C targets despite statin therapy **(Ib/A)**.

The remaining second-line agents have various mechanisms of action and can be added on or used as initial therapy when statin intolerance or contraindications exist **(IV/C)**. Fibrates, which are weak peroxisome proliferator-activated receptor (PPAR)-α agonists, can decrease LDL-C and TG levels by ~10% and 50%, respectively [26]. In two open-label trials of FH patients, bezafibrate reduced LDL-C by an additional 6-9% when added to statin therapy [27, 28] **(IIb/B)**. However, co-administration of a fibrate with a statin should be undertaken cautiously; fenofibrate might be preferable to gemfibrozil, since there has been fewer reports of rhabdomyolysis with fenofibrate compared to gemfibrozil in combination with a statin [29] **(IV/C)**.

BAS, such as colestipol, colesevelam, colestimide, and cholestyramine, interfere with enterohepatic circulation, leading to excretion of bound bile acids in the faeces, thereby stimulating bile acid synthesis from intra-hepatic cholesterol stores. The resultant increase in LDLR expression increases LDL particle clearance and lowers LDL-C by ~15% [30]. Although BAS can raise TG levels and interfere with the absorption of certain medications, BAS appear safe, even in children with FH [31]. The addition of cholestyramine (8g/day) to fluvastatin plus bezafibrate in 22 FH patients reduced LDL-C by an additional 15% after 54 weeks [27]. Similarly, a 20% LDL-C reduction was observed when colestimide (3g/d) was added to atorvastatin (20-40mg/d) in 15 patients with HeFH [32]. In a randomized cross-over trial of 17 HeFH patients who had not achieved their target LDL-C level on 20mg/d atorvastatin, the addition of 3g/d of colestimide resulted in ~25% LDL-C reduction, a magnitude similar to doubling atorvastatin to 40mg/d [33]. Thus, as per the NICE guidelines [25] and the International Panel on Management of Familial Hypercholesterolemia [4], BAS may be an effective alternative to statins in the case of intolerance or contraindications [25] **(IV/C)** or as add-on therapy [4, 25] **(Ib/A)**.

Niacin has manifold effects on lipid parameters, reducing TG, LDL-C, and lipoprotein (a) (Lp(a)) levels by 28-44%, 14-21%, and 17-26%, respectively, while increasing HDL-C levels by 22-30% [34]. However, tolerability has been limited primarily due to flushing. Despite this, niacin effectively lowers LDL-C levels in HeFH patients without [35] or with [36] statins (Figure 2). Thus, niacin may be effective in statin intolerance or contraindications [25] **(IV/C)** as well as in combination therapy as needed [4, 25] **(III/B)**.

Special mention should be made regarding the treatment of children and adolescents with HeFH. Meta-analysis of short-term trials (12-104 weeks in duration) has demonstrated safety

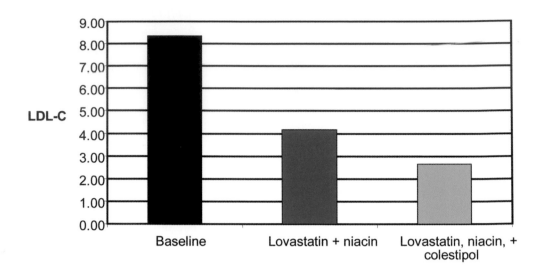

Figure 2. Combination therapy in heterozygous FH. *Adapted from Malloy MJ, et al [36].*

and efficacy of statins in children [37-42] **(Ia/A)**. The position statement by the American Heart Association (AHA) and American Academy of Pediatrics recommends lifestyle intervention [43]. In those with significantly elevated LDL-C levels despite lifestyle intervention, statin therapy may be undertaken for males ≥10 years old and females after the onset of menses [43] **(IV/C)**. Bile acid sequestrants and intestinal cholesterol absorption inhibitors may be employed as add-on therapy, since randomized trials support their efficacy and safety [44-47] **(Ib/A)**. However, the position statement suggests that statin therapy may be initiated at a younger age in the context of a particularly worrisome family history [43] **(IV/C)**. As yet, no RCTs have demonstrated reduced CVD outcomes with statin therapy in children, and data from a recent long-term HeFH cohort study [20] questions whether very early intervention in children is required.

Therapeutic strategies for HoFH

The above pharmacologic strategies are often ineffective at reducing LDL-C levels in HoFH patients. Thus, the main therapy in HoFH is LDL apheresis, which refers to the removal of LDL from blood using one of three methods: plasmapheresis (plasma exchange), dextran sulphate adsorption (DSA), or heparin-mediated extracorporeal LDL precipitation (HELP). Regardless of the method, LDL apheresis can reduce LDL-C by ~53-68% [48] with improved angiographic outcomes [49] and functional improvement [50]. Moreover, plasmapheresis in five HoFH patients prolonged survival by an average of 5.5 years compared to their five respective HoFH siblings who had not previously received plasmapheresis [51]. The cardiovascular benefits from apheresis also seem to extend to HeFH patients. In a non-randomized trial of 130 HeFH patients with CVD in which 87 received medical therapy alone while the remaining 43 received both medical therapy and apheresis, there was a two-fold decrease in LDL-C levels as well as a 72% reduction in total coronary events in the apheresis group compared to the medical therapy group [52].

Several authorities have therefore made recommendations regarding LDL apheresis **(IV/C)**. The Food and Drug Administration (FDA) has approved DSA or HELP in HoFH patients with LDL-C >13mmol/L, HeFH patients with LDL-C >7.8mmol/L, and HeFH patients with CVD and LDL-C >5.2mmol/L if these elevations persist despite adequate treatment for 6 months using the AHA Step 2 diet and maximum tolerated drug therapy. The International Panel on the Management of FH recognizes LDL apheresis as the standard of care for HoFH and also recommends its use for HeFH with symptomatic CVD and LDL-C >4.2mmol/L or reduction in LDL-C <40% despite maximal medical therapy [4, 53]. Most recently, the HEART-UK LDL Apheresis Working Group [53] recommended LDL apheresis for all HoFH ≥7 years old unless their serum cholesterol had been reduced by ≥50% and/or to ≤9mmol/L by drug therapy, and in HeFH with objective progression of CVD and with LDL-C >5.0mmol/L or a decrease in LDL-C by <40% with maximal drug therapy. Despite the variable recommendations, the current mainstay of treatment in HoFH is LDL apheresis **(IIa/B)**.

Liver transplantation (with or without concomitant heart transplantation) has been successfully reported in HoFH and HeFH [54-56]. However, the risks associated with lifelong immunosuppression, together with the sparse availability of donor organs preclude its widespread use. Although liver transplantation is theoretically curative in HoFH, it should be attempted only after careful consideration and after all other options have been exhausted **(IV/C)**. Another theoretically curative treatment is gene therapy using a vector expressing the normal *LDLR* gene. In five HoFH patients who underwent *ex vivo* gene therapy, only three showed sustained and prolonged reduction in LDL-C [57], indicating that the technique requires further improvements.

Based on the fact that certain loss-of-function mutations in either *APOB* or *PCSK9* are associated with significantly reduced LDL-C levels, biological treatments based on RNA interference or monoclonal antibodies directed against *APOB* and *PCSK9* are under development for FH patients who are refractory to statin-based regimens or who cannot tolerate existing treatments. There is no evidence at present for the long-term efficacy or safety of these approaches. ISIS 301012 currently represents the first molecule in the class of antisense oligonucleotides (ASOs) to be approved for clinical trials. ISIS 301012 is directed against apoB, the major apolipoprotein in LDL, thereby reducing expression and synthesis of apoB. Dose-dependent reductions in LDL-C up to 45% were seen in a phase I study [58] of ISIS 301012; the major side effects were injection-site erythema and liver aminotransferase elevations. However, ongoing trials in FH are pending before making recommendations regarding the use of ISIS 301012. A related unproven strategy is inhibition – either by antibodies or by ASO – of the protease PCSK9.

Another emerging therapy for HoFH is the microsomal triglyceride transfer protein (MTP) inhibitor BMS-201038. A dose-escalation study of BMS-201038 among six HoFH patients revealed a significant 51% LDL-C reduction, but was associated with liver aminotransferase elevation and hepatic fat accumulation [59]. Further trials of BMS-201038 in FH are pending.

Primary hypertriglyceridemia

Primary disorders causing hypertriglyceridemia include lipoprotein lipase (LPL) or apoCII deficiency (hyperlipoproteinemia [HLP] type 1; OMIM 238600), mixed hyperlipoproteinemia (HLP type 5; OMIM 207750), familial hypertriglyceridemia (HLP type 4; OMIM 145750), and familial dysbetalipoproteinemia (HLP type 3; OMIM 107741).

LPL deficiency and apoCII deficiency are both autosomal recessive disorders, resulting in chylomicronemia. LPL deficiency has an estimated prevalence of 1 in 10^6 although the carrier frequency may be as high as 1 in 40 persons in some regions of Quebec [60, 61]. Meanwhile, apoCII deficiency affects <1 in 10^6 individuals. Patients with LPL or apoCII deficiency typically present in childhood with marked hypertriglyceridemia (TG >11.3mmol/L) together with clinical features such as recurrent abdominal pain, failure to thrive, hepatosplenomegaly, and frequent bouts of acute pancreatitis. Clinical manifestations such as eruptive xanthomas or lipemia retinalis are typically observed with plasma TG levels >22.6mmol/L [62]. Although the diagnosis between these two disorders relies heavily on specialized biochemical testing – post-heparin lipolytic assay – as well as genetic testing if available, the treatment of these two disorders is identical and depends heavily on dietary intervention. However, in apoCII deficiency, plasma transfusions, which contain apoCII, may be considered [62].

In familial hypertriglyceridemia, TG levels are typically 2.3 to 5.6mmol/L, with 'normal' LDL-C levels, and are often only noted once in adulthood [62, 63]. The hallmark is an increased concentration of TG-rich very-low-density lipoprotein (VLDL), attributed to overproduction of VLDL TGs in the context of near-normal apoB production [62, 64, 65]. Although typically mild, TG elevations with familial hypertriglyceridemia may be exacerbated by secondary factors such as alcohol ingestion. Importantly, most individuals do not demonstrate any particular clinical manifestations, unless their TG levels are >11.3mmol/L, at which time eruptive xanthomas or pancreatitis may occur. The genetic basis for familial hypertriglyceridemia remains to be determined [62].

Familial dysbetalipoproteinemia has a prevalence of 1 in 10^4 and is associated with homozygosity for the apoE2 isoform. Although the prevalence of E2/E2 homozygosity is ~1 in 100, only ~1 in 10 to ~1 in 100 homozygotes will develop dyslipidemia [62]. Similar to familial hypertriglyceridemia, individuals with familial dysbetalipoproteinemia are typically detected in adulthood and demonstrate only modest elevations in TG levels (3.4-4.5mmol/L), which can be further exacerbated by secondary factors [62]. Unlike familial hypertriglyceridemia with its isolated VLDL elevation, familial dysbetalipoproteinemia is characterized by accumulation of cholesterol-rich remnants of VLDL, intermediate-density lipoproteins (IDL), and chylomicrons due to ineffective clearance by variant apoE [62]. Furthermore, familial dysbetalipoproteinemia can be characterized by the presence of pathognomonic palmar xanthomas, and tuberous, tubero-eruptive, and tendon xanthomas. Importantly, premature CVD is common [62]. Diagnosis can be aided by determination of the APOE genotype.

Therapeutic strategies for primary hypertriglyceridemia

Non-pharmacologic management

Non-pharmacologic control of hypertriglyceridemia is crucial. In general, since primary disorders of hypertriglyceridemia can be exacerbated by secondary modifiable factors, non-pharmacologic interventions such as strict glycemic control in diabetics, treatment with levothyroxine in hypothyroidism, avoidance of medications that increase TGs (such as β-blockers or thiazide diuretics), limitation or abstinence of alcohol, avoidance of high sugar or simple carbohydrates, and weight loss (in those overweight or obese) are recommended **(IV/C)** [66].

Dietary recommendations in LPL deficiency are very stringent, consisting of a low fat diet with <10-15% of daily caloric intake from fat [67, 68] **(IV/C)**. Medium chain fatty acids, which are directly absorbed into the portal circulation and do not rely on chylomicron formation, can provide an alternate source of dietary fat [69] **(IV/C)**. Furthermore, due to this stringent dietary regimen, supplementation with essential fatty acids (such as walnut oil, or sunflower oil topically) [70] and fat-soluble vitamins should also be considered **(IV/C)**.

Pharmacologic management

In addition to non-pharmacologic therapy, pharmacologic intervention using fibrates, statins, niacin, ezetimibe, or fish oil is often required. Fibrates represent the initial choice in individuals with primary hypertriglyceridemia unresponsive to non-pharmacologic interventions **(Ib/A)**. Several RCTs have been conducted in primary hypertriglyceridemic disorders, demonstrating the efficacy of fibrates [71-75]. Most recently, among 75 individuals with HLP type 4, those randomized to receive ciprofibrate demonstrated greater TG reductions (38.0% vs. 21.6%, p<0.0007) and HDL-C increases (25.6% vs. 9.4%, p<0.02) than controls [76]. These results reflect those seen in other clinical trials in HLP types 4 and 5 [71, 72] as well as HLP type 3 [73-75].

Statins can reduce TG levels by 10-30% [77, 78]. Statins tend to be most efficacious in HLP type 3 since both TG and IDL are elevated. In a RCT comparing gemfibrozil to simvastatin in ten HLP type 3 patients, gemfibrozil resulted in greater TG reductions while simvastatin was associated with greater LDL-C reductions [75]. Thus, due to the potential for treatment gaps with monotherapy in HLP type 3, combination therapy with a statin and fibrate has demonstrated beneficial effects and is currently recommended for those who do not respond to monotherapy [79, 80] **(IIb/B)**. However, the combination of statin and fibrate should preferentially involve fenofibrate since gemfibrozil has been associated with a higher risk of rhabdomyolysis compared to fenofibrate when combined with a statin [29].

Because niacin has multiple lipid-lowering effects, it is a suitable adjunct therapy in primary hypertriglyceridemia **(Ib/A)**. In a randomized cross-over trial of clofibrate and nicotinic acid among five patients with HLP type 3, similar TG reductions (~40%) and HDL-C increases (~25%) were seen [81]. The efficacy of niacin was demonstrated in uncontrolled trials of patients with HLP type 3 [81]. Meanwhile, no clinical trials to date have evaluated ezetimibe in the context of primary hypertriglyceridemia. Among 576 individuals with mixed hyperlipidemia assigned to fenofibrate 160mg or combination therapy of ezetimibe with fenofibrate, significantly greater TG reductions were noted in combination therapy vs. the fenofibrate only group (46.0% vs. 41.8%, p=0.002) [82]. Thus, based on extrapolation of this data, the addition of ezetimibe may be useful to the management of primary hypertriglyceridemia **(IV/C)**.

Omega-3 fatty acids have demonstrated significant TG reductions in patients with familial hypertriglyceridemia: 45% after 12 weeks [83] and 34% after 11 months [84]. Twelve-week treatment with 6g/d omega-3 fatty acids resulted in TG reductions of 57% and 55% among HLP type 3 and 4 patients, respectively [85]. Thus, omega-3 fatty acids could be used in the management of hypertriglyceridemia **(III/B)**.

No randomized trials have been performed in patients with HLP types 1 and 5. Although pharmacotherapy with fibrates can be attempted in HLP types 1 and 5, these agents may not affect TG levels since they primarily work by upregulating LPL activity and enhancing VLDL clearance from the plasma [86, 87]. Gemfibrozil has been reported in HLP type 1 in pregnancy [88, 89]. Statins and niacin may also be similarly ineffective since they work on LDL uptake and endogenous free fatty acid production, respectively. Thus, the mainstay of treatment for both disorders remains dietary modification **(IV/C)**. Omega-3 fatty acids may help lower TG levels although no RCTs exist to support this statement **(IV/C)**. In cases of pancreatitis in apoCII deficiency, transfusions may be considered since plasma contains apoCII, which can activate LPL. For HLP type 1 patients with homozygous mutations in LPL, the efficacy and safety of LPL-based gene therapies are currently being examined [87, 90].

Abetalipoproteinemia

Abetalipoproteinemia is an autosomal recessive disorder occurring in <1 in 10^6 individuals [62]. It is caused by a deficiency in MTP, leading to insufficient transfer of TG to nascent apoB-containing lipoproteins, which in turn impairs the metabolism of these particles, including chylomicrons. Since chylomicrons are essential for absorption of fats and fat-soluble vitamins, fat malabsorption and deficiency of fat-soluble vitamins (A, D, E and K) are common. Progressive neurologic deterioration related to vitamin E deficiency, retinitis pigmentosa due to vitamin A deficiency, and acanthocytosis due to altered erythrocyte lipid content are classic manifestations. However, other manifestations can include vitamin K deficiency with bleeding [91] and hepatic steatosis [92]. Patients have extremely low plasma total cholesterol (<1.3mmol/L) with low levels of LDL-C and TG. The diagnosis can be genetically confirmed by sequencing the *MTP* gene [62]. Homozygous mutations in the *APOB* gene can produce a similar phenotype.

Therapeutic strategies for abetalipoproteinemia

Management

Diet is the mainstay of therapy in abetalipoproteinemia. A low-fat diet (<20g/d) supplemented with medium-chain fatty acids is helpful in managing the associated steatorrhea and hepatic steatosis while still providing a source of fat in the diet **(III/B)** [93-95]. High oral doses of vitamins A and E can attenuate retinal and neurologic deterioration **(III/B)**. Although some individuals develop retinal lesions on vitamin A supplementation, their progression was halted after treatment with high doses of vitamin E [96]. The retinal and neurological complications may be prevented with high-dose vitamins shortly after birth or in early childhood [97] and progression may be halted or reversed if neurologic manifestations are of new onset [93, 95, 98-100]. Thus, early vitamin replacement is warranted **(III/B)**. A recent review recommended daily doses of 2400 to 12000IU with monitoring of compliance and adequacy of treatment using serum vitamin E levels [100] **(IV/C)**. Furthermore, 100-400IU/kg/day of vitamin A were recommended in patients with abetalipoproteinemia, with titration of the dose guided by serum carotene levels [100] **(IV/C)**.

Furthermore, low serum calcium and vitamin D levels have been described in abetalipoproteinemia [101]; thus, routine vitamin D replacement (1000IU/day) has been recommended [100] **(IV/C)**. Similarly, vitamin K deficiency, manifested as elevated prothrombin time [91] or as bleeding [91], warrants oral vitamin K replacement (5mg/day) [100] **(IV/C)**. It is also important to ensure that other vitamins involved in the development of neuropathy, such as B6 and B12, are also followed and treated in these patients if necessary **(IV/C)**.

Hypoalphalipoproteinemia

The primary disorders resulting in hypoalphalipoproteinemia include familial hypoalphalipoproteinemia (OMIM 604091), familial apoAI deficiency (OMIM 107680), Tangier disease (OMIM 205400), and lecithin:cholesterol acyltransferase (LCAT) deficiency (OMIM 245900). Familial hypoalphalipoproteinemia is an autosomal dominant disorder while both LCAT deficiency and Tangier disease are autosomal recessive disorders. Each tends to be associated with early CVD and a family history of low HDL-C levels. In familial hypoalphalipoproteinemia, HDL-C levels are typically <10th percentile (<0.8mmol/L in men and <1.0mmol/L in premenopausal women). In many patients, the genetic basis of familial hypoalphalipoproteinemia remains unsolved [62].

Unlike familial hypoalphalipoproteinemia, which has few clinical manifestations, LCAT deficiency is associated with corneal opacities, normochromic anemia, and renal failure [62]. A variant of LCAT deficiency, known as 'fish-eye disease', has similar clinical manifestations except for premature CVD, which has been attributed to decreased LCAT activity occurring only in HDL rather than in both HDL and apoB-containing lipoproteins. Plasma HDL-C levels are typically <0.3mmol/L in both forms [62]. Meanwhile, Tangier disease is characterized by significant reductions of both HDL-C (typically <0.1mmol/L) and LDL-C. Clinical manifestations of Tangier disease result from cholesteryl ester accumulation, including corneal opacities, orange tonsils, hepatosplenomegaly, peripheral neuropathy and perhaps early CVD. Mutations in ABCA1, the cholesterol efflux transporter important for reverse cholesterol transport, cause Tangier disease [62].

Since apoAI is the major apolipoprotein of HDL particles, apoAI deficiency can lead to low plasma HDL-C levels (<0.3mmol/L) [62]. Furthermore, individuals with apoAI deficiency may demonstrate corneal opacities, xanthomas, and premature CVD [62]. However, one apoAI mutation known as apoAIMilano, although associated with low HDL-C levels, is not associated with premature CVD [62] and is being considered as a novel therapy to reduce CVD in those with low HDL-C levels.

Therapeutic strategies for hypoalphalipoproteinemia

Non-pharmacologic management

Although non-pharmacologic measures, such as exercise, weight loss, smoking cessation, and moderate alcohol consumption may raise HDL-C levels by up to 6% [102], this may not be clinically meaningful in individuals with primary low HDL syndromes. Thus, reducing LDL-C levels through dietary and pharmacologic interventions discussed above as well as pharmacologic interventions to raise HDL-C levels are emphasized.

Pharmacologic management

Niacin increases HDL-C levels by 15- 30% [103]. Several clinical trials using niacin such as the Coronary Drug Project (CDP), Familial Atherosclerosis Treatment Study (FATS), HDL Atherosclerosis Treatment Intervention Study (HATS), UC-San Francisco Specialized Center of Research (UCSF-SCOR) trial, Cholesterol Lowering Atherosclerosis Study (CLAS), and Arterial Biology for the Investigation of the Treatment Effects of Reducing cholesterol trials (ARBITER 2 and 3) have demonstrated improvements in either surrogate or hard outcomes [104-110]. The CDP is the only RCT evaluating clinical outcomes in niacin therapy. Among the 8341 men aged 30-64 years with a history of MI, niacin decreased MI risk by 26%, coronary revascularisation by 67% and stroke by 24% after 6 years of follow-up and reduced all-cause mortality by 11% after 15 years of follow-up [110, 111]. Among 19 males with genetic or familial HDL-deficiency, niacin therapy (2g/day) was associated with a 22% increase in HDL-C levels compared to only a 6% increase with fenofibrate (200mg/day) and 6% decrease with atorvastatin (20mg/day) [112] (Figure 3). Given niacin's manifold beneficial biochemical effects, the question of whether these benefits are solely due to raising HDL-C levels still remains. Regardless, niacin effectively raises HDL-C levels and can be considered for the treatment of genetic hypoalphalipoproteinemia (IIb/B).

Fibrates also raise HDL-C levels from 5% to 50%, and also lower TG, total cholesterol, and LDL-C levels [26]. Among men with familial HDL deficiency, treatment with fenofibrate was associated with a 6% increase in HDL-C levels [112]. Moreover, earlier RCTs such as the Helsinki Heart Study [113] and Veterans Affairs HDL Intervention Trial (VA-HIT)[114] demonstrated increases in HDL-C and decreases in CVD outcomes. In particular, gemfibrozil increased HDL-C by 6% and reduced CHD death or non-fatal MI by 22% [114] and each 0.13mmol/L increase in HDL-C was associated with an 11% reduction in CVD events [115]. However, such positive outcomes were not seen in two more recent fibrate RCTs – the Bezafibrate Infarction Prevention (BIP) [116] and Fenofibrate Intervention and Event Lowering in Diabetes (FIELD) trials [117]. The lack of benefit in BIP and FIELD could have been due to high numbers of patients in the placebo groups who received additional 'drop-in' lipid-lowering treatment, mainly statins [116, 117]. Furthermore, in FIELD, fenofibrate therapy

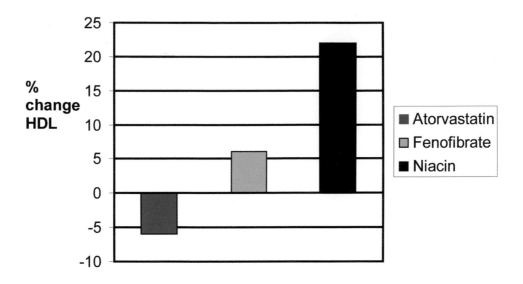

Figure 3. Change in HDL in response to different therapies among men with severe HDL deficiency. *Adapted from Alrasadi K, et al [112].*

increased HDL-C by only 3%, which may have been too small for any clinical benefit [117]. Yet, despite conflicting evidence regarding the benefits of HDL-C raising for CVD outcomes, fibrates have been shown to raise HDL-C levels in non-genetic HDL-deficiency states. Therefore, fibrates can be considered as a therapeutic option for primary hypoalphalipoproteinemia **(IIb/B)**.

Statins such as pravastatin, lovastatin, simvastatin, and rosuvastatin have demonstrated increases in HDL-C levels by 3-8% [118, 119]. Other pharmacologic strategies are being actively pursued to raise HDL-C levels particularly in the context of CVD prevention. Notably leading the pack are the cholesteryl ester transfer protein (CETP) inhibitors, which include torcetrapib, dalcetrapib, and anacetrapib. While torcetrapib raised HDL-C levels by as much as 72%, it was associated with adverse cardiovascular outcomes [120] and was pulled from further trials. The adverse outcomes were possibly mediated by molecule-specific pressor effects rather than through the mechanism of CETP inhibition [121]. As yet, both dalcetrapib and anacetrapib do not demonstrate adverse pressor effects [121-124]. However, these newer therapies cannot be recommended without convincing CVD endpoint data. Similarly, clinical trials are still pending regarding the efficacy of other HDL-based therapies including phospholipids [125], reconstituted HDL [126-128], apolipoprotein AI mimetic peptides [129-132], and apoAIMilano [133]. Of all these latter therapies, only reconstituted HDL has been evaluated in a genetic HDL-deficiency state, with a substantial 225% increase in HDL-C levels noted [126].

Conclusions

Primary disorders of lipid metabolism are relatively rare. Evidence for particular treatment strategies is stronger for attenuating CVD outcomes in FH and certain primary hypertriglyceridemias, compared to improvement of multisystem deterioration in abetalipoproteinemia and both multisystem disease and CVD in hypoalphalipoproteinemia. In the case of abetalipoproteinemia, the strongest level of evidence is based on case reports. Meanwhile, for hypoalphalipoproteinemia, treatment is primarily guided by clinical trial data in non-genetic states of HDL deficiency. Several new targets for treatment, such as inhibition of MTP and PCSK9, have resulted from understanding the biochemical genetics of these rare disorders. Several questions remain unanswered such as the actual benefit of statin treatment in HeFH children in terms of clinical outcomes despite RCT evidence demonstrating short-term efficacy and safety. Thus, the treatment of primary lipid disorders is an evolving field that requires the ongoing commitment of both physicians and patients.

Key points	Evidence level
Familial hypercholesterolemia	
◆ Although a low-fat diet is recommended as initial therapy, statins represent the first line of pharmacologic intervention.	Ib/A
◆ When adequate LDL-C lowering has not been achieved with statin monotherapy, combination therapy to lower LDL-C further can be achieved using:	
o ezetimibe;	Ib/A
o fibrates;	IIb/B
o niacin;	III/B
o bile acid sequestrant.	Ib/A
◆ In FH patients with intolerance or contraindications to statins, alternative medications include ezetimibe, fibrates, niacin, and/or bile acid sequestrants.	IV/C
◆ Early statin treatment of children with heterozygous FH is controversial, but is supported by short-term studies of efficacy and safety. However, the long-term effects including any increased benefit in CVD events with earlier treatment are not yet known.	Ia/A
◆ Treatment of children with heterozygous FH with bile acid sequestrants or ezetimibe may be used as add-on therapy.	Ib/A
◆ In homozygous FH, the mainstay of treatment is LDL apheresis.	IIa/B
Continued overleaf	

Key points *continued*	Evidence level
Primary hypertriglyceridemia	
◆ Non-pharmacologic strategies such as weight loss, reduction/abstinence of alcohol, and strict glycemic control may be helpful in reducing triglyceride levels.	IV/C
◆ Although pharmacologic intervention may be attempted, the first-line treatment for LPL or apoCII deficiency is a strict dietary regimen of <10-15% of calories derived from fat with supplementation from medium-chain triglycerides and essential fatty acids.	IV/C
◆ First-line pharmacologic therapy for all other primary hypertriglyceridemic disorders is fibrates.	Ib/A
◆ The addition of a statin to fibrate therapy may be helpful in controlling the mixed dyslipidemia of type III hyperlipoproteinemia.	IIb/B
◆ Niacin is a suitable addition to fibrate therapy in primary hypertriglyceridemia.	Ib/A
◆ Ezetimibe can be helpful in lowering triglycerides further when added to fibrate therapy.	IV/C
◆ Omega-3 fatty acids have been shown to decrease TGs in types III and IV hyperlipoproteinemia.	III/B
Abetalipoproteinemia	
◆ First-line treatment includes dietary modification for a very low-fat diet (<20g/d) together with high-dose vitamins A and E to prevent or retard retinal and neurologic complications.	III/B
◆ Routine vitamin D and K replacement should also be considered.	IV/C
Hypoalphalipoproteinemia	
◆ Although non-pharmacologic measures may result in some minor increase in HDL-C levels, the pharmacologic strategy with the greatest demonstrated increase in HDL-C levels is niacin.	IIb/B
◆ Fibrates can also cause minor increases in HDL-C levels.	IIb/B

References

1. Wong ND, Lopez V, Tang S, Williams GR. Prevalence, treatment, and control of combined hypertension and hypercholesterolemia in the United States. *Am J Cardiol* 2006; 98(2): 204-8
2. Brown MS, Goldstein JL. A receptor-mediated pathway for cholesterol homeostasis. *Science* 1986; 232(4746): 34-47
3. Yuan G, Wang J, Hegele RA. Heterozygous familial hypercholesterolemia: an underrecognized cause of early cardiovascular disease. *CMAJ* 2006; 174(8): 1124-9

4.   Civeira F. Guidelines for the diagnosis and management of heterozygous familial hypercholesterolemia. *Atherosclerosis* 2004; 173(1): 55-68.

5.   Connor WE, Connor SL. Importance of diet in the treatment of familial hypercholesterolemia. *Am J Cardiol* 1993; 72(10): 42D-53D.

6.   Chisholm A, Sutherland W, Ball M. The effect of dietary fat content on plasma noncholesterol sterol concentrations in patients with familial hypercholesterolemia treated with simvastatin. *Metabolism* 1994; 43(3): 310-4.

7.   Galvan AQ, Natali A, Baldi S, *et al.* Effect of a reduced-fat diet with or without pravastatin on glucose tolerance and insulin sensitivity in patients with primary hypercholesterolemia. *J Cardiovasc Pharmacol* 1996; 28(4): 595-602.

8.   Moruisi KG, Oosthuizen W, Opperman AM. Phytosterols/stanols lower cholesterol concentrations in familial hypercholesterolemic subjects: a systematic review with meta-analysis. *J Am Coll Nutr* 2006; 25(1): 41-8.

9.   Stein EA, Strutt K, Southworth H, Diggle PJ, Miller E. Comparison of rosuvastatin versus atorvastatin in patients with heterozygous familial hypercholesterolemia. *Am J Cardiol* 2003; 92(11): 1287-93.

10.   Nozue T, Michishita I, Ito Y, Hirano T. Effects of statin on small dense low-density lipoprotein cholesterol and remnant-like particle cholesterol in heterozygous familial hypercholesterolemia. *J Atheroscler Thromb* 2008; 15(3): 146-53.

11.   Kastelein JJ, Akdim F, Stroes ES, *et al.* Simvastatin with or without ezetimibe in familial hypercholesterolemia. *N Engl J Med* 2008; 358(14): 1431-43.

12.   Kawashiri MA, Nohara A, Tada H, *et al.* Comparison of effects of pitavastatin and atorvastatin on plasma coenzyme Q10 in heterozygous familial hypercholesterolemia: results from a crossover study. *Clin Pharmacol Ther* 2008; 83(5): 731-9.

13.   van Tits LJ, Smilde TJ, van Wissen S, de Graaf J, Kastelein JJ, Stalenhoef AF. Effects of atorvastatin and simvastatin on low-density lipoprotein subfraction profile, low-density lipoprotein oxidizability, and antibodies to oxidized low-density lipoprotein in relation to carotid intima media thickness in familial hypercholesterolemia. *J Investig Med* 2004; 52(3): 177-84.

14.   Bo M, Nicolello MT, Fiandra U, Mercadante G, Piliego T, Fabris F. Treatment of heterozygous familial hypercholesterolemia: atorvastatin vs simvastatin. *Nutr Metab Cardiovasc Dis* 2001; 11(1): 17-24.

15.   Olsson AG, Pauciullo P, Soska V, *et al.* Comparison of the efficacy and tolerability of fluvastatin extended-release and immediate-release formulations in the treatment of primary hypercholesterolemia: a randomized trial. *Clin Ther* 2001; 23(1): 45-61.

16.   Illingworth DR, Bacon S, Pappu AS, Sexton GJ. Comparative hypolipidemic effects of lovastatin and simvastatin in patients with heterozygous familial hypercholesterolemia. *Atherosclerosis* 1992; 96(1): 53-64.

17.   Smilde TJ, van Wissen S, Wollersheim H, Trip MD, Kastelein JJ and Stalenhoef AF. Effect of aggressive versus conventional lipid lowering on atherosclerosis progression in familial hypercholesterolaemia (ASAP): a prospective, randomised, double-blind trial. *Lancet* 2001; 357(9256): 577-81.

18.   Mortality in treated heterozygous familial hypercholesterolaemia: implications for clinical management. Scientific Steering Committee on behalf of the Simon Broome Register Group. *Atherosclerosis* 1999; 142(1): 105-12.

19.   Mills EJ, Rachlis B, Wu P, Devereaux PJ, Arora P, Perri D. Primary prevention of cardiovascular mortality and events with statin treatments: a network meta-analysis involving more than 65,000 patients. *J Am Coll Cardiol* 2008; 52(22): 1769-81.

20.   Versmissen J, Oosterveer DM, Yazdanpanah M, *et al.* Efficacy of statins in familial hypercholesterolaemia: a long-term cohort study. *BMJ* 2008; 337: a2423.

21.   Pearson TA, Denke MA, McBride PE, Battisti WP, Brady WE, Palmisano J. A community-based, randomized trial of ezetimibe added to statin therapy to attain NCEP ATP III goals for LDL cholesterol in hypercholesterolemic patients: the ezetimibe add-on to statin for effectiveness (EASE) trial. *Mayo Clin Proc* 2005; 80(5): 587-95.

22.   Knopp RH, Gitter H, Truitt T, *et al.* Effects of ezetimibe, a new cholesterol absorption inhibitor, on plasma lipids in patients with primary hypercholesterolemia. *Eur Heart J* 2003; 24(8): 729-41.

23.   Dujovne CA, Ettinger MP, McNeer JF, *et al.* Efficacy and safety of a potent new selective cholesterol absorption inhibitor, ezetimibe, in patients with primary hypercholesterolemia. *Am J Cardiol* 2002; 90(10): 1092-7.

24. Stein E, Stender S, Mata P, *et al*. Achieving lipoprotein goals in patients at high risk with severe hypercholesterolemia: efficacy and safety of ezetimibe co-administered with atorvastatin. *Am Heart J* 2004; 148(3): 447-55.

25. NICE Clinical Guideline 71: Identification and management of familial hypercholesterolaemia. 2008. Accessed March 9, 2009, at http://www.nice.org.uk/nicemedia/pdf/CG071NICEGuidelineWord.doc.

26. Chapman MJ. Fibrates in 2003: therapeutic action in atherogenic dyslipidaemia and future perspectives. *Atherosclerosis* 2003; 171(1): 1-13.

27. Leitersdorf E, Muratti EN, Eliav O, Peters TK. Efficacy and safety of triple therapy (fluvastatin-bezafibrate-cholestyramine) for severe familial hypercholesterolemia. *Am J Cardiol* 1995; 76(2): 84A-8.

28. Eliav O, Schurr D, Pfister P, Friedlander Y, Leitersdorf E. High-dose fluvastatin and bezafibrate combination treatment for heterozygous familial hypercholesterolemia. *Am J Cardiol* 1995; 76(2): 76A-9.

29. Jones PH, Davidson MH. Reporting rate of rhabdomyolysis with fenofibrate + statin versus gemfibrozil + any statin. *Am J Cardiol* 2005; 95(1): 120-2.

30. Einarsson K, Ericsson S, Ewerth S, *et al*. Bile acid sequestrants: mechanisms of action on bile acid and cholesterol metabolism. *Eur J Clin Pharmacol* 1991; 40 Suppl 1: S53-8.

31. Hoeg JM. Pharmacologic and surgical treatment of dyslipidemic children and adolescents. *Ann N Y Acad Sci* 1991; 623: 275-84

32. Kawashiri MA, Higashikata T, Nohara A, *et al*. Efficacy of colestimide coadministered with atorvastatin in Japanese patients with heterozygous familial hypercholesterolemia (FH). *Circ J* 2005; 69(5): 515-20.

33. Tasaki H, Miyamoto M, Kubara T, *et al*. Cross-over trial of intensive monotherapy with atorvastatin and combined therapy with atorvastatin and colestimide for Japanese familial hypercholesterolemia. *Circ J* 2006; 70(1): 14-20.

34. Goldberg A, Alagona P, Jr., Capuzzi DM, *et al*. Multiple-dose efficacy and safety of an extended-release form of niacin in the management of hyperlipidemia. *Am J Cardiol* 2000; 85(9): 1100-5.

35. Illingworth DR, Phillipson BE, Rapp JH, Connor WE. Colestipol plus nicotinic acid in treatment of heterozygous familial hypercholesterolaemia. *Lancet* 1981; 1(8215): 296-8.

36. Malloy MJ, Kane JP, Kunitake ST, Tun P. Complementarity of colestipol, niacin, and lovastatin in treatment of severe familial hypercholesterolemia. *Ann Intern Med* 1987; 107(5): 616-23.

37. Avis HJ, Vissers MN, Stein EA, *et al*. A systematic review and meta-analysis of statin therapy in children with familial hypercholesterolemia. *Arterioscler Thromb Vasc Biol* 2007; 27(8): 1803-10.

38. McCrindle BW, Ose L, Marais AD. Efficacy and safety of atorvastatin in children and adolescents with familial hypercholesterolemia or severe hyperlipidemia: a multicenter, randomized, placebo-controlled trial. *J Pediatr* 2003; 143(1): 74-80.

39. Knipscheer HC, Boelen CC, Kastelein JJ, *et al*. Short-term efficacy and safety of pravastatin in 72 children with familial hypercholesterolemia. *Pediatr Res* 1996; 39(5): 867-71.

40. Stein EA, Illingworth DR, Kwiterovich PO, Jr., *et al*. Efficacy and safety of lovastatin in adolescent males with heterozygous familial hypercholesterolemia: a randomized controlled trial. *JAMA* 1999; 281(2): 137-44.

41. Lambert M, Lupien PJ, Gagne C, *et al*. Treatment of familial hypercholesterolemia in children and adolescents: effect of lovastatin. Canadian Lovastatin in Children Study Group. *Pediatrics* 1996; 97(5): 619-28.

42. de Jongh S, Ose L, Szamosi T, *et al*. Efficacy and safety of statin therapy in children with familial hypercholesterolemia: a randomized, double-blind, placebo-controlled trial with simvastatin. *Circulation* 2002; 106(17): 2231-7.

43. Kavey RE, Allada V, Daniels SR, *et al*. Cardiovascular risk reduction in high-risk pediatric patients: a scientific statement from the American Heart Association Expert Panel on Population and Prevention Science; the Councils on Cardiovascular Disease in the Young, Epidemiology and Prevention, Nutrition, Physical Activity and Metabolism, High Blood Pressure Research, Cardiovascular Nursing, and the Kidney in Heart Disease; and the Interdisciplinary Working Group on Quality of Care and Outcomes Research: endorsed by the American Academy of Pediatrics. *Circulation* 2006; 114(24): 2710-38.

44. Tonstad S, Knudtzon J, Sivertsen M, Refsum H, Ose L. Efficacy and safety of cholestyramine therapy in peripubertal and prepubertal children with familial hypercholesterolemia. *J Pediatr* 1996; 129(1): 42-9.

45. McCrindle BW, O'Neill MB, Cullen-Dean G, Helden E. Acceptability and compliance with two forms of cholestyramine in the treatment of hypercholesterolemia in children: a randomized, crossover trial. *J Pediatr* 1997; 130(2): 266-73.

46. Schlierf G, Mrozik K, Heuck CC, *et al.* 'Low dose' colestipol in children, adolescents and young adults with familial hypercholesterolemia. *Atherosclerosis* 1982; 41(1): 133-8.

47. van der Graaf A, Cuffie-Jackson C, Vissers MN, *et al.* Efficacy and safety of coadministration of ezetimibe and simvastatin in adolescents with heterozygous familial hypercholesterolemia. *J Am Coll Cardiol* 2008; 52(17): 1421-9.

48. Thompsen J, Thompson PD. A systematic review of LDL apheresis in the treatment of cardiovascular disease. *Atherosclerosis* 2006; 189(1): 31-8.

49. Thompson GR, Maher VM, Matthews S, *et al.* Familial Hypercholesterolaemia Regression Study: a randomised trial of low-density-lipoprotein apheresis. *Lancet* 1995; 345(8953): 811-6.

50. Kroon AA, Aengevaeren WR, van der Werf T, *et al.* LDL-Apheresis Atherosclerosis Regression Study (LAARS). Effect of aggressive versus conventional lipid lowering treatment on coronary atherosclerosis. *Circulation* 1996; 93(10): 1826-35.

51. Thompson GR, Miller JP, Breslow JL. Improved survival of patients with homozygous familial hypercholesterolaemia treated with plasma exchange. *Br Med J* (Clin Res Ed) 1985; 291(6510): 1671-3.

52. Mabuchi H, Koizumi J, Shimizu M, *et al.* Long-term efficacy of low-density lipoprotein apheresis on coronary heart disease in familial hypercholesterolemia. Hokuriku-FH-LDL-Apheresis Study Group. *Am J Cardiol* 1998; 82(12): 1489-95.

53. Thompson GR. Recommendations for the use of LDL apheresis. *Atherosclerosis* 2008; 198(2): 247-55.

54. Kawagishi N, Satoh K, Akamatsu Y, *et al.* Long-term outcome after living donor liver transplantation for two cases of homozygous familial hypercholesterolemia from a heterozygous donor. *J Atheroscler Thromb* 2007; 14(2): 94-8.

55. Alkofer BJ, Chiche L, Khayat A, *et al.* Liver transplant combined with heart transplant in severe heterozygous hypercholesterolemia: report of the first case and review of the literature. *Transplant Proc* 2005; 37(5): 2250-2.

56. Revell SP, Noble-Jamieson G, Johnston P, Rasmussen A, Jamieson N, Barnes ND. Liver transplantation for homozygous familial hypercholesterolaemia. *Arch Dis Child* 1995; 73(5): 456-8.

57. Grossman M, Rader DJ, Muller DW, *et al.* A pilot study of *ex vivo* gene therapy for homozygous familial hypercholesterolaemia. *Nat Med* 1995; 1(11): 1148-54.

58. Kastelein JJ, Wedel MK, Baker BF, *et al.* Potent reduction of apolipoprotein B and low-density lipoprotein cholesterol by short-term administration of an antisense inhibitor of apolipoprotein B. *Circulation* 2006; 114(16): 1729-35.

59. Cuchel M, Bloedon LT, Szapary PO, *et al.* Inhibition of microsomal triglyceride transfer protein in familial hypercholesterolemia. *N Engl J Med* 2007; 356(2): 148-56.

60. Hayden MR, Ma Y. Molecular genetics of human lipoprotein lipase deficiency. *Mol Cell Biochem* 1992; 113(2): 171-6.

61. Gagne C, Brun LD, Julien P, Moorjani S, Lupien PJ. Primary lipoprotein-lipase-activity deficiency: clinical investigation of a French Canadian population. *CMAJ* 1989; 140(4): 405-11.

62. Mahley RW, Weisgraber KH, Farese Jr RV. Disorders of Lipid Metabolism. In: *Williams' Textbook of Endocrinology*, 10th ed. Larsen PR, Kronenberg HM, Melmed S, Polonsky KS, Eds. Philadelphia, PA, USA: Elsevier Science, 2003: 1642-705.

63. Schaefer EJ. Familial lipoprotein disorders and premature coronary artery disease. *Med Clin North Am* 1994; 78(1): 21-39.

64. Chait A, Albers JJ, Brunzell JD. Very low density lipoprotein overproduction in genetic forms of hypertriglyceridaemia. *Eur J Clin Invest* 1980; 10(1): 17-22.

65. Janus ED, Nicoll AM, Turner PR, Magill P, Lewis B. Kinetic bases of the primary hyperlipidaemias: studies of apolipoprotein B turnover in genetically defined subjects. *Eur J Clin Invest* 1980; 10(2 Pt 1): 161-72.

66. Brunzell JD, Deeb SS. Familial lipoprotein deficiency, apo C-II deficiency, and hepatic lipase deficiency. In: *Metabolic and Molecular Bases of Inherited Disease*, 8th ed. Scriver CR, Beaudet AL, Sly WS, Valle D, Eds. New York: McGraw-Hill, 2001: 2789-816.

67. Yuan G, Al-Shali KZ, Hegele RA. Hypertriglyceridemia: its etiology, effects and treatment. *CMAJ* 2007; 176(8): 1113-20.

68. Davignon J, DuFour R. *Primary Hyperlipidemias: An Atlas of Investigation and Diagnosis.* Oxford: Clinical Publishing, 2007.

69. Rouis M, Dugi KA, Previato L, *et al*. Therapeutic response to medium-chain triglycerides and omega-3 fatty acids in a patient with the familial chylomicronemia syndrome. *Arterioscler Thromb Vasc Biol* 1997; 17(7): 1400-6.

70. Press M, Hartop PJ, Prottey C. Correction of essential fatty-acid deficiency in man by the cutaneous application of sunflower-seed oil. *Lancet* 1974; 1(7858): 597-8.

71. Leaf DA, Connor WE, Illingworth DR, Bacon SP, Sexton G. The hypolipidemic effects of gemfibrozil in type V hyperlipidemia. A double-blind, crossover study. *JAMA* 1989; 262(22): 3154-60.

72. Goldberg AC, Schonfeld G, Feldman EB, *et al*. Fenofibrate for the treatment of type IV and V hyperlipoproteinemias: a double-blind, placebo-controlled multicenter US study. *Clin Ther* 1989; 11(1): 69-83.

73. Lussier-Cacan S, Bard JM, Boulet L, *et al*. Lipoprotein composition changes induced by fenofibrate in dysbetalipoproteinemia type III. *Atherosclerosis* 1989; 78(2-3): 167-82.

74. Baggio G, Gasparotto A, Ciuffetti G, *et al*. Long term-effect of fenofibrate on lipoprotein level and composition in different types of genetic hyperlipidemias. *Pharmacol Res Commun* 1986; 18(5): 471-80.

75. Civeira F, Cenarro A, Ferrando J, *et al*. Comparison of the hypolipidemic effect of gemfibrozil versus simvastatin in patients with type III hyperlipoproteinemia. *Am Heart J* 1999; 138(1 Pt 1): 156-62.

76. Bermudez-Pirela V, Souki A, Cano-Ponce C, *et al*. Ciprofibrate treatment decreases non-high density lipoprotein cholesterol and triglycerides and increases high density lipoprotein cholesterol in patients with Frederickson type IV dyslipidemia phenotype. *Am J Ther* 2007; 14(2): 213-20.

77. Knopp RH. Drug treatment of lipid disorders. *N Engl J Med* 1999; 341(7): 498-511.

78. Saito Y, Yamada N, Shirai K, *et al*. Effect of rosuvastatin 5-20mg on triglycerides and other lipid parameters in Japanese patients with hypertriglyceridemia. *Atherosclerosis* 2007; 194(2): 505-11.

79. Feussner G, Eichinger M, Ziegler R. The influence of simvastatin alone or in combination with gemfibrozil on plasma lipids and lipoproteins in patients with type III hyperlipoproteinemia. *Clin Investig* 1992; 70(11): 1027-35.

80. Illingworth DR, O'Malley JP. The hypolipidemic effects of lovastatin and clofibrate alone and in combination in patients with type III hyperlipoproteinemia. *Metabolism* 1990; 39(4): 403-9.

81. Hoogwerf BJ, Bantle JP, Kuba K, Frantz ID, Jr., Hunninghake DB. Treatment of type III hyperlipoproteinemia with four different treatment regimens. *Atherosclerosis* 1984; 51(2-3): 251-9.

82. McKenney JM, Farnier M, Lo KW, *et al*. Safety and efficacy of long-term co-administration of fenofibrate and ozetimibe in patients with mixed hyperlipidemia. *J Am Coll Cardiol* 2006; 47(8): 1584-7.

83. Richter WO, Jacob BG, Ritter MM, Schwandt P. Treatment of primary chylomicronemia due to familial hypertriglyceridemia by omega-3 fatty acids. *Metabolism* 1992; 41(10): 1100-5.

84. Pschierer V, Richter WO, Schwandt P. Primary chylomicronemia in patients with severe familial hypertriglyceridemia responds to long-term treatment with (n-3) fatty acids. *J Nutr* 1995; 125(6): 1490-4.

85. Dallongeville J, Boulet L, Davignon J, Lussier-Cacan S. Fish oil supplementation reduces beta very-low-density lipoprotein in type III dysbetalipoproteinemia. *Arterioscler Thromb* 1991; 11(4): 864-71.

86. Grundy SM, Vega GL. Fibric acids: effects on lipids and lipoprotein metabolism. *Am J Med* 1987; 83(5B): 9-20.

87. Nierman MC, Rip J, Twisk J, *et al*. Gene therapy for genetic lipoprotein lipase deficiency: from promise to practice. *Neth J Med* 2005; 63(1): 14-9.

88. Al-Shali K, Wang J, Fellows F, Huff MW, Wolfe BM, Hegele RA. Successful pregnancy outcome in a patient with severe chylomicronemia due to compound heterozygosity for mutant lipoprotein lipase. *Clin Biochem* 2002; 35(2): 125-30.

89. Keilson LM, Vary CP, Sprecher DL, Renfrew R. Hyperlipidemia and pancreatitis during pregnancy in two sisters with a mutation in the lipoprotein lipase gene. *Ann Intern Med* 1996; 124(4): 425-8.

90. Rip J, Nierman MC, Sierts JA, *et al*. Gene therapy for lipoprotein lipase deficiency: working toward clinical application. *Hum Gene Ther* 2005; 16(11): 1276-86.

91. Caballero FM, Buchanan GR. Abetalipoproteinemia presenting as severe vitamin K deficiency. *Pediatrics* 1980; 65(1): 161-3.

92. Collins JC, Scheinberg IH, Giblin DR, Sternlieb I. Hepatic peroxisomal abnormalities in abetalipoproteinemia. *Gastroenterology* 1989; 97(3): 766-70.

93. Azizi E, Zaidman JL, Eshchar J, Szeinberg A. Abetalipoproteinemia treated with parenteral and oral vitamins A and E, and with medium chain triglycerides. *Acta Paediatr Scand* 1978; 67(6): 796-801.

94. Triantafillidis JK, Kottaras G, Sgourous S, *et al*. A-beta-lipoproteinemia: clinical and laboratory features, therapeutic manipulations, and follow-up study of three members of a Greek family. *J Clin Gastroenterol* 1998; 26(3): 207-11.

95. MacGilchrist AJ, Mills PR, Noble M, Foulds WS, Simpson JA, Watkinson G. Abetalipoproteinaemia in adults: role of vitamin therapy. *J Inherit Metab Dis* 1988; 11(2): 184-90.

96. Runge P, Muller DP, McAllister J, Calver D, Lloyd JK, Taylor D. Oral vitamin E supplements can prevent the retinopathy of abetalipoproteinaemia. *Br J Ophthalmol* 1986; 70(3): 166-73.

97. Muller DP, Lloyd JK. Effect of large oral doses of vitamin E on the neurological sequelae of patients with abetalipoproteinemia. *Ann N Y Acad Sci* 1982; 393: 133-44.

98. Illingworth DR, Connor WE, Miller RG. Abetalipoproteinemia. Report of two cases and review of therapy. *Arch Neurol* 1980; 37(10): 659-62.

99. Hegele RA, Angel A. Arrest of neuropathy and myopathy in abetalipoproteinemia with high-dose vitamin E therapy. *Can Med Assoc J* 1985; 132(1): 41-4.

100. Zamel R, Khan R, Pollex RL, Hegele RA. Abetalipoproteinemia: two case reports and literature review. *Orphanet J Rare Dis* 2008; 3: 19.

101. Triantafillidis JK, Kottaras G, Peros G, *et al*. Endocrine function in abetalipoproteinemia: a study of a female patient of Greek origin. *Ann Ital Chir* 2004; 75(6): 683-90.

102. Rosenson RS. Low HDL-C: a secondary target of dyslipidemia therapy. *Am J Med* 2005; 118(10): 1067-77.

103. Malik S, Kashyap ML. Niacin, lipids, and heart disease. *Curr Cardiol Rep* 2003; 5(6): 470-6.

104. Taylor AJ, Lee HJ and Sullenberger LE. The effect of 24 months of combination statin and extended-release niacin on carotid intima-media thickness: ARBITER 3. *Curr Med Res Opin* 2006; 22(11): 2243-50.

105. Taylor AJ, Sullenberger LE, Lee HJ, Lee JK, Grace KA. Arterial Biology for the Investigation of the Treatment Effects of Reducing Cholesterol (ARBITER) 2: a double-blind, placebo-controlled study of extended-release niacin on atherosclerosis progression in secondary prevention patients treated with statins. *Circulation* 2004; 110(23): 3512-7.

106. Blankenhorn DH, Nessim SA, Johnson RL, Sanmarco ME, Azen SP, Cashin-Hemphill L. Beneficial effects of combined colestipol-niacin therapy on coronary atherosclerosis and coronary venous bypass grafts. *JAMA* 1987; 257(23): 3233-40.

107. Kane JP, Malloy MJ, Ports TA, Phillips NR, Diehl JC, Havel RJ. Regression of coronary atherosclerosis during treatment of familial hypercholesterolemia with combined drug regimens. *JAMA* 1990; 264(23): 3007-12.

108. Brown BG, Zhao XQ, Chait A, *et al*. Simvastatin and niacin, antioxidant vitamins, or the combination for the prevention of coronary disease. *N Engl J Med* 2001; 345(22): 1583-92.

109. Brown G, Albers JJ, Fisher LD, *et al*. Regression of coronary artery disease as a result of intensive lipid-lowering therapy in men with high levels of apolipoprotein B. *N Engl J Med* 1990; 323(19): 1289-98.

110. The Coronary Drug Project Research Group. Clofibrate and niacin in coronary heart disease. *JAMA* 1975; 231(4): 360-81.

111. Canner PL, Berge KG, Wenger NK, *et al*. Fifteen year mortality in Coronary Drug Project patients: long-term benefit with niacin. *J Am Coll Cardiol* 1986; 8(6): 1245-55.

112. Alrasadi K, Awan Z, Alwaili K, *et al*. Comparison of treatment of severe high-density lipoprotein cholesterol deficiency in men with daily atorvastatin (20mg) versus fenofibrate (200mg) versus extended-release niacin (2g). *Am J Cardiol* 2008; 102(10): 1341-7.

113. Frick MH, Elo O, Haapa K, *et al*. Helsinki Heart Study: primary-prevention trial with gemfibrozil in middle-aged men with dyslipidemia. Safety of treatment, changes in risk factors, and incidence of coronary heart disease. *N Engl J Med* 1987; 317(20): 1237-45.

114. Rubins HB, Robins SJ, Collins D, *et al*. Gemfibrozil for the secondary prevention of coronary heart disease in men with low levels of high-density lipoprotein cholesterol. Veterans Affairs High-Density Lipoprotein Cholesterol Intervention Trial Study Group. *N Engl J Med* 1999; 341(6): 410-8.

115. Robins SJ, Collins D, Wittes JT, *et al*. Relation of gemfibrozil treatment and lipid levels with major coronary events: VA-HIT: a randomized controlled trial. *JAMA* 2001; 285(12): 1585-91.

116. Secondary prevention by raising HDL cholesterol and reducing triglycerides in patients with coronary artery disease: the Bezafibrate Infarction Prevention (BIP) study. *Circulation* 2000; 102(1): 21-7.

117. Keech A, Simes RJ, Barter P, *et al*. Effects of long-term fenofibrate therapy on cardiovascular events in 9795 people with type 2 diabetes mellitus (the FIELD study): randomised controlled trial. *Lancet* 2005; 366(9500): 1849-61.

118. Bermudez V, Cano R, Cano C, *et al*. Pharmacologic management of isolated low high-density lipoprotein syndrome. *Am J Ther* 2008; 15(4): 377-88.

119. Kostapanos MS, Milionis HJ, Filippatos TD, *et al*. Dose-dependent effect of rosuvastatin treatment on HDL-subfraction phenotype in patients with primary hyperlipidemia. *J Cardiovasc Pharmacol Ther* 2009; 14(1): 5-13.

120. Barter PJ, Caulfield M, Eriksson M, *et al*. Effects of torcetrapib in patients at high risk for coronary events. *N Engl J Med* 2007; 357(21): 2109-22.

121. Forrest MJ, Bloomfield D, Briscoe RJ, *et al*. Torcetrapib-induced blood pressure elevation is independent of CETP inhibition and is accompanied by an increase in circulating aldosterone levels. *Br J Pharm* 2008; 154(7): 1465-73.

122. Kuivenhoven JA, de Grooth GJ, Kawamura H, *et al*. Effectiveness of inhibition of cholesteryl ester transfer protein by JTT-705 in combination with pravastatin in type II dyslipidemia. *Am J Cardiol* 2005; 95(9): 1085-8.

123. Krishna R, Anderson MS, Bergman AJ, *et al*. Effect of the cholesteryl ester transfer protein inhibitor, anacetrapib, on lipoproteins in patients with dyslipidaemia and on 24-h ambulatory blood pressure in healthy individuals: two double-blind, randomised placebo-controlled phase I studies. *Lancet* 2007; 370(9603): 1907-14.

124. de Grooth GJ, Kuivenhoven JA, Stalenhoef AF, *et al*. Efficacy and safety of a novel cholesteryl ester transfer protein inhibitor, JTT-705, in humans: a randomized phase II dose-response study. *Circulation* 2002; 105(18): 2159-65.

125. Burgess JW, Neville TA, Rouillard P, Harder Z, Beanlands DS, Sparks DL. Phosphatidylinositol increases HDL-C levels in humans. *J Lipid Res* 2005; 46(2): 350-5.

126. Bisoendial RJ, Hovingh GK, Levels JH, *et al*. Restoration of endothelial function by increasing high-density lipoprotein in subjects with isolated low high-density lipoprotein. *Circulation* 2003; 107(23): 2944-8.

127. Spieker LE, Sudano I, Hurlimann D, *et al*. High-density lipoprotein restores endothelial function in hypercholesterolemic men. *Circulation* 2002; 105(12): 1399-402.

128. Tardif JC, Gregoire J, L'Allier PL, *et al*. Effects of reconstituted high-density lipoprotein infusions on coronary atherosclerosis: a randomized controlled trial. *JAMA* 2007; 297(15): 1675-82.

129. Garber DW, Datta G, Chaddha M, *et al*. A new synthetic class A amphipathic peptide analogue protects mice from diet-induced atherosclerosis. *J Lipid Res* 2001; 42(4): 545-52.

130. Navab M, Anantharamaiah GM, Hama S, *et al*. Oral administration of an Apo A-I mimetic peptide synthesized from D-amino acids dramatically reduces atherosclerosis in mice independent of plasma cholesterol. *Circulation* 2002; 105(3): 290-2.

131. Ou J, Wang J, Xu H, *et al*. Effects of D-4F on vasodilation and vessel wall thickness in hypercholesterolemic LDL receptor-null and LDL receptor/apolipoprotein A-I double-knockout mice on Western diet. *Circ Res* 2005; 97(11): 1190-7.

132. Ou J, Ou Z, Jones DW, *et al*. L-4F, an apolipoprotein A-1 mimetic, dramatically improves vasodilation in hypercholesterolemia and sickle cell disease. *Circulation* 2003; 107(18): 2337-41.

133. Nissen SE, Tsunoda T, Tuzcu EM, *et al*. Effect of recombinant ApoA-I Milano on coronary atherosclerosis in patients with acute coronary syndromes: a randomized controlled trial. *JAMA* 2003; 290(17): 2292-300.

Chapter 6

Does raising HDL protect against atherosclerosis?

Menno Vergeer MD, Resident, Internal Medicine and Vascular Medicine
G. Kees Hovingh MD PhD, Resident, Internal Medicine and Vascular Medicine
Department of Vascular Medicine, Academic Medical Center
Amsterdam, The Netherlands

Introduction

Despite revolutionary advances allowing early detection and aggressive therapeutic intervention, atherosclerosis remains a major cause of mortality and morbidity in the industrialized world [1]. Reduction of low-density lipoprotein cholesterol (LDL-C) is the primary target for cardiovascular prevention, and statin-induced lowering of LDL-C has been shown to reduce the cardiovascular disease (CVD) risk by approximately 30%. The substantial residual risk of 70% has resulted in the endeavour to create additional risk-decreasing strategies. Raising plasma high-density lipoprotein cholesterol (HDL-C) levels or increasing the functionality of the HDL particle is commonly regarded as an attractive goal to reduce the residual risk. However, a series of disappointing results in intervention studies have been published recently, of which most notable was the dramatic failure of the HDL-C increasing cholesteryl ester transfer protein (CETP) inhibitor, torcetrapib [2]. Consequently, the consensus on HDL's protective capacity has become subject to debate amongst researchers and physicians.

In this chapter we will briefly discuss the epidemiological and biological data, which formed the foundation of the rationale to strive for HDL-directed therapeutic interventions. We will then focus on the outcome of currently available drugs that increase HDL-C levels followed by a description of a number of potential novel therapies.

Epidemiology

A low plasma level of HDL-C has consistently been shown to be an independent risk factor for CVD in large epidemiological studies [3]. In the Framingham Heart Study it was found that individuals with an HDL-C level below 35mg/dL (0.91mmol/L) were at an eight-fold increased risk for coronary artery disease (CAD) compared to subjects with plasma levels above 65mg/dL (1.68mmol/L) [4]. These findings were in line with the results of the European PROCAM (PROspective CArdiovascular Munster) study where a plasma HDL-C level above 35mg/dL was associated with a 70% reduced CVD risk during the 6-year follow-up compared to HDL-C levels below 35mg/dL [5]. The INTERHEART study, which comprised over 30,000 individuals from 52 countries, identified the apoB/apoAI ratio as an important risk factor for CAD, which emphasizes the pivotal role in atherosclerosis of apolipoprotein AI, the major protein constituent of HDL-particles [6].

Low plasma HDL-C levels are amongst the most common risk phenotypes encountered in patients presenting with clinical manifestations of CVD, such as acute myocardial infarction (AMI) [7]. This has led to awareness that low HDL-C levels (below 40mg/dL or 1.03mmol/L for men and below 50mg/dL or 1.23mmol/L for women) should be taken into account while assessing CVD risk in patients (PROCAM and Framingham risk score). The association between HDL-C levels and CVD risk is not restricted to apparently healthy subjects (i.e. in the Framingham study), but was also found in secondary prevention trials, where, despite the reduction in LDL-C levels, low HDL-C levels remained significantly associated with cardiovascular endpoints [8].

Low HDL-C is not only a widely recognized risk factor, but current guidelines from the National Cholesterol Education Program (NCEP) Adult Treatment Panel (ATP) III and the American Diabetes Association even emphasize that increasing HDL-C levels in high-risk patients should be aimed for, after primarily focusing on low-density lipoprotein cholesterol (LDL-C) and non-HDL cholesterol [9, 10]. This is largely based on the findings derived from studies like the ones described above, and the anticipated net effect of HDL-C increase is commonly extrapolated from these studies. The potential effect of HDL-C increase is described in a widely cited meta-analysis of four large American cross-sectional studies, where a 1mg/dL increase of HDL-C levels was reported to be associated with a 2-3% decreased CVD risk [11]. Based on these results one would expect a huge CVD risk reduction by means of HDL-C increase. However, direct extrapolation of this cross-sectional finding to an interventional setting is probably an oversimplification. While the associations between elevated LDL-C and blood pressure and increased CVD risk are close-to-perfect examples of causal relationships, such a connection between low HDL-C levels and increased CVD is not universally acknowledged [12]. An important argument to question direct causality is the fact that HDL-C levels are heavily influenced by other CVD risk factors, which makes dissecting the exact role of HDL-C in atherosclerosis very hard, if at all possible.

Men, for example, have on average lower HDL-C levels compared to women [13] and this is related to hormonal differences, which, by itself, might also be causal for a higher risk for CVD in men. Smoking reduces HDL-C levels by over 10%, and the relationship between smoking and HDL-C appears to be dose-dependent [14]. Physical activity represents another important factor that influences HDL-C levels. Cross-sectional studies show that physical activity is associated with higher HDL-C levels [15] and a recent meta-analysis of 25 studies showed that regular aerobic exercise increased HDL-C levels with an average of 2.5mg/dL [16]. Obesity, especially abdominal obesity, is also associated with low HDL-C levels [17]. Type 2 diabetes mellitus and the metabolic syndrome are characterized by low HDL-C levels [18] and hypertriglyceridemia. In close relation to this, (post-prandial) hypertriglyceridemia by itself results in low HDL-C levels [19]. In fact, more than half the patients with low HDL-C levels have increased fasting triglycerides as well [20].

Systemic inflammatory diseases have also been shown to be associated with low HDL-C levels [21]. And finally, a low socioeconomic status is an independent predictor of lower HDL-C levels [22]. All these factors – gender, smoking, physical activity, obesity, diabetes, hypertriglyceridemia, inflammatory state and socioeconomic status – do not only affect HDL-C levels, but also CVD risk.

Although HDL-C levels remain a strong, significant predictor after statistical adjustment for these variables, this does not guarantee the absence of residual confounding [23]. As a consequence, predictions about the effect of HDL-C increase based on large epidemiological studies are highly likely to be imprecise or even completely false, because of the complex interplay between all HDL-C level influencing factors.

HDL metabolism – reverse cholesterol transport as a rationale for HDL increasing therapy

The concept of reverse cholesterol transport was first described decades ago [24] and it encompasses the removal and transport of excess cholesterol from peripheral tissues (including foam cells) by HDL towards the liver for catabolism and excretion in the bile. The current knowledge regarding HDL metabolism and reverse cholesterol transport is summarized in Figure 1.

Apolipoprotein AI (apoAI), the key protein in this process, is synthesized by the liver and the intestine, and subsequently lipidated with cholesterol and phospholipids by ATP-binding cassette protein A1 (ABCA1) to yield nascent, disc-shaped high-density lipoprotein (HDL) particles. These particles grow larger under the influence of ATP-binding cassette protein G1 (ABCG1), which further lipidates HDL, and lecithin:cholesterol-acyl transferase (LCAT), an HDL-bound enzyme, which esterifies free cholesterol to cholesteryl ester (CE) [25]. HDL particles can acquire cholesterol from peripheral cells, such as macrophages in the vessel wall, through a transport process facilitated by ABCA1, ABCG1 and scavenger receptor class B type 1 (SR-BI) [26]. This cholesterol is then returned to the liver. In humans it is not fully known which mechanisms regulate the hepatic uptake of CE transported by HDL. In mice, CE is selectively taken up by the liver through SR-BI [27], which uses apoAI as ligand. Holoparticle uptake of the HDL particle by the recently described novel hepatic receptor (ectopic β-chain of ATP synthase) might play a role in this process as well [28]. Alternatively, CE can also be transferred to apolipoprotein B (apoB)-containing particles in exchange for

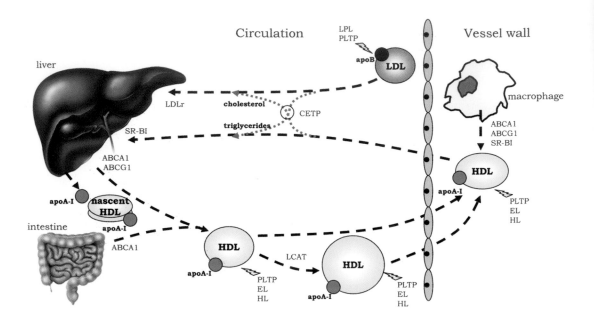

Figure 1. HDL metabolism.

triglycerides, a process that is mediated via cholesteryl ester transfer protein (CETP). These particles can subsequently be cleared by the hepatic LDL receptor (LDLR). Conversely, phospholipids can be transferred from apoB-containing particles to HDL by phospholipid transfer protein (PLTP), a shuttle protein that plays a key role in HDL remodelling [29]. While LCAT, CETP and PLTP primarily act directly on HDL, lipoprotein lipase (LPL) acts on triglyceride-rich lipoproteins. This enzyme hydrolyzes triglycerides resulting in the generation of free fatty acids and surface remnants that contribute to the HDL pool. Another lipase, hepatic lipase (HL), hydrolyzes HDL phospholipids but also triglycerides, generating smaller lipid-depleted HDL particles. Finally, the most recently identified member of the lipase family, endothelial lipase (EL), hydrolyzes HDL phospholipids and promotes HDL catabolism, at least in mice [30]. Reverse cholesterol transport is considered one of the most important anti-atherogenic characteristics of HDL, but several studies have been published questioning the role of HDL in this process [31, 32].

A large number of proteins is involved in HDL metabolism, and all might serve as a potential target for HDL-increasing therapy. However, precise information about the exact impact of these factors on both HDL levels and the extent of atherosclerosis is lacking and has thus far hampered the identification of suitable targets. Human carriers of molecular defects in the genes encoding the above mentioned proteins suffer from either hypo- or hyperalphalipoproteinemia. Insight into the progression of atherosclerotic vascular disease in subjects with such monogenetic disorders of HDL metabolism is of particular interest since it might reveal which proteins are attractive targets for future compounds to intervene in HDL metabolism [33].

Other, non-RCT-related atheroprotective roles of HDL

Apart from its assumed role in RCTs, HDL is considered to have anti-inflammatory and anti-oxidant activities. HDL has been shown *in vitro* to inhibit the expression of the endothelial adhesion molecules, vascular cell adhesion molecule-1 (VCAM-1), intercellular adhesion molecule-1 (ICAM-1) and E-selectin after induction with interleukin-1 or tumor necrosis factor α (TNFα) [34]. The anti-oxidative activity of HDL is typically characterized by its ability to specifically inhibit the oxidation of LDL [35], but it has also been shown to inhibit the formation of reactive oxygen species in rabbit smooth muscle or human endothelial cells [36]. These *in vitro* findings were confirmed in animal studies as well [37]. The exact role of the above mentioned anti-atherogenic capacities of the HDL particle in human physiology is largely unknown and subject to debate. The question remains whether assessment of the functionality of the HDL particle accurately reflects its role in the patient from whom it is derived.

Non-pharmacological interventions to increase HDL-C levels

Apart from pharmacological interventions, lifestyle changes can also be instituted to increase HDL-C levels.

Tobacco cessation

Smoking cessation has been shown to result in an approximately 4mg/dL (0.10mmol/L) increase in HDL-C levels, without significantly affecting other lipids and lipoproteins [38] and smokers who quit smoking have been shown to have similar HDL-C levels compared to non-smokers [39]. Apart from its direct role on levels of HDL-C, smoking is considered to result in the formation of dysfunctional HDL particles by its virtue to induce oxidative stress [40].

Aerobic exercise

In their study, Kraus and co-workers showed that in a relatively small cohort comprising 111 healthy, but sedentary individuals, regular aerobic training for a period of 2 months resulted in a 5% increase in HDL-C levels [41]. Most benefit was shown in males with low HDL-C and high TG levels [42]. Based on a meta-analysis, five 30-minute sessions of aerobic exercise are recommended [9, 16].

Weight loss

Low HDL-C levels are found in subjects with visceral obesity and a 10kg weight reduction has been shown to result in a 20% increase in HDL-C levels [43]. A rather dated meta-analysis showed that every kilogram reduction in weight is associated with a 0.07mmol/L HDL-C increase [44], and the findings in a more recent analysis did not support a strong effect of weight loss on HDL-C levels [45].

Alcohol consumption

Moderate amounts of alcohol (1-3 drinks per day) result in a 12% increase in HDL-C, irrespective of the type of alcoholic beverage [46]. Guidelines do state that more than two drinks for men and one drink for women should not be encouraged and that those who are non-drinkers should not be advised to start drinking alcohol [9].

Dietary changes

High intake of n-3 polyunsaturated fats can elevate levels of HDL-C by up to 20% [47] and result in an improvement of HDL anti-inflammatory capacity [48], which might be the reason for the finding that ingestion of n-3 polyunsaturated fatty acids results in cardiovascular benefits [49].

It is hard to dissect the exact role of HDL-C increase in lifestyle intervention studies. The HDL-C increase may actually contribute to a better CVD outcome, or, alternatively, it may simply be a reflection of the improvement in lifestyle.

Clinical trials

Different therapies are being developed with the aim to prevent atherosclerosis by increasing levels of circulating HDL. A summary of the largest intervention trials studying the effects of HDL-C increasing drugs is depicted in Table 1.

Nicotinic acid

Nicotinic acid, or niacin, can increase HDL-C levels up to 23%, and lower TG and LDL-C by 20% and 12%, respectively [50]. Niacin is believed to have multiple effects on lipid metabolism. Firstly, it reduces triglyceride synthesis, thereby decreasing plasma apoB-containing lipoproteins. Secondly, by inhibiting the surface expression of hepatic ATP synthase β chain, it decreases hepatic holoparticle HDL uptake, thereby raising HDL levels. Thirdly, ABCA1-mediated transport might be upregulated upon niacin treatment [51]. Finally, experiments with APOE*3-Leiden/CETPtg mice showed that the HDL increasing effect of niacin is at least partly mediated by inhibition of hepatic CETP expression [52]. In small trials niacin has been reported to beneficially affect subclinical measures of atherosclerosis as well as cardiovascular event rates **(Ib/A)**.

In the mid 1950s, Altschul and co-workers published the effects of nicotinic acids on serum cholesterol levels [53] and it was not until the 1970s and 1980s that endpoint trials were published.

One of the first large clinical trials with cardiovascular endpoints was the Coronary Drug Prevention trial. Long-term follow-up of this study showed a 21% reduction in non-fatal MI and an 11% reduction in death in niacin-treated subjects. Stroke was reduced by 24% [54]. The HDL Atherosclerosis Treatment Study (HATS) showed in 160 patients that niacin/simvastatin combination therapy led to a lower cardiovascular event rate compared with placebo [55]. The subsequent Arterial Biology for the Investigation of the Treatment Effects of Reducing Cholesterol (ARBITER 2) study examined the impact on carotid intima-media thickness (cIMT) progression of the addition of extended-release niacin to statin therapy in patients with established coronary heart disease and low HDL-C. No significant difference in cIMT progression was found between both treatment arms, but a significant cIMT progression occurred in the statin-only arm versus baseline, in the absence of a significant progression in the niacin arm. The authors concluded from this that niacin slowed cIMT progression [56]. In the open-label extension trial, the ARBITER 3 study, 104 participants were treated with extended-release niacin and these subjects showed cIMT regression. However, in this case the open-label design and the lack of a control arm obviously constitute serious limitations [57]. Two recent carotid imaging studies provided additional evidence of vascular benefit conferred by extended-release niacin on top of statins [58, 59].

Fibrates

Fibrates were designed to reduce plasma triglyceride levels by means of agonizing the peroxisome proliferator-activator receptor-alpha (PPAR-α), which is mostly expressed in muscle and liver. Fibrates induce lipoprotein lipolysis and hepatic fatty acid uptake, reduce hepatic triglyceride production, increase the removal of LDL particles from the plasma, reduce neutral lipid exchange between HDL and VLDL (i.e. reduce CETP activity) and increase the production of ApoAI and ApoAII in the liver [60]. Fibrates have been reported to reduce TG levels by 18-48% and LDL cholesterol levels by 8-13% while increasing HDL cholesterol with up to 10% [50, 61].

The initial study showing the effect of one of the fibrates was the Helsinki Heart Study, where 4081 healthy men (non-HDL-C >5.2mmol/L [200mg/dL]) were treated with gemfibrozil, resulting in a 34% reduction of major coronary events [62, 63].

In the subsequent VA-HIT trial, which studied the atheroprotective effect of gemfibrozil in 2531 men with coronary heart disease, the cardiovascular event rate was reported to be inversely associated with on-trial HDL-C levels, which might be interpreted as evidence in favour of a causal relationship between HDL-C and cardiovascular disease [61]. However, in light of the much stronger triglyceride-lowering effect of fibrates, the inverse biological relationship between HDL-C and triglycerides, and the much higher variability of triglyceride measurements, this interpretation deserves criticism. By whatever mechanism, fibrates have shown efficacy on cardiovascular endpoints: in a recent meta-analysis, fibrates were shown

Table 1. Studies on HDL increasing drugs, their reported effect on HDL-C levels and their impact on clinical and intermediate endpoints.

	Drug	Publication	Participants	Patients in the active arm	Follow-up (yrs)	% HDL increase	Endpoint(s)	Endpoint results
NIACIN								
CLINICAL OUTCOME								
Coronary Drug Project (CDP) follow-up	Niacin	Canner PL JACC 1986; 8: 1245-55	8341	1119	15	NR	death	11% reduced death
Stockholm Ischemic Heart Disease Secondary Prevention Study	Niacin	Carlson LA Acta Med Scand 1988; 223: 405-18	555	279	5	NR	CAD-related death	36% reduction in CAD-related death, 26% overall reduction in deaths
HDL-atherosclerosis Treatment Study (HATS)	Niacin and simvastatin	Brown BG NEJM 2001; 345:1583-92	160	38	3	26	composite	90% reduction in composite endpoint (MI, stroke, revascularization, death); 24% in placebo, 3% in treated patients
Armed Forces Regression Study (AFREGS)	Niacin and gemfibrozil and cholestyramine and diet and counselling	Whitney EJ Ann Intern Med 2005; 142: 95-104	143	71	2.5	36	composite	50% decrease in composite endpoint (angina, stroke, MI, TIA and cardio-vascular procedures): 26% in placebo vs 13% in treated subjects
INTERMEDIATE ENDPOINT, IMAGING								
Cholesterol Lowering Atherosclerosis Study (CLAS I and II) follow-up	Niacin and colestipol	Cashin-Hemphill L JAMA 1990; 264: 3013-7	138	75	4	37	qCAG	52% of treated patients non-progression of coronary lesions by angiography after 4 years vs. 15% in placebo group
CLAS IMT	Niacin and colestipol	Blankenhorn DH Circulation 1993; 88: 20-8	78	39	4	38	IMT and qCAG	Decrease in carotid IMT progression amongst treated subjects; correlation with coronary angiography data (n=46)

Table 1. Studies on HDL increasing drugs, their reported effect on HDL-C levels and their impact on clinical and intermediate endpoints continued.

	Drug	Publication	Participants	Patients in the active arm	Follow-up (yrs)	% HDL increase	Endpoint(s)	Endpoint results
Familial Atherosclerosis Treatment Study (FATS)	Niacin and colestipol	Brown G NEJM 1990; 323;1289	120	48	2.5	43	qCAG	Less progression of atherosclerosis on qCAG in niacin and colestipol treated patients vs placebo (46% vs 25%) and less events (death, MI or revascularization): 10 of 52 in placebo and 2 of 48 in treated patients
Coronary Risk Intervention Project (SCRIP)	Niacin and colestipol and gemfibrozil and lovastatin and lifestyle counselling	Haskell WL Circulation 1994; 89: 975-90	300	145	4	12	qCAG	Decrease in coronary luminal narrowing and less hospitalization compared to placebo (25 in treated vs. 44 in placebo). No differences in death
Arterial Biology for the Investigation of the Treatment Effects of Reducing Cholesterol (ARBITER 2 and 3)	Niacin (extended release) and statin	Taylor AJ Curr Med Res Opin 2006; 22: 2243-50	104	57	2	23	cIMT	Decrease in cIMT progression compared to placebo
Arterial Biology for the Investigation of the Treatment Effects of Reducing Cholesterol 6-HDL and LDL Treatment Strategies (ARBITER-HALTS)	Niacin (extended release) and statin	Taylor AJ NEJM 2009; 361: 2113-22	208	97	1.2	17	cIMT	Decrease in cIMT progression compared to ezetimibe
Oxford Niaspan Study	Niacin (extended release) and statin	Lee JM JACC 2009; 54: 1787-94	54	24	1	23	carotid MRI	Decrease in carotid wall areas compared to placebo

Table 1. Studies on HDL increasing drugs, their reported effect on HDL-C levels and their impact on clinical and intermediate endpoints continued.

	Drug	Publication	Participants	Patients in the active arm	Follow-up (yrs)	% HDL increase	Endpoint(s)	Endpoint results
FIBRATES								
CLINICAL OUTCOME								
Scottish prevention trial	Clofibrate	Scottish Society of Physicians *Br Med J* 1971; 4: 775-84	717	350	6	NR	death and MI	62% reduction in death and 53% reduction MI
Coronary Drug Project (CDP)	Clofibrate	The Coronary Drug Project *JAMA* 1975; 231: 360-81	8341	1103	6	NR	composite	9% reduction in non-fatal MI or death due to CAD (NS)
WHO Cooperative Trial follow-up	Clofibrate	Investigators CoP *Lancet* 1984; 2: 600-4	15745	5331	13	NR	death	Initial increased death rate amongst treated subjects (47% increase, non-ischemic cardiac deaths) was found to be decreased to a 11% excess of deaths in the formerly treated subjects (NS)
Helsinki Heart Study (HHS)	Gemfibrozil	Frick MH *NEJM* 1987; 317: 1237-45	4081	2051	5	11	composite	34% reduction in CAD death or non-fatal MI
Veterans Affairs HDL-C Intervention Trial (VA-HIT)	Gemfibrozil	Rubins HB *NEJM* 1999; 341: 410-8	2531	1264	5	6	composite	22% reduction in CAD death or non-fatal MI
Bezafibrate Infarction Prevention (BIP) study	Bezafibrate	The BIP Study Group *Circulation* 2000; 102: 21-27	3090	1548	6	18	composite	7% reduction in fatal and non-fatal MI or sudden death
Lower Extremity Arterial Disease Event Reduction (LEADER) trial	Bezafibrate	Meade T *BMJ* 2002; 325: 1139	1568	783	5	11	composite	4% decrease in combined endpoint (stroke and CAD) (NS)
Fenofibrate Intervention and Event Lowering in Diabetes (FIELD) study	Fenofibrate	Keech A *Lancet* 2005; 366: 1849-61	9795	4895	5	1.2	CHD death or non-fatal MI	11% relative risk reduction of coronary event (288 [5.9%] in placebo and 256 [5.2%] in treated patients) (NS)

Table 1. Studies on HDL increasing drugs, their reported effect on HDL-C levels and their impact on clinical and intermediate endpoints continued.

	Drug	Publication	Participants	Patients in the active arm	Follow-up (yrs)	% HDL increase	Endpoint(s)	Endpoint results
INTERMEDIATE ENDPOINT, IMAGING								
Bezafibrate Coronary Atherosclerosis Intervention Trial (BECAIT)	Bezafibrate	Ericsson CG *Lancet* 1996; 347: 849-53	92	42	5	9	qCAG	Less progression in bezafibrate treated subjects (vs. placebo)
Lopid Coronary Angiography Trial (LOCAT) Study	Gemfibrozil	Frick MH *Circulation* 1997; 96: 2137-43	395	197	2.5	21	qCAG	Less progression in gemfibrozil treated subjects (vs. placebo)
Diabetes Atherosclerosis Intervention Study (DAIS)	Fenofibrate	Diabetes Atherosclerosis Intervention Study Investigators *Lancet* 2001; 357: 905-10	418	207	3	8	qCAG	Less progression in fenofibrate treated diabetic subjects (vs. placebo)
CETP INHIBITORS *CLINICAL OUTCOME*								
Investigation of Lipid Level Management to Understand its Impact in Atherosclerotic Events (ILLUMINATE)	Torcetrapib	Barter P *N Engl J Med* 2007; 357: 2109-22	15067	7533	1	72	composite	Torcetrapib therapy resulted in an increased risk of mortality and morbidity of unknown mechanism
INTERMEDIATE ENDPOINT, IMAGING								
Investigation of Lipid Level Management Using Coronary Ultrasound to Assess Reduction of Atherosclerosis by CETP Inhibition and HDL Elevation (Illustrate)	Atorvastatin and torcetrapib	Nissen SE *N Engl J Med* 2007; 356: 1304-16	1188	591	2	61	IVUS	No significant decrease in the progression of coronary atherosclerosis

Table 1. Studies on HDL increasing drugs, their reported effect on HDL-C levels and their impact on clinical and intermediate endpoints continued.

	Drug	Publication	Participants	Patients in the active arm	Follow-up (yrs)	% HDL increase	Endpoint(s)	Endpoint results
Rating Atherosclerotic Disease Change by Imaging with a New CETP Inhibitor Trial 1 (RADIANCE 1)	Atorvastatin and torcetrapib	Bots ML Lancet 2007; 370: 153-60	904	450	2	54	cIMT	No decrease in c-IMT
Rating Atherosclerotic Disease Change by Imaging with a New CETP Inhibitor Trial 2 (RADIANCE 2)	Atorvastatin and torcetrapib	Kastelein N Engl J Med 2007; 356:1620	752	377	1.8	63	cIMT	No reduction of atherosclerosis in FH patients
APOA-I MIMETICS *INTERMEDIATE ENDPOINT, IMAGING*								
ApoAI Milano	ETC216	Nissen SE JAMA 2003; 290: 2292-300	57	45	5 wks	NR	IVUS	Decrease in coronary atheroma volume
Effect of rHDL on Atherosclerosis- Safety and Efficacy (ERASE)	rHDL (CSL111)	Tardif JC JAMA 2007; 297: 1675	183	111	6 wks	NR	IVUS	No significant decrease in atheroma volume, but significant improvement of plaque characteristics

to reduce the risk of non-fatal myocardial infarction by 25% in the absence of effects on mortality, cancer or stroke **(Ia/A)** [64].

The development of fibrates and nicotinic acid derivatives was not grounded in the HDL-hypothesis; their potential to increase HDL was rather heralded as a welcome side effect. Given their broad spectrum of effects, it is difficult to confidently ascribe their atheroprotective potential to the conferred increase in HDL levels.

HDL-like particles

In contrast, the rationale for the application of HDL-like particles directly strongly relies on a causal role for HDL in atheroprotection. In a study performed by Eriksson *et al*, the intravenous infusion of human proapoAI liposome complexes in four subjects with heterozygous familial hypercholesterolemia was shown to increase faecal cholesterol excretion [65]. These data lent support to the concept of reverse cholesterol transport and served as the basis for this entire field of research. In 2003, a widely-cited study reported regression of coronary plaque atheroma volume compared to baseline after infusion of recombinant apoAIMilano/phospholipid complexes [66]. Although this study was of a large conceptual importance, it only comprised 45 patients in the active arm and 12 patients in the placebo arm, leaving it underpowered for a formal direct comparison between treatment arms **(IIb/B)**. In addition, the investigators did not observe a dose-effect relation [67]. A larger study to address these issues would therefore be of substantial interest.

A similar HDL-like particle is reconstituted HDL (rHDL), consisting of apoAI from human plasma combined with soybean phosphatidylcholine (CSL-111). Based on the encouraging results of the aforementioned study, hopes for this compound to show efficacy versus placebo in a larger trial were running high. However, in a placebo-controlled trial in 145 patients, published in 2007, four weekly infusions of rHDL proved ineffective in reducing coronary plaque atheroma volume versus placebo, although plaque regression relative to baseline in the active arm of the study was observed [68]. Upon rHDL infusion, the atheroma was found to change morphologically, which was considered beneficial.

ApoAI mimetic peptides are another potential therapy in the category of HDL-like particles. One of these peptides, orally administered D-4F, has been shown to be safe and well-tolerated in a first trial in humans [69]. Data on efficacy of these compounds are at this point unavailable.

A successful reduction of atherosclerosis in humans through the infusion of HDL-like particles would constitute strong proof for the atheroprotective capacity of HDL. Unfortunately, results so far cause these therapies to remain a promise rather than established therapeutic tools and, hence, do not unequivocally support a causal relationship between HDL and cardiovascular disease.

CETP inhibition

Another means to increase HDL levels is through the inhibition of CETP. By inhibiting CETP, the normal exchange of cholesteryl esters from HDL and triglycerides from apoB-containing lipoproteins is blocked, which results in higher HDL cholesterol and lower LDL cholesterol levels [70]. Administration of CETP inhibitors, dalcetrapib (previously denoted as JTT-705), torcetrapib and anacetrapib, has been shown to potently increase HDL-C levels in humans [71]. Although phase III trials with dalcetrapib and anacetrapib were recently initiated, similar studies with torcetrapib were prematurely halted in 2006; the large phase III mortality and morbidity trial ILLUMINATE was terminated because of significantly higher cardiovascular and non-cardiovascular mortality rates in the atorvastatin/torcetrapib arm [2]. Concurrent imaging trials did not show positive effects of torcetrapib treatment on cIMT [72, 73] or on coronary percent atheroma volume [74].

An important question was whether the failure of torcetrapib could be attributed to CETP inhibition in general or to off-target toxicity of the torcetrapib molecule. Torcetrapib use has consistently been associated with increased blood pressure, plasma aldosterone levels and electrolyte changes [75]. These effects appear to be specific to torcetrapib since other CETP inhibitors have no effect on blood pressure [71].

Although these findings clearly indicate off-target toxicity for torcetrapib, they leave the question whether CETP inhibition constitutes a viable strategy for atheroprotection unanswered. Results from future trials are therefore eagerly awaited.

In summary, there is a paucity of data regarding the effects of specific HDL-increasing drugs on cardiovascular endpoints. Fibrates and niacin have shown to reduce cardiovascular disease, but since these therapies have broad effects on lipid metabolism it is difficult to assess how much of this atheroprotection is mediated by the increase in HDL. Interventions with HDL-like particles have shown promise in preclinical studies and small-scale clinical trials, but have thus far not improved patient outcomes on a larger scale. In order to draw definitive conclusions, these compounds require careful evaluation and follow-up.

Conclusions

A considerable body of evidence has been generated to support the hypothesis that HDL protects against the development of atherosclerosis, which has resulted in a quest for drugs targeting HDL.

The evidence that HDL-C increase would be beneficial is, however, primarily generated in *in vitro* experiments and in several animal models. Direct evidence from human intervention studies is scarce. This is largely due to the difficulty to disentangle HDL-related effects from those that are related to other key factors in atherosclerosis.

The causality of the relationship between HDL and human cardiovascular disease remains, in our view, to be proven by intervention trials where specific HDL-C increase is established.

The counterintuitive results of recent HDL-C-increasing trials (i.e. ILLUMINATE) should, however, not be regarded as a moratorium against HDL-C increase *per se*, but should be interpreted as a reflection of the complexity of HDL metabolism and the unpredictable outcome associated with medical intervention in these pathways.

Key points	Evidence level
◆ Based on multiple different lines of evidence, it has been proposed that raising HDL, or improving HDL functionality, will result in cardiovascular benefit. However, criticism has intensified in light of recent unexpected and disappointing results.	III/B
◆ A low HDL-C is an important risk factor for cardiovascular disease but this association is not necessarily causal, given confounding by smoking, physical activity, obesity, diabetes, hypertriglyceridemia, inflammatory status, gender and socio-economic status.	III/B
◆ *In vitro* experiments support numerous atheroprotective roles for HDL, including a central role in reverse cholesterol transport as well as anti-inflammatory, anti-thrombotic, anti-apoptotic and anti-oxidative effects, but how this translates into clinical benefit is not known.	III/B
◆ Clinical endpoint trials with HDL-modulating therapies have thus far provided ambiguous results with regard to reduction of CVD. Fibrates (Ia/A) and nicotinic acid (Ib/A) raise HDL-C and reduce CVD, but these drugs were not developed to raise HDL-C and also have a strong impact on LDL-C and triglyceride levels.	Ia/A & Ib/A
◆ Several features of HDL biology should guide a cautious development of novel anti-atherosclerotic drugs, appropriately reflecting the considerable remaining uncertainties.	IV/C
◆ Patients at risk for CVD should receive lifestyle counselling and treatment with statins to achieve LDL-C goals (Ia/A); in patients with a low HDL-C, additional treatment with a fibrate or nicotinic acid can be considered (IIb/B).	Ia/A & IIb/B

References

1. Lewis SJ. Prevention and treatment of atherosclerosis: a practitioner's guide for 2008. *Am J Med* 2009; 122(1 Suppl): S38-S50.
2. Barter PJ, Caulfield M, Eriksson M, *et al*. Effects of torcetrapib in patients at high risk for coronary events. *N Engl J Med* 2007; 357(21): 2109-22.
3. Gordon T, Castelli WP, Hjortland MC, Kannel WB, Dawber TR. High density lipoprotein as a protective factor against coronary heart disease: The Framingham study. *Am J Med* 1977; 62(5): 707-14.

4. Castelli WP, Garrison RJ, Wilson PW, Abbott RD, Kalousdian S, Kannel WB. Incidence of coronary heart disease and lipoprotein cholesterol levels. The Framingham Study. *JAMA* 1986; 256(20): 2835-8.

5. Assmann G, Schulte H, von Eckardstein A, Huang Y. High-density lipoprotein cholesterol as a predictor of coronary heart disease risk. The PROCAM experience and pathophysiological implications for reverse cholesterol transport. *Atherosclerosis* 1996; 124 Suppl: S11-20.

6. Yusuf S, Hawken S, Ounpuu S, *et al.* Effect of potentially modifiable risk factors associated with myocardial infarction in 52 countries (the INTERHEART study): case-control study. *Lancet* 2004; 364(9438): 937-52.

7. Genest JJ, Corbett HM, McNamara JR, Schaefer MM, Salem DN, Schaefer EJ. Effect of hospitalization on high-density lipoprotein cholesterol in patients undergoing elective coronary angiography. *Am J Cardiol* 1988; 61(13): 998-1000.

8. Sacks FM, Tonkin AM, Shepherd J, *et al.* Effect of pravastatin on coronary disease events in subgroups defined by coronary risk factors: the Prospective Pravastatin Pooling Project. *Circulation* 2000; 102(16): 1893-1900.

9. Executive Summary of The Third Report of The National Cholesterol Education Program (NCEP) Expert Panel on Detection, Evaluation, And Treatment of High Blood Cholesterol In Adults (Adult Treatment Panel III). *JAMA* 2001; 285(19): 2486-97.

10. Haffner SM. Dyslipidemia management in adults with diabetes. *Diabetes Care* 2004; 27 Suppl 1: S68-71.

11. Gordon DJ, Probstfield JL, Garrison RJ, *et al.* High-density lipoprotein cholesterol and cardiovascular disease. Four prospective American studies. *Circulation* 1989; 79(1): 8-15.

12. Wild S, Byrne CD. Time to rethink high-density lipoprotein? *Heart* 2008; 94(6): 692-4.

13. Hansel B, Kontush A, Giral P, Bonnefont-Rousselot D, Chapman MJ, Bruckert E. One third of the variability in HDL-cholesterol level in a large dyslipidaemic population is predicted by age, sex and triglyceridaemia: The Paris La Pitie Study. *Curr Med Res Opin* 2006; 22(6): 1149-60.

14. Criqui MH, Wallace RB, Heiss G, Mishkel M, Schonfeld G, Jones GT. Cigarette smoking and plasma high-density lipoprotein cholesterol. The Lipid Research Clinics Program Prevalence Study. *Circulation* 1980; 62(4 Pt 2): IV70-6.

15. Williams PT. High-density lipoprotein cholesterol and other risk factors for coronary heart disease in female runners. *N Engl J Med* 1996; 334(20): 1298-304.

16. Kodama S, Tanaka S, Saito K, *et al.* Effect of aerobic exercise training on serum levels of high-density lipoprotein cholesterol: a meta-analysis. *Arch Intern Med* 2007; 167(10): 999-1008.

17. Rashid S, Genest J. Effect of obesity on high-density lipoprotein metabolism. *Obesity* 2007; 15(12): 2875-8.

18. Chahil TJ, Ginsberg HN. Diabetic dyslipidemia. *Endocrinol Metab Clin North Am* 2006; 35(3): 491-510.

19. Hayek T, Azrolan N, Verdery RB, *et al.* Hypertriglyceridemia and cholesteryl ester transfer protein interact to dramatically alter high density lipoprotein levels, particle sizes, and metabolism. Studies in transgenic mice. *J Clin Invest* 1993; 92(3): 1143-52.

20. Tai ES, Emmanuel SC, Chew SK, Tan BY, Tan CE. Isolated low HDL cholesterol: an insulin-resistant state only in the presence of fasting hypertriglyceridemia. *Diabetes* 1999; 48(5): 1088-92.

21. Khovidhunkit W, Memon RA, Feingold KR, Grunfeld C. Infection and inflammation-induced proatherogenic changes of lipoproteins. *J Infect Dis* 2000; 181(s3): S462-S472.

22. Heiss G, Haskell W, Mowery R, Criqui MH, Brockway M, Tyroler HA. Plasma high-density lipoprotein cholesterol and socioeconomic status. The Lipid Research Clinics Program Prevalence Study. *Circulation* 1980; 62(4 Pt 2): IV108-15.

23. Becher H. The concept of residual confounding in regression models and some applications. *Stat Med* 1992; 11(13): 1747-58.

24. Glomset JA. The plasma lecithin:cholesterol acyltransferase reaction. *J Lipid Res* 1968; 9(2): 155-67.

25. Kuivenhoven JA, Pritchard H, Hill J, Frohlich J, Assmann G, Kastelein J. The molecular pathology of lecithin:cholesterol acyltransferase (LCAT) deficiency syndromes. *J Lipid Res* 1997; 38(2): 191-205.

26. Fielding CJ, Fielding PE. Cellular cholesterol efflux. *Biochim Biophys Acta* 2001; 1533(3): 175-89.

27. Acton S, Rigotti A, Landschulz KT, Xu S, Hobbs HH, Krieger M. Identification of scavenger receptor SR-BI as a high density lipoprotein receptor. *Science* 1996; 271(5248): 518-20.

28. Martinez LO, Jacquet S, Esteve JP, *et al.* Ectopic beta-chain of ATP synthase is an apolipoprotein A-I receptor in hepatic HDL endocytosis. *Nature* 2003; 421(6918): 75-9.

29. Vergeer M, Dallinga-Thie GM, Dullaart RPF, van Tol A. Evaluation of phospholipid transfer protein as a therapeutic target. *Future Lipidology* 2008; 3(3): 327-35.

30. Jaye M, Lynch KJ, Krawiec J, *et al*. A novel endothelial-derived lipase that modulates HDL metabolism. *Nat Genet* 1999; 21(4): 424-8.

31. Alam K, Meidell RS, Spady DK. Effect of up-regulating individual steps in the reverse cholesterol transport pathway on reverse cholesterol transport in normolipidemic mice. *J Biol Chem* 2001; 276(19): 15641-9.

32. Groen AK, Bloks VW, Bandsma RH, Ottenhoff R, Chimini G, Kuipers F. Hepatobiliary cholesterol transport is not impaired in Abca1-null mice lacking HDL. *J Clin Invest* 2001; 108(6): 843-50.

33. Rader DJ. Molecular regulation of HDL metabolism and function: implications for novel therapies. *J Clin Invest* 2006; 116(12): 3090-100.

34. Cockerill GW, Rye KA, Gamble JR, Vadas MA, Barter PJ. High-density lipoproteins inhibit cytokine-induced expression of endothelial cell adhesion molecules. *Arterioscler Thromb Vasc Biol* 1995; 15(11): 1987-94.

35. Navab M, Berliner JA, Subbanagounder G, *et al*. HDL and the inflammatory response induced by LDL-derived oxidized phospholipids. *Arterioscler Thromb Vasc Biol* 2001; 21(4): 481-8.

36. Lee CM, Chien CT, Chang PY, *et al*. High-density lipoprotein antagonizes oxidized low-density lipoprotein by suppressing oxygen free-radical formation and preserving nitric oxide bioactivity. *Atherosclerosis* 2005; 183(2): 251-8.

37. Puranik R, Bao S, Nobecourt E, *et al*. Low dose apolipoprotein A-I rescues carotid arteries from inflammation *in vivo*. *Atherosclerosis* 2008; 196(1): 240-7.

38. Maeda K, Noguchi Y, Fukui T. The effects of cessation from cigarette smoking on the lipid and lipoprotein profiles: a meta-analysis. *Prev Med* 2003; 37(4): 283-90.

39. Garrison RJ, Kannel WB, Feinleib M, Castelli WP, McNamara PM, Padgett SJ. Cigarette smoking and HDL cholesterol: the Framingham offspring study. *Atherosclerosis* 1978; 30(1): 17-25.

40. Ansell BJ, Fonarow GC, Fogelman AM. High-density lipoprotein: is it always atheroprotective? *Curr Atheroscler Rep* 2006; 8(5): 405-11.

41. Kraus WE, Houmard JA, Duscha BD, *et al*. Effects of the amount and intensity of exercise on plasma lipoproteins. *N Engl J Med* 2002; 347(19): 1483-92.

42. Couillard C, Despres JP, Lamarche B, *et al*. Effects of endurance exercise training on plasma HDL cholesterol levels depend on levels of triglycerides: evidence from men of the Health, Risk Factors, Exercise Training and Genetics (HERITAGE) Family Study. *Arterioscler Thromb Vasc Biol* 2001; 21(7): 1226-32.

43. James WP, Astrup A, Finer N, *et al*. Effect of sibutramine on weight maintenance after weight loss: a randomised trial. STORM Study Group. Sibutramine Trial of Obesity Reduction and Maintenance. *Lancet* 2000; 356(9248): 2119-25.

44. Dattilo AM, Kris-Etherton PM. Effects of weight reduction on blood lipids and lipoproteins: a meta-analysis. *Am J Clin Nutr* 1992; 56(2): 320-8.

45. Poobalan A, Aucott L, Smith WC, *et al*. Effects of weight loss in overweight/obese individuals and long-term lipid outcomes - a systematic review. *Obes Rev* 2004; 5(1): 43-50.

46. Gaziano JM, Buring JE, Breslow JL, *et al*. Moderate alcohol intake, increased levels of high-density lipoprotein and its subfractions, and decreased risk of myocardial infarction. *N Engl J Med* 1993; 329(25): 1829-34.

47. Lichtenstein AH. Dietary fat and cardiovascular disease risk: quantity or quality? *J Womens Health* (Larchmt) 2003; 12(2): 109-14.

48. Nicholls SJ, Lundman P, Harmer JA, *et al*. Consumption of saturated fat impairs the anti-inflammatory properties of high-density lipoproteins and endothelial function. *J Am Coll Cardiol* 2006; 48(4): 715-20.

49. Kromhout D, Bosschieter EB, de Lezenne CC. The inverse relation between fish consumption and 20-year mortality from coronary heart disease. *N Engl J Med* 1985; 312(19): 1205-9.

50. Birjmohun RS, Hutten BA, Kastelein JJP, Stroes ESG. Efficacy and safety of high-density lipoprotein cholesterol-increasing compounds: a meta-analysis of randomized controlled trials. *J Am Coll Cardiol* 2005; 45(2): 185-97.

51. Rubic T, Trottmann M, Lorenz RL. Stimulation of CD36 and the key effector of reverse cholesterol transport ATP-binding cassette A1 in monocytoid cells by niacin. *Biochem Pharmacol* 2004; 67(3): 411-9.

52. van der Hoorn JW, de Haan W, Berbee JF *et al*. Niacin increases HDL by reducing hepatic expression and plasma levels of cholesteryl ester transfer protein in APOE*3Leiden.CETP mice. *Arterioscler Thromb Vasc Biol* 2008; 28(11): 2016-22.

53. Altschul R, Hoffer A, Stephen JD. Influence of nicotinic acid on serum cholesterol in man. *Arch Biochem* 1955; 54(2): 558-9.

54. Canner PL, Berge KG, Wenger NK, *et al.* Fifteen year mortality in Coronary Drug Project patients: long-term benefit with niacin. *J Am Coll Cardiol* 1986; 8(6): 1245-55.

55. Brown BG, Zhao XQ, Chait A, *et al.* Simvastatin and niacin, antioxidant vitamins, or the combination for the prevention of coronary disease. *N Engl J Med* 2001; 345(22): 1583-92.

56. Taylor AJ, Sullenberger LE, Lee HJ, Lee JK, Grace KA. Arterial Biology for the Investigation of the Treatment Effects of Reducing Cholesterol (ARBITER) 2: a double-blind, placebo-controlled study of extended-release niacin on atherosclerosis progression in secondary prevention patients treated with statins. *Circulation* 2004; 110(23): 3512-7.

57. Taylor AJ, Lee HJ, Sullenberger LE. The effect of 24 months of combination statin and extended-release niacin on carotid intima-media thickness: ARBITER 3. *Curr Med Res Opin* 2006; 22(11): 2243-50.

58. Taylor AJ, Villines TC, Stanek EJ, *et al.* Extended-release niacin or ezetimibe and carotid intima-media thickness. *N Engl J Med* 2009; 361(22): 2113-22.

59. Lee JMS, Robson MD, Yu LM, *et al.* Effects of high-dose modified-release nicotinic acid on atherosclerosis and vascular function: a randomized, placebo-controlled, magnetic resonance imaging study. *J Am Coll Cardiol* 2009; 54(19): 1787-94.

60. Staels B, Dallongeville J, Auwerx J, Schoonjans K, Leitersdorf E, Fruchart JC. Mechanism of action of fibrates on lipid and lipoprotein metabolism. *Circulation* 1998; 98(19): 2088-93.

61. Robins SJ, Collins D, Wittes JT, *et al.* Relation of gemfibrozil treatment and lipid levels with major coronary events: VA-HIT: a randomized controlled trial. *JAMA* 2001; 285(12): 1585-91.

62. Manninen V, Elo MO, Frick MH, *et al.* Lipid alterations and decline in the incidence of coronary heart disease in the Helsinki Heart Study. *JAMA* 1988; 260(5): 641-51.

63. Frick MH, Elo O, Haapa K, *et al.* Helsinki Heart Study: primary-prevention trial with gemfibrozil in middle-aged men with dyslipidemia. Safety of treatment, changes in risk factors, and incidence of coronary heart disease. *N Engl J Med* 1987; 317(20): 1237-45.

64. Saha SA, Kizhakepunnur LG, Bahekar A, Arora RR. The role of fibrates in the prevention of cardiovascular disease - a pooled meta-analysis of long-term randomized placebo-controlled clinical trials. *Am Heart J* 2007; 154(5): 943-53.

65. Eriksson M, Carlson LA, Miettinen TA, Angelin B. Stimulation of fecal steroid excretion after infusion of recombinant proapolipoprotein A-I: potential reverse cholesterol transport in humans. *Circulation* 1999; 100(6): 594-8.

66. Nissen SE, Tsunoda T, Tuzcu EM, *et al.* Effect of recombinant ApoA-I Milano on coronary atherosclerosis in patients with acute coronary syndromes: a randomized controlled trial. *JAMA* 2003; 290(17): 2292-300.

67. Rader DJ. High-density lipoproteins as an emerging therapeutic target for atherosclerosis. *JAMA* 2003; 290(17): 2322-4.

68. Tardif JC, Gregoire J, L'Allier PL, *et al.* Effects of reconstituted high-density lipoprotein infusions on coronary atherosclerosis: a randomized controlled trial. *JAMA* 2007; 297(15): 1675-82.

69. Bloedon LT, Dunbar R, Duffy D, *et al.* Safety, pharmacokinetics, and pharmacodynamics of oral apoA-I mimetic peptide D-4F in high-risk cardiovascular patients. *J Lipid Res* 2008; 49(6): 1344-52.

70. Tall AR. CETP inhibitors to increase HDL cholesterol levels. *N Engl J Med* 2007; 356(13): 1364-6.

71. Vergeer M, Stroes ES. The pharmacology and off-target effects of some cholesterol ester transfer protein inhibitors. *Am J Cardiol* 2009; 104(10 Suppl): 32E-38E.

72. Bots ML, Visseren FL, Evans GW, *et al.* Torcetrapib and carotid intima-media thickness in mixed dyslipidaemia (RADIANCE 2 study): a randomised, double-blind trial. *Lancet* 2007; 370(9582): 153-60.

73. Kastelein JJP, van Leuven SI, Burgess L, *et al.* Effect of torcetrapib on carotid atherosclerosis in familial hypercholesterolemia. *N Engl J Med* 2007; 356(16): 1620-30.

74. Nissen SE, Tardif JC, Nicholls SJ, *et al.* Effect of torcetrapib on the progression of coronary atherosclerosis. *N Engl J Med* 2007; 356(13): 1304-16.

75. Vergeer M, Bots ML, van Leuven SI, *et al.* Cholesteryl ester transfer protein inhibitor torcetrapib and off-target toxicity: a pooled analysis of the rating atherosclerotic disease change by imaging with a new CETP inhibitor (RADIANCE) trials. *Circulation* 2008; 118(24): 2515-22.

Chapter 7

How do we diagnose hypertriglyceridemia in clinical practice and what are the consequences for treatment?

Adie Viljoen MBBS FRCPath, Consultant Chemical Pathologist
Lister Hospital, Stevenage, Hertfordshire, UK

Anthony S. Wierzbicki DM DPhil FRCPath FAHA
Consultant Metabolic Physician & Chemical Pathologist
Guy's & St Thomas' Hospitals, London, UK

Introduction

Triglycerides (also referred to as triacylglycerols) are formed from a single molecule of glycerol combined with three fatty acids. They are transported in the blood in lipoprotein particles allied with specific proteins – apolipoproteins which are also responsible for cholesterol transport. The two main sources of plasma triglycerides are exogenous (i.e. from dietary fat) carried in chylomicrons (CM), and endogenous (synthesized in the liver from fatty acids released from adipose tissue) and carried in very-low-density lipoprotein (VLDL) particles (Figure 1)[1]. In addition, cholesteryl ester transfer protein (CETP) shunts triglycerides to HDL particles in exchange for cholesterol from VLDL and other triglyceride-rich lipoproteins as part of the process involved in creation of the atherogenic lipid profile of insulin resistance/diabetes, as these triglyceride-rich particles are potent substrates for hepatic lipase and subsequent degradation. Triglyceride-rich particles also contain substantial amounts of apolipoprotein CIII, an inhibitor of lipoprotein lipase which releases fatty acids from triglycerides and apolipoprotein E which is the main apolipoprotein involved in clearance of these particles by the apoB100/E (low-density lipoprotein) receptor [2]. Additional mechanisms for clearance of triglyceride-rich particles include the LDL-related receptor, the heparin sulphate proteoglycans and the GP1HBP1 receptor for lipoprotein lipase which can be adsorbed onto these particles [1-3].

Several epidemiological studies have reported on the association of elevated serum triglyceride levels and the risk of coronary heart disease (CHD) [4-8] (Figure 2). All analyses are complicated by the skewed distribution of triglycerides which necessitates log transformation. Meta-analysis of the studies suggests a cardiovascular disease (CVD) risk

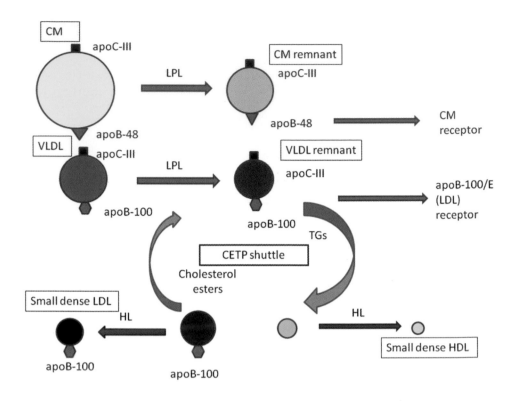

Figure 1. Metabolism of lipoproteins in atherogenic dyslipidemia. Apo = apolipoprotein; CETP = cholesteryl ester transfer protein; CM = chylomicron; HL = hepatic lipase; LPL = lipoprotein lipase; VLDL = very low density lipoprotein.

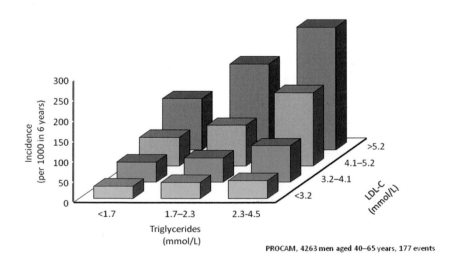

PROCAM, 4263 men aged 40–65 years, 177 events

Figure 2. Relationship of triglycerides to CHD risk in the Munster Heart Study (PROCAM). *Reproduced with permission from Assmann G, et al[8]. Copyright © 1996, Elsevier.*

attenuated after analysis for other factors of 1.72 (1.56-1.90) for each log elevation or 1.26 (116-1.39) per 1mmol/L elevation [9] **(Ia/A)**. However, the relevance of triglycerides to cardiovascular disease remains uncertain. Lipoprotein metabolism is integrally linked, and elevations of serum triglycerides can be confounded by significant correlations with total cholesterol, low-density lipoprotein cholesterol (LDL-C), and high-density lipoprotein cholesterol (HDL-C) levels. Non-lipid risk factors of obesity, hypertension, diabetes, inflammation (C-reactive protein) and cigarette smoking are also interrelated with triglycerides. Although there is consistent evidence that raised triglyceride levels are associated with increased CHD risk, adjustment for established coronary risk factors, especially HDL-C, substantially attenuates the magnitude of this association. Despite several reports and meta-analyses [10, 11] suggesting that triglycerides are an independent risk factor for CVD, the latest conclusion from the American National Cholesterol Education Program - Adult Treatment Panel (NCEP-ATP III) [12] is that there is insufficient evidence to regard triglycerides as an independent coronary risk factor **(IIa/B)**. It is, however, concluded that the link between serum triglycerides and CHD is stronger than previously recognized **(IV/C)**.

Diagnosing hypertriglyceridemia

Triglycerides form one of the bases of the Fredrickson classification of hyperlipidemia [13] with type I (>20mmol/L; CM), type V (>20mmol/L), type IV (>10mmol/L), type III (triglycerides cholesterol) and type IIb (>2.5mmol/L) defined on the basis of various degrees of hypertriglyceridemia. These classifications indirectly reflect the five different types of lipoproteins, which vary in their triglyceride content:

- chylomicrons (CM): 85% to 90% triglycerides;
- very-low-density lipoproteins (VLDL): 50% to 60%;
- intermediate-density lipoproteins (IDL): 20% to 25%;
- low-density lipoproteins (LDL): ≤10%;
- high-density lipoproteins (HDL): ≤10%.

The main triglyceride-rich lipoproteins are therefore CM, VLDL and IDL. These triglyceride-rich lipoproteins encompass a heterogeneous spectrum which differs in terms of size, density, and lipid and apolipoprotein composition.

The triglyceride concentration is also dependent on the relative fasting state. After a meal, most of the circulating triglycerides originate in the intestine and are secreted in CM, whereas during periods of fasting, endogenous triglycerides secreted by the liver as VLDL predominate. In the non-fasting state, plasma triglyceride concentrations can vary considerably, with concentrations rising fairly rapidly, reaching peak concentrations about 4 hours after ingestion of a fat-containing meal. They remain above fasting concentrations for approximately 8 hours or more as CM are removed from the circulation [14]. As opposed to fasting triglyceride levels, non-fasting triglyceride concentrations may be a superior marker to predict CHD [5, 6], as post-prandial measurements capture additional physiological risk

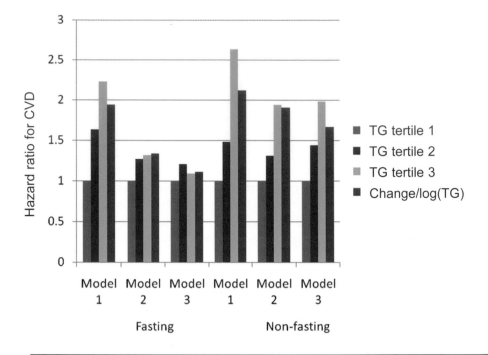

Model 1 = adjusted for age, blood pressure, smoking and use of hormone therapy
Model 2 = model 1 plus total cholesterol and HDL-C
Model 3 = model 2 plus diabetes mellitus, BMI, and CRP

Figure 3. Relationship of fasting and non-fasting triglycerides (TG) to CVD risk. *Adapted from Bansal S, et al [5].*

information (Figure 3). In practice, as fasting and post-prandial triglyceride levels show a correlation of 0.67-0.80 they are used interchangeably [15, 16]. Furthermore, because most humans find themselves in the non-fasting state for the majority of a 24-hour period it may therefore be more useful to measure triglycerides in the non-fasting state. In fact the hypertriglyceridemia of insulin resistance simply represents the delayed clearance of triglyceride-rich particles even after a 12-14-hour fast. The use of non-fasting measurements has several technical drawbacks such as the lack of standardised non-fasting protocols as well as the lack of reference values and therefore it is currently recommended that measurements are taken after a 12-hour fast [17]. In practice the primary risk factor for cardiovascular disease is LDL-cholesterol and the main requirement for fasting lipid levels is due to confounding of the Friedewald equation for calculation of LDL-cholesterol by triglyceride-rich particles [18]. This problem is not seen when LDL-cholesterol levels are measured by direct assays though the specificity of the various methods remains to be fully confirmed. However, recent data which included more than 30,000 individuals has shown that triglyceride concentrations differ only slightly (increasing at most by 0.3mmol/L) following normal food intake making an argument against the dogma of fasting lipid profiles [16].

Classification of hypertriglyceridemia

Hypertriglyceridemia can be divided into primary and secondary causes (Table 1) . Primary causes are rare and most clinical hypertriglyceridemia occurs secondary to other causes. The commonest of these associated with severe hypertriglcyeridemia (>10mmol/L) are poorly controlled diabetes, excess alcohol intake, chronic renal failure on peritoneal dialysis and HIV-

Table 1. Primary and secondary causes of elevated triglycerides.

TG>1000mg/dL (>10mmol/L)		TG 200-1000mg/dL (2-10mmol/L)	
Primary	**Secondary**	**Primary**	**Secondary**
Familial hyperchylomicronemia	Type I diabetes (poor glycemic control)	Remnant hyperlipidemia	Type 2 diabetes (poor glycemic control)
Familial lipodystrophy	Type 2 diabetes (very poor glycemic control)	Familial combined hyperlipidemia	Excess alcohol
Primary myopathies	Gross alcohol excess	Primary myopathies	Chronic renal failure (on peritoneal dialysis)
	Glucocorticoids (high dose)		HIV disease (on protease inhibitors)
	HIV lipodystrophy (with certain drug treatments, e.g. ddI, ddC)		Retinoid therapy for psoriasis
	Anti-psychotics, e.g olanzapine		Calcineurin inhibiting immunosuppressants, (e.g. cyclosporine > sirolimus)
	Lymphoma – Bexarotene therapy		Tamoxifen therapy
			Systemic sex steroids (androgens, progestagens, oestrogens)
			Thiazide diuretics or β-blockers (high dose)

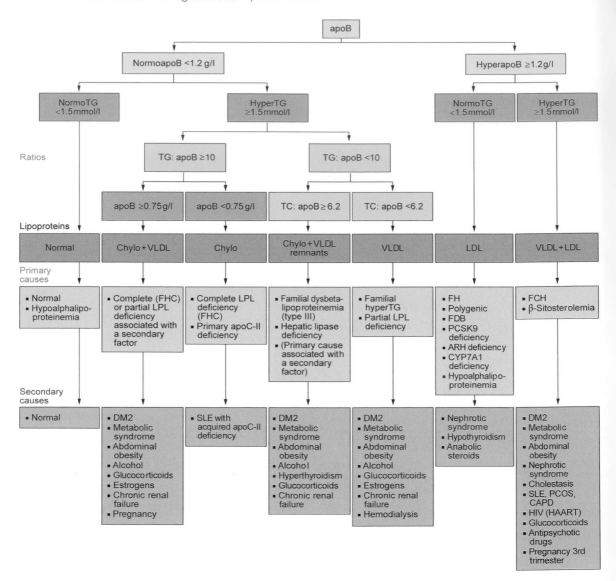

Figure 4. Algorithm for diagnosis of hypertriglyceridemia using apolipoprotein B, triglyceride and cholesterol concentrations. Total cholesterol and triglyceride are expressed as mmol/L and apoB as g/L. The triglyceride:apoB ratio of 10:1 is 8.8:1 if triglyceride and apoB are expressed in mg/dL. The equivalent total cholesterol:apoB ratio of 6.2:1 is 2.4:1 if cholesterol and apoB are expressed in mg/dL. apo = apolipoprotein; ARH = autosomal recessive hypercholesterolemia; CAPD = continuous ambulatory peritoneal dialysis; chylo = chylomicrons; CYP7A1 = cytochrome P450 7A1; DM2 = diabetes mellitus type 2; FCH = familial combined hyperlipidemia; FDB = familial defective apoB; FH = familial hypercholesterolemia; FHC = familial hyperchylomicronemia; HAART = highly active antiretroviral therapy; LPL = lipoprotein lipase; PCOS = polycystic ovary syndrome; SLE = systemic lupus erythematosus; TC = total cholesterol; TG = triglyceride. *Reproduced with permission from de Graaf J, et al. A diagnostic algorithm for the atherogenic apolipoprotein B dyslipoproteinemias. Nat Clin Pract Endocrinol Metab 2008; 4(11): 608-18. Copyright © 2008, Nature Publishing Group.*

associated hyperlipidemia and lipodystrophy. In milder hypertriglyceridemia (2-10mmol/L), the presence of the metabolic syndrome is a common feature and the causes are often the result of an interaction between a disease process, genetics and medications. One method for determining the cause of these abnormalities is to use a clinical algorithm combining measurement of triglycerides and apolipoprotein B (Figure 4) [19].

Methodological issues in the measurement of triglycerides

Triglycerides are used clinically as indices of principally VLDL levels with lesser contributions in most cases from CM or intermediate-density lipoprotein (IDL). There is no universal definition of hypertriglyceridemia. There are several reasons for this which include high biological variation (>20%), measurement techniques, the complexity and the heterogeneity of the lipoprotein particles which carry triglycerides in the blood as well as the heterogeneity of triglyceride molecules themselves. If the triglyceride: total cholesterol ratio (expressed as mmol/L) exceeds two then CM are likely to be present. Reference methods for lipoprotein analysis use density-based ultracentrifugation to determine VLDL and CM levels with particles with a density <1.066g/L being classed as triglyceride-rich. Measurement of VLDL-TG shows a greater correlation with plasma levels than VLDL-cholesterol [20]. Alternatively, VLDL and CM levels can be determined by capillary isotachophoresis [21] or fast pressure liquid chromatography (FPLC) [22]. All these methods are used for research and reference purposes only as they are not practical. The only direct practical measurement methods for VLDL/CM is the use of gradient electrophoresis on denaturing gradient gels [23] or by nuclear magnetic resonance spectroscopy (NMR) to determine particle sizes and numbers [24].

Routine clinical laboratory measurements using the common CHOD-PAP method do not take into account the fatty acid composition of triglycerides and actually determine the glycerol concentration which is measured as a surrogate for these heterogeneous molecules. Individual fatty acid levels can be measured by gas chromatography allied with mass spectrometry though the only measurement that is made in cardiovascular research practice is to compare the relative concentrations of the omega-3 and omega-6 fatty acid families.

The NCEP ATP III guidelines defined normal fasting plasma triglycerides as <1.7mmol/L (150mg/dL) [12]. The preceding NCEP ATP II guidelines had a higher cut-off point of <2.2mmol/L (200mg/dL) to define normality [25]. This shift came with the recognition that the link between serum triglycerides and CHD is stronger than was previously recognized. In similar fashion, all the other categories also have lower concentrations compared to the preceding ATP II report. The ATP III guidelines include the following concentration categories: borderline high (1.6-2.2mmol/L, 150-299mg/dL), high (2.2-5.6mmol/L, 300-499mg/dL) and very high (>5.6mmol/L, >500mg/L).

The American Diabetes Association recommends a triglyceride target of <1.7mmol/L [26] and the Joint British Societies' (JBS) Guidelines state that a fasting triglyceride >1.7mmol/L indicates increased CVD risk and this should be incorporated in the risk assessment [27, 28]. By these definitions hypertriglyceridemia is common. Data from the third National Health and Nutrition Examination Survey (NHANES) in the United States report the prevalence of fasting serum triglycerides of >1.7mmol/L to be approximately 30% in individuals >20 years of age [29] **(IIb/B)**.

Treating hypertriglyceridemia – the risk of CHD

Two questions about triglycerides persist:

* whether they constitute an independent risk factor for CHD; and
* whether they should be a direct target for therapy (ATPIII).

Triglycerides are related to CHD in many ways. This relationship is due to the fact that elevated triglycerides tend to 'keep bad company', being associated with abnormal lipoprotein metabolism, as well as with other cardiovascular risk factors including obesity, insulin resistance, diabetes mellitus, and lowered levels of HDL-C. The abnormal lipoprotein metabolism leads to what is referred to as atherogenic dyslipidemia which includes small dense LDL particles and low HDL-C [30]. The elevated triglyceride levels reflect the elevation in triglyceride-rich remnant lipoproteins. The pathophysiology of this process is complex and is related to adverse changes in the quality of LDL and HDL molecules. With high triglycerides the plasma residence time of triglyceride-rich lipoproteins rises with a subsequent increased interchange of triglyceride from CM and VLDL into LDL and HDL in exchange for cholesterol via cholesteryl ester transfer protein (CETP) [31]. The triglyceride-enriched LDL is converted to small dense LDL which is cleared less rapidly from the circulation. The small dense LDL particle is known to be more atherogenic and estimation of the LDL-C may therefore be misleading as there will be more LDL particles for any cholesterol concentration [32]. In contrast the cholesterol-depleted small HDL is cleared more rapidly in the kidney. Triglyceride in HDL is a substrate for plasma lipases especially hepatic lipase that converts HDL to a smaller particle.

Some causes of hypertriglyceridemia have no apparent effect on the risk of atherosclerotic vascular disease [33] but other data show a consistent effect. Establishing a triglyceride threshold as a risk factor for CVD is also not clear cut. Whereas the JBS2 guidelines report on the increased CVD risk with concentrations >1.7mmol/L, in the Munster Heart Study (PROCAM) the risk of non-fatal myocardial infarction and sudden cardiac death rose with triglyceride levels up to 9mmol/L (800mg/dL), but fell off at higher levels [8]. One of the most confounding variables in assessing the role of hypertriglyceridemia in atherosclerosis is its close and inverse relation with HDL-C. In most studies, HDL-C is reduced when triglycerides are increased and increases when the triglyceride increase is treated, whether by diet or drug. Specifically the drug classes that target hypertriglyceridemia have an inverse effect on HDL-C concentrations. Taking all this into account it is unsurprising that there is no clear consensus on the benefits of directly targeting hypertriglyceridemia *per se* and neither is there agreement or sufficient evidence on target concentrations [34].

Non-pharmacological intervention

Triglycerides respond particularly well to lifestyle changes, which should always form part of all therapeutic interventions. Two randomized controlled studies in obese patients found that low-carbohydrate diets respectively lowered triglyceride levels by 20% [35] and 28% [36] and that weight loss and assignment to a low-carbohydrate diet independently predicted

lower triglycerides. The Finnish Diabetes Prevention Study reported an 18% decline in serum
triglyceride levels with lifestyle changes [37] **(Ib/A)**.

Statins

Statins are the first-line therapy for lipoprotein disorders in the majority of cardiovascular
disease [12, 27, 38] **(Ia/A)**. There are considerable data that statins reduce triglycerides with the
effect being proportional to the LDL-C lowering capacity of the statin and baseline triglyceride
levels [39, 40] **(Ia/A)**. The mechanism of the effect occurs through increased clearance of
triglyceride-rich lipoproteins probably mediated through their apolipoprotein E content [41]. The
evidence that statins decrease cardiovascular events is overwhelming for both primary and
secondary prevention [42]. In these trials where patients with triglycerides >4-6mmol/L are
usually excluded there is no heterogeneity with respect to the relative efficacy of statin therapy
when analysed by medians or tertiles though patients with higher triglycerides (and lower
HDL-C) always have a higher baseline event rate. The only exceptions seem to relate to
patients with established grade 2-3 heart failure [43, 44] and in patients with diabetes undergoing
renal dialysis [45], both conditions in which hypertriglyceridemia is common, where reductions of
LDL-C of 42-50% were associated with minimal (and non-significant) reductions in
cardiovascular events but in some trials a beneficial statin response in heart failure was
associated with lower levels of inflammation as measured by C-reactive protein [46].

Fibrates

The fibrate class of lipid-lowering drugs is useful for lowering elevated triglyceride levels.
These drugs can reduce triglyceride levels by 25% to 50%, and up to 70% in severe
hypertriglyceridemia [47, 48]. Clinical trials of these drugs have reported mixed results. No
fibrate reduces all-cause mortality though meta-analysis suggests that they reduce non-fatal
myocardial infarcts [49] **(Ia/A)**. The World Health Organisation trial found reduced coronary
events but a significant increase in all-cause mortality with clofibrate monotherapy [50] which
did not persist after the trial [51]. The Helsinki Heart Study in primary prevention found reduced
coronary events but an (insignificant) increase in all-cause mortality in patients taking
gemfibrozil achieving a 34% reduction in CHD and up to 71% in patients with increased
body mass index, low HDL-cholesterol and elevated triglycerides >2.3mmol/L but
<7.6mmol/L [52, 53]. The Veterans Affairs High-Density Lipoprotein Cholesterol Intervention
Trial (VA-HIT) evaluated the potential benefits of gemfibrozil in 2531 men who suffered from
an acute myocardial infarction [54]. A significant reduction in the primary endpoint (fatal and
non-fatal MI) of 22% was achieved. These outcomes were achieved despite relatively small
changes in HDL-C (8%) and no change in LDL-C. The effects of gemfibrozil were
independent of baseline and change in triglycerides despite a 31% reduction [55] (Figure 5).
However, the enthusiasm for fibrates has been considerably dampened by results of the
Fenofibrate Intervention and Event Lowering in Diabetes (FIELD) study [56]. This trial
randomized 9795 type 2 DM subjects to fenofibrate (200mg daily) or placebo who were not
on statin treatment at the beginning of the study and participants were treated for 5 years. A
non-significant 11% reduction in the primary endpoint of CHD independent of baseline

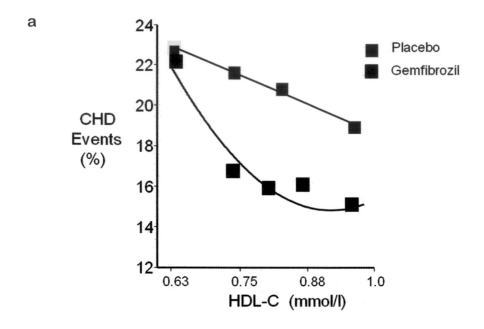

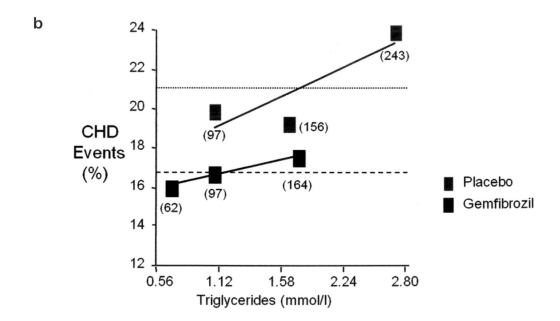

Figure 5. a) Prospective relationship of on-trial HDL achieved to CHD events in the VA-HIT study; b) Prospective relationship of on-trial triglycerides to CHD events in the VA-HIT trial. *Reproduced with permission from Robins SJ, et al [55]. © 2001 American Medical Association. All rights reserved.*

triglycerides was found. However, total cardiovascular events were reduced with fenofibrate therapy (p=0.035). The study was confounded by asymmetrical statin drop-in and other factors but as triglyceride concentrations (median 1.73mmol/L) were not raised, the effects of fenofibrate were predictably independent of triglycerides. A subsequent re-analysis for metabolic syndrome for triglycerides >2.3mmol/L did show benefits for fibrate therapy in this group [57]. It is difficult to compare fibrate trials as they seem to give disparate results depending on the compound used as might be expected from their PPAR selectivity [58]. Importantly no fibrate trials have shown to reduce all-cause mortality [59]. Fibrates can be added to statins to induce further reductions in triglycerides [60, 61] **(Ib/A)**. However, the recent Action to Control Cardiovascular Risk in Diabetes (ACCORD) trial substantiated that fenofibrate on top of statins did not reduce the rate of fatal cardiovascular events, non-fatal myocardial infarction, or non-fatal stroke [62] **(Ia/A)**.

Niacin (nicotinic acid)

Niacin (nicotinic acid) reduces triglyceride levels by 20% to 40% [63]. Due to its other favourable effects on HDL-C and LDL-C it has been referred to as the 'broad-spectrum' lipid drug [64]. Niacin was the first lipid-lowering agent to show a significant reduction in cardiovascular events but not mortality. The Coronary Drug Project randomized 3908 men with previous myocardial infarction (MI) to either nicotinic acid or placebo [65]. Major CHD events, non-fatal MI and cerebrovascular events were reduced by 22% but there was no effect on mortality. However, in the 15-year post-trial follow-up, nearly 9 years after termination of the trial, mortality from all causes was 11% lower in the nicotinic acid group [66]. Several long-term clinical studies with niacin have since demonstrated a reduction in CHD events and mortality when used in combination with other lipid-modifying drugs which include: colestipol (a bile acid sequestrant) [67], clofibrate [68] and statins [69] **(Ia/A)**. Ongoing trials include the Atherothrombosis Intervention in Metabolic syndrome with low HDL-C / High triglyceride and Impact on Global Health outcomes trial (AIM-HIGH) [70], which hopes to report in 2011, the large Oxford-based outcome trial with extended release niacin/laropiprant (an inhibitor of prostaglandin receptor D1 which reduces flushing), and the Heart Protection Study 2 – Treatment of HDL to Reduce the Incidence of Vascular Events (HPS2-THRIVE), which includes 28,000 patients with cardiovascular disease or at high risk of developing it which hopes to report in around 2013 [71].

Omega-3 fatty acids

Omega-3 fatty acids are also a heterogeneous group of molecules which are poorly synthesized in man but found in plants and fish, the latter recommended to be the primary source [72]. The common forms include eicosapentaenoic (EPA) and docosahexaenoic (DHA) acids. Apart from having a triglyceride-lowering effect, several other beneficial effects such as reducing sympathetic overactivity, enhancing nitric oxide-mediated vasodilatation, reducing levels of arachidonic acid-derived mediators and reducing insulin resistance, have been reported [72, 73]. Their triglyceride-lowering effect is most likely via their interaction with peroxisomal proliferator-activator activating receptor (PPAR). Apart from their ability to activate PPAR-α, PPAR-δ and PPAR-γ, they also interact with the farnesoid-X and the liver-x receptors [74]. Several studies have demonstrated the ability of EPA and DHA to lower triglyceride levels at high doses [75] **(Ia/A)**. This is amplified in patients with hypertriglyceridemia and also occurs in a dose-dependent manner. In the Gruppo Italiano per lo Studio della Sopravvivenza nell'Infarto miocardico Prevenzione (GISSI-P) trial including 11,324 participants, 1g DHA-EPA reduced triglycerides by 3.4% [76]. In a smaller, shorter Norwegian study, triglycerides were lowered by 18.56% by 1.7g/day EPA-DHA [77]. In 40 patients with severe hypertriglyceridemia (5.6-22mmol/L; 500-2000mg/dL), 3.4g/day EPA-DHA given for 4 months, reduced triglycerides by 45%, as compared with patients randomized to placebo [78] **(Ia/A)**. It is currently unclear whether there is a difference in the triglyceride-lowering abilities of EPA vs. DHA [79].

Numerous observational studies have documented an inverse relationship between questionnaire-assessed omega-3 fatty acid concentrations with reduced rates of cardiovascular disease [80, 81]. The GISSI-P trial randomized 11,324 patients with recent myocardial infarction (<3 months) to 1g omega-3 fatty acids (50% EPA and 50% DHA) or 300mg vitamin E in a 2 x 2 open label design, with a 42-month follow-up. Two-way analysis showed no effect for vitamin E and a 10% (1-18%) reduction in the primary endpoint from 13.9% to 12.6% (p=0.048) giving a number needed to treat (NNT) of 263 patients/year [76]. There was an increase in statin therapy from ~5% at baseline to 28% at 6 months and 45% at 42 months. In the GISSI heart failure study, 1g DHA-EPA in 7975 patients with heart failure reduced events by 9% in a 2 x 2 design using a primary endpoint of total mortality and hospital admission compared to no effect with a 42% reduction in LDL-C with a statin [44]. The Japan EPA lipid intervention study (JELIS) [82] investigated the effect of 1.8g of EPA added to 10-20mg pravastatin or 5-10mg simvastatin in 18,645 patients at least 6 months post-myocardial infarction with total cholesterol >6.5mmol/L (LDL-C >4.4mmol/L). The results showed a 19% reduction in events (3.5% to 2.8%, p=0.01), driven by a 24% reduction in unstable angina. On the basis of GISSI-P, omega-3 fatty acid supplements are recommended in many guidelines [12, 27, 38] and in the UK NICE guidelines if <6 portions / fish are consumed weekly in the first 3 months post-MI [83] **(Ia/A)**. The effect of omega-3 fatty acids added to optimal statin therapy in a high-risk group is unknown but calculations suggest that the NNT will rise to 480 / year (i.e. 97 for a typical 5-year period) [73]. On-going studies include the OMEGA trial which has randomized 3800 patients within 2-5 days of MI to 1g DHA-EPA or placebo with a primary endpoint of sudden cardiac death at 1 year [84]. In patients with diabetes, the ASCEND trial, 10,000 patients are being randomized to 1g DHA-EPA or aspirin in a 2 x 2 design to investigate the effects of omega-3 fatty acids on major adverse cardiac events [85]. The results are expected in 2012.

Other lipid-lowering drugs

Ezetimibe has only a small effect on triglycerides (10%) [86] while bile acid sequestrants raise triglycerides **(Ia/A)**. Among more novel agents microsomal transfer protein inhibitors are potent reducers of triglycerides by up to 70% but are hepatotoxic while anti-apoB antisense RNA therapy reduces triglycerides by 20-30% [87]. Many other agents with triglyceride-lowering potential such as combined PPAR α-γ agonists and PPAR-δ agonists have either failed in development or are still in early phase trials.

Combination therapy

An increasing literature addresses the role of combination therapy for the treatment of hypertriglyceridemia. The usual starting point is the use of initial statin therapy to which fibrates [60, 61, 88] (Figure 6), niacin [89] or omega-3 fatty acids [90] are added **(Ib/A)**. Triple therapy may be necessary [91] **(Ib/A)**. All of these interventions are additive and mostly seem to work by increasing the clearance of triglyceride-rich particles (statin-fibrate [92, 93] and statin-niacin [94]), while omega-3 fatty acid therapy may reduce secretion of VLDL. However, the recent ACCORD trial has reported that fenofibrate in combination with statins did not reduce the rate of fatal cardiovascular events, non-fatal myocardial infarction, or non-fatal stroke. These results do not support the routine use of fibrates on top of statins in high-risk type 2 diabetes mellitus patients, except possibly in patients with TG >2.3mmol/L and HDL-C <0.88mmol/L [62] **(Ia/A)**. Other additive therapies that can benefit triglyceride levels include the use of weight-loss drugs (orlistat, sibutramine, rimonabant), and some hypoglycemic drugs (e.g. pioglitazone) [95].

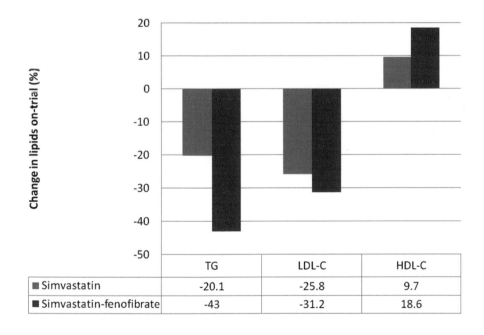

	TG	LDL-C	HDL-C
■ Simvastatin	-20.1	-25.8	9.7
■ Simvastatin-fenofibrate	-43	-31.2	18.6

Figure 6. Statin-fibrate combination therapy: changes in lipids with simvastatin 20mg-fenofibrate 160mg in the SAFARI trial. HDL-C = high-density lipoprotein-cholesterol; LDL-C = low-density lipoprotein cholesterol; TG = triglycerides. *Reproduced with permission from Grundy SM, et al [60]. Copyright © 2005, Elsevier.*

Treating severe hypertriglyceridemia – the risk of pancreatitis

Apart from its association with cardiovascular disease, elevated triglyceride levels are also a risk factor for pancreatitis [17, 96]. Hypertriglyceridemia-induced pancreatitis rarely occurs unless triglyceride levels exceed 20mmol/L [17, 97]. The recommended treatment threshold is not universal. The ATPIII guidelines recommend preventative treatment at levels >5.6mmol/L (>500mg/dL). More recently it has been recommended that levels greater than 11.3-16.0mmol/L (1000 to 1500mg/dL) require treatment with fibrates or nicotinic acid (niacin) to reduce the risk of pancreatitis [17] but this is still being debated [98] **(IV/C)**.

Patients with type I or type V hyperlipidemia present with gross lipemia often but not always associated with pancreatitis or eruptive xanthomata. Additional risk factors for lipemia in these patients include the presence of insulin resistance, obesity, pregnancy, lipid-raising drug therapies (usually high-dose glucocorticoids, HIV anti-retrovirals, sex steroids, retinoids or tamoxifen) and smoking [17]. Patients with type 2 diabetes often have extreme lipemia (>100mmol/L). A rare group of patients with familial lipodystrophy syndromes including juvenile dermatomyositis show a similar clinical phenotype of gross hypertriglyceridemia and pancreatitis but also signs of lipodystrophy [99].

Management is supportive with analgesia, fluid replacement, therapy for comorbidities and restriction of food intake. Acute lipid management consists of total food restriction to reduce CM and VLDL levels allied with an insulin sliding scale infusion if hyperglycemia is present [100]. Patients typically halve triglyceride levels every 24 hours and the initial profound insulin resistance rapidly disappears when plasma triglycerides fall to <20mmol/L. Once patients are able to eat they are started on fibrate therapy which may be continued long term in addition to a diet low in saturated fat. Many authorities recommend the use of ultra-low-fat diets (<10g/day) but adherence with these ultra-strict diets tends to be poor so more relaxed regimes (<20g/day) are generally used. In some patients it is necessary to combine fibrates with omega-3 fatty acids, niacin, statins or even orlistat to keep triglyceride levels <5mmol/L [101-103].

In gross hypertriglyceridemia of pregnancy the first-line therapy is omega-3 fatty acids which are preferably commenced at the beginning of the third trimester. Regular monitoring is required for gestational diabetes given the positive feedback between glucose and triglyceride levels seen in these patients. Acute management of pancreatitis may be necessary [104]. Labour often has to be induced early **(IV/C)** .

Conclusions

Elevated triglyceride concentrations are undoubtedly associated with risk of CHD. This link is stronger than was previously recognized. As lipoprotein metabolism is integrally linked, it is difficult to ascertain whether they constitute an independent risk factor for CHD. The clinician should be prompted to look at the other lipid and non-lipid risk factors to which elevated triglycerides are intimately linked.

Key points	Evidence level
◆ Diagnostic cut-points to categorise hypertriglyceridemia are not universal and have changed over the last decade.	IV/C
◆ A 12-hour fast is recommended when assessing triglyceride concentrations.	IV/C
◆ Elevated serum triglycerides are associated with increased risk for CHD.	Ia/A
◆ Elevated triglycerides are commonly associated with other lipid and non-lipid risk factors.	Ia/A
◆ Lifestyle intervention is effective in lowering triglyceride levels.	Ia/A
◆ Statins reduce triglycerides in proportion to their efficacy on LDL-C and baseline triglyceride levels.	Ia/A
◆ Statins reduce cardiovascular events in patients with moderately raised triglycerides.	Ia/A
◆ Fibrates are effective in lowering serum triglycerides.	Ia/A
◆ Fibrate therapy moderately reduces risk for non-fatal CHD events.	Ia/A
◆ Fibrates also can be combined with LDL-lowering drugs in the treatment of combined hyperlipidemia to improve the lipoprotein profile (Ib/A). However, combination therapy has no additive impact on cardiovascular event rate compared to statin treatment alone (Ia/A).	Ib/A & Ia/A
◆ Niacin is effective at lowering serum triglycerides.	Ia/A
◆ Niacin therapy produces a moderate reduction in CHD risk, either when used alone or in combination with other lipid-lowering drugs.	Ia/A
◆ Omega-3 fatty acids modestly reduce serum triglyceride concentrations in a dose-dependent manner.	Ib/A
◆ Omega-3 fatty acids modestly reduce CHD risk.	Ia/A
◆ Hypertriglyceridemia requires treatment to reduce the risk of pancreatitis.	IV/C

References

1.   Ginsberg HN. Lipoprotein physiology. *Endocrinol Metab Clin North Am* 1998; 27(3): 503-19.
2.   van Dijk KW, Hofker MH, Havekes LM. Dissection of the complex role of apolipoprotein E in lipoprotein metabolism and atherosclerosis using mouse models. *Curr Atheroscler Rep* 1999; 1(2): 101-7.
3.   Bishop JR, Stanford KI, Esko JD. Heparan sulfate proteoglycans and triglyceride-rich lipoprotein metabolism. *Curr Opin Lipidol* 2008; 19(3): 307-13.
4.   Criqui MH, Heiss G, Cohn R, *et al*. Plasma triglyceride level and mortality from coronary heart disease. *N Engl J Med* 1993; 328(17): 1220-5.
5.   Bansal S, Buring JE, Rifai N, *et al*. Fasting compared with nonfasting triglycerides and risk of cardiovascular events in women. *JAMA* 2007; 298(3): 309-16.
6.   Nordestgaard BG, Benn M, Schnohr P, *et al*. Nonfasting triglycerides and risk of myocardial infarction, ischemic heart disease, and death in men and women. *JAMA* 2007; 298(3): 299-308.

7.   Castelli WP. Epidemiology of triglycerides: a view from Framingham. *Am J Cardiol* 1992; 70(19): 3H-9H.

8.   Assmann G, Schulte H, von Eckardstein A. Hypertriglyceridemia and elevated lipoprotein(a) are risk factors for major coronary events in middle-aged men. *Am J Cardiol* 1996; 77(14): 1179-84.

9.   Sarwar N, Danesh J, Eiriksdottir G, *et al.* Triglycerides and the risk of coronary heart disease: 10,158 incident cases among 262,525 participants in 29 Western prospective studies. *Circulation* 2007; 115(4): 450-8.

10.   Assmann G, Schulte H, Funke H, *et al.* The emergence of triglycerides as a significant independent risk factor in coronary artery disease. *Eur Heart J* 1998; 19 Suppl M: M8-14.

11.   Hokanson JE, Austin MA. Plasma triglyceride level is a risk factor for cardiovascular disease independent of high-density lipoprotein cholesterol level: a meta-analysis of population-based prospective studies. *J Cardiovasc Risk* 1996; 3(2): 213-9.

12.   Expert Panel on Detection Evaluation and Treatment of High Blood Cholesterol In Adults (Adult Treatment Panel III). Executive Summary of The Third Report of The National Cholesterol Education Program (NCEP). *JAMA* 2001; 285(19): 2486-97.

13.   Fredrickson DS, Lees RS. A system for phenotyping hyperlipoproteinemia. *Circulation* 1965; 31: 321-7.

14.   Stein EA, Myers GL. National Cholesterol Education Program recommendations for triglyceride measurement: executive summary. The National Cholesterol Education Program Working Group on Lipoprotein Measurement. *Clin Chem* 1995; 41(10): 1421-6.

15.   Brown SA, Chambless LE, Sharrett AR, *et al.* Postprandial lipemia: reliability in an epidemiologic field study. *Am J Epidemiol* 1992; 136(5): 538-45.

16.   Langsted A, Freiberg JJ, Nordestgaard BG. Fasting and nonfasting lipid levels: influence of normal food intake on lipids, lipoproteins, apolipoproteins, and cardiovascular risk prediction. *Circulation* 2008; 118(20): 2047-56.

17.   Brunzell JD. Clinical practice. Hypertriglyceridemia. *N Engl J Med* 2007; 357(10): 1009-17.

18.   Friedewald WT, Levy RI, Fredrickson DS. Estimation of the concentration of low-density lipoprotein cholesterol in plasma, without use of the preparative ultracentrifuge. *Clin Chem* 1972; 18(6): 499-502.

19.   Sniderman AD. Applying apoB to the diagnosis and therapy of the atherogenic dyslipoproteinemias: a clinical diagnostic algorithm. *Curr Opin Lipidol* 2004; 15(4): 433-8.

20.   Fredrickson DS, Morganroth J, Levy RI. Type III hyperlipoproteinemia: an analysis of two contemporary definitions. *Ann Intern Med* 1975; 82(2): 150-7.

21.   Schmitz G, Borgmann U, Assmann G. Analytical capillary isotachophoresis: a routine technique for the analysis of lipoproteins and lipoprotein subfractions in whole serum. *J Chromatogr* 1985; 320(1): 253-62.

22.   Le NA, Innis-Whitehouse W, Li X, *et al.* Lipid and apolipoprotein levels and distribution in patients with hypertriglyceridemia: effect of triglyceride reductions with atorvastatin. *Metabolism* 2000; 49(2): 167-77.

23.   Ensign W, Hill N, Heward CB. Disparate LDL phenotypic classification among 4 different methods assessing LDL particle characteristics. *Clin Chem* 2006; 52(9): 1722-7.

24.   Tsai MY, Georgopoulos A, Otvos JD, *et al.* Comparison of ultracentrifugation and nuclear magnetic resonance spectroscopy in the quantification of triglyceride-rich lipoproteins after an oral fat load. *Clin Chem* 2004; 50(7): 1201-4.

25.   Expert Panel on Detection Evaluation and Treatment of High Blood Cholesterol In Adults (Adult Treatment Panel II). Summary of the second report of the National Cholesterol Education Program (NCEP) Expert Panel on Detection, Evaluation, and Treatment of High Blood Cholesterol in Adults (Adult Treatment Panel II). *JAMA* 1993; 269(23): 3015-23.

26.   American Diabetes Association. Standards of medical care in diabetes - 2009. *Diabetes Care* 2009; 32 Suppl 1: S13-61.

27.   British Cardiac Society, British Hypertension Society, Diabetes UK, *et al.* JBS 2: the Joint British Societies' guidelines for prevention of cardiovascular disease in clinical practice. *Heart* 2005; 91 (suppl V): v1-v52.

28.   National Institute for Health and Clinical Excellence. Type 2 diabetes: the management of type 2 diabetes (update). London: National Institute for Health and Clinical Excellence, 2008 Dec 5. Report No.: CG66.

29.   Ford ES, Giles WH, Dietz WH. Prevalence of the metabolic syndrome among US adults: findings from the third National Health and Nutrition Examination Survey. *JAMA* 2002; 287(3): 356-9.

30.   Durrington PN. Diabetic dyslipidaemia. *Baillieres Best Pract Res Clin Endocrinol Metab* 1999; 13(2): 265-78.

31.   Austin MA. Triglyceride, small, dense low-density lipoprotein, and the atherogenic lipoprotein phenotype. *Curr Atheroscler Rep* 2000; 2(3): 200-7.

32. St-Pierre AC, Cantin B, Dagenais GR, *et al*. Low-density lipoprotein subfractions and the long-term risk of ischemic heart disease in men: 13-year follow-up data from the Quebec Cardiovascular Study. *Arterioscler Thromb Vasc Biol* 2005; 25(3): 553-9.

33. Austin MA, McKnight B, Edwards KL, *et al*. Cardiovascular disease mortality in familial forms of hypertriglyceridemia: a 20-year prospective study. *Circulation* 2000; 101(24): 2777-82.

34. Garg A, Simha V. Update on dyslipidemia. *J Clin Endocrinol Metab* 2007; 92(5): 1581-9.

35. Samaha FF, Iqbal N, Seshadri P, *et al*. A low-carbohydrate as compared with a low-fat diet in severe obesity. *N Engl J Med* 2003; 348(21): 2074-81.

36. Foster GD, Wyatt HR, Hill JO, *et al*. A randomized trial of a low-carbohydrate diet for obesity. *N Engl J Med* 2003; 348(21): 2082-90.

37. Tuomilehto J, Lindstrom J, Eriksson JG, *et al*. Prevention of type 2 diabetes mellitus by changes in lifestyle among subjects with impaired glucose tolerance. *N Engl J Med* 2001; 344(18): 1343-50.

38. Graham I, Atar D, Borch-Johnsen K, *et al*. European guidelines on cardiovascular disease prevention in clinical practice: full text. Fourth Joint Task Force of the European Society of Cardiology and other societies on cardiovascular disease prevention in clinical practice (constituted by representatives of nine societies and by invited experts). *Eur J Cardiovasc Prev Rehabil* 2007;14 Suppl 2: S1-113.

39. Stein EA, Lane M, Laskarzewski P. Comparison of statins in hypertriglyceridemia. *Am J Cardiol* 1998; 81(4A): 66B-9B.

40. Wierzbicki AS, Lumb PJ, Chik G, *et al*. High-density lipoprotein cholesterol and triglyceride response with simvastatin versus atorvastatin in familial hypercholesterolemia. *Am J Cardiol* 2000; 86(5): 547-9, A9.

41. Forster LF, Stewart G, Bedford D, *et al*. Influence of atorvastatin and simvastatin on apolipoprotein B metabolism in moderate combined hyperlipidemic subjects with low VLDL and LDL fractional clearance rates. *Atherosclerosis* 2002; 164(1): 129-45.

42. Baigent C, Keech A, Kearney PM, *et al*. Efficacy and safety of cholesterol-lowering treatment: prospective meta-analysis of data from 90,056 participants in 14 randomised trials of statins. *Lancet* 2005; 366(9493): 1267-78.

43. Kjekshus J, Apetrei E, Barrios V, *et al*. Rosuvastatin in older patients with systolic heart failure. *N Engl J Med* 2007; 357(22): 2248-61.

44. Gissi-HF I, Tavazzi L, Maggioni AP, *et al*. Effect of rosuvastatin in patients with chronic heart failure (the GISSI-HF trial): a randomised, double-blind, placebo-controlled trial. *Lancet* 2008; 372(9645): 1231-9.

45. Wanner C, Krane V, Marz W, *et al*. Atorvastatin in patients with type 2 diabetes mellitus undergoing hemodialysis. *N Engl J Med* 2005; 353(3): 238-48.

46. Krum H, Latini R, Maggioni AP, *et al*. Statins and symptomatic chronic systolic heart failure: a post-hoc analysis of 5010 patients enrolled in Val-HeFT. *Int J Cardiol* 2007; 119(1): 48-53.

47. Staels B, Dallongeville J, Auwerx J, *et al*. Mechanism of action of fibrates on lipid and lipoprotein metabolism. *Circulation* 1998; 98(19): 2088-93.

48. Chapman MJ. Fibrates in 2003: therapeutic action in atherogenic dyslipidaemia and future perspectives. *Atherosclerosis* 2003; 171(1): 1-13.

49. Saha SA, Kizhakepunnur LG, Bahekar A, *et al*. The role of fibrates in the prevention of cardiovascular disease - a pooled meta-analysis of long-term randomized placebo-controlled clinical trials. *Am Heart J* 2007; 154(5): 943-53.

50. Committee of Principal Investigators. A co-operative trial in the primary prevention of ischaemic heart disease using clofibrate. Report from the Committee of Principal Investigators. *Br Heart J* 1978; 40(10): 1069-118.

51. Committee of Principal Investigators. WHO cooperative trial on primary prevention of ischaemic heart disease with clofibrate to lower serum cholesterol: final mortality follow-up. Report of the Committee of Principal Investigators. *Lancet* 1984; 2(8403): 600-4.

52. Frick MH, Elo O, Haapa K, *et al*. Helsinki Heart Study: primary-prevention trial with gemfibrozil in middle-aged men with dyslipidemia. Safety of treatment, changes in risk factors, and incidence of coronary heart disease. *N Engl J Med* 1987; 317(20): 1237-45.

53. Manninen V, Tenkanen L, Koskinen P, *et al*. Joint effects of serum triglyceride and LDL cholesterol and HDL cholesterol concentrations on coronary heart disease risk in the Helsinki Heart Study. Implications for treatment. *Circulation* 1992; 85(1): 37-45.

54. Rubins HB, Robins SJ, Collins D, *et al.* Gemfibrozil for the secondary prevention of coronary heart disease in men with low levels of high-density lipoprotein cholesterol. Veterans Affairs High-Density Lipoprotein Cholesterol Intervention Trial Study Group. *N Engl J Med* 1999; 341(6): 410-8.

55. Robins SJ, Collins D, Wittes JT, *et al.* Relation of gemfibrozil treatment and lipid levels with major coronary events: VA-HIT: a randomized controlled trial. *JAMA* 2001; 285(12): 1585-91.

56. Keech A, Simes RJ, Barter P, *et al.* Effects of long-term fenofibrate therapy on cardiovascular events in 9795 people with type 2 diabetes mellitus (the FIELD study): randomised controlled trial. *Lancet* 2005; 366(9500): 1849-61.

57. Scott R, O'Brien R, Fulcher G, *et al.* Effects of fenofibrate treatment on cardiovascular disease risk in 9,795 individuals with type 2 diabetes and various components of the metabolic syndrome: the Fenofibrate Intervention and Event Lowering in Diabetes (FIELD) study. *Diabetes Care* 2009; 32(3): 493-8.

58. Rubenstrunk A, Hanf R, Hum DW, *et al.* Safety issues and prospects for future generations of PPAR modulators. *Biochim Biophys Acta* 2007; 1771(8): 1065-81.

59. Wierzbicki AS. Fibrates after the FIELD study: some answers, more questions. *Diab Vasc Dis Res* 2006; 3(3): 166-71.

60. Grundy SM, Vega GL, Yuan Z, *et al.* Effectiveness and tolerability of simvastatin plus fenofibrate for combined hyperlipidemia (the SAFARI trial). *Am J Cardiol* 2005; 95(4): 462-8.

61. Wierzbicki AS, Mikhailidis DP, Wray R, *et al.* Statin-fibrate combination: therapy for hyperlipidemia: a review. *Curr Med Res Opin* 2003; 19(3): 155-68.

62. The ACCORD Study Group. Effects of combination lipid therapy in type 2 diabetes mellitus. *N Engl J Med* 2010; 362(17): 1563-74.

63. Knopp RH, Alagona P, Davidson M, *et al.* Equivalent efficacy of a time-release form of niacin (Niaspan) given once-a-night versus plain niacin in the management of hyperlipidemia. *Metabolism* 1998; 47(9): 1097-104.

64. Carlson LA. Nicotinic acid: the broad-spectrum lipid drug. A 50th anniversary review. *J Intern Med* 2005; 258(2): 94-114.

65. The Coronary Drug Project Research Group. Clofibrate and niacin in coronary heart disease. *JAMA* 1975; 231(4): 360-81.

66. Canner PL, Berge KG, Wenger NK, *et al.* Fifteen year mortality in Coronary Drug Project patients: long-term benefit with niacin. *J Am Coll Cardiol* 1986; 8(6): 1245-55.

67. Blankenhorn DH, Nessim SA, Johnson RL, *et al.* Beneficial effects of combined colestipol-niacin therapy on coronary atherosclerosis and coronary venous bypass grafts. *JAMA* 1987; 257(23): 3233-40.

68. Carlson LA, Rosenhamer G. Reduction of mortality in the Stockholm Ischaemic Heart Disease Secondary Prevention Study by combined treatment with clofibrate and nicotinic acid. *Acta Med Scand* 1988; 223(5): 405-18.

69. Brown BG, Zhao XQ, Chait A, *et al.* Simvastatin and niacin, antioxidant vitamins, or the combination for the prevention of coronary disease. *N Engl J Med* 2001; 345(22): 1583-92.

70. National Heart LaBIN. Niacin Plus Statin to Prevent Vascular Events: AIM-HIGH. ClinicalTrials gov 2006 [cited 2006 Jul 18]; Available from: URL: http://www.clinicaltrials.gov/ct/show/NCT00120289.

71. A Randomized Trial of the Long-Term Clinical Effects of Raising HDL Cholesterol With Extended Release Niacin/Laropiprant. ClinicalTrials Gov 2007 April 17 [cited 2009 Jan 26]; Available from: URL: http://clinicaltrials.gov/ct2/show/NCT00461630.

72. Harris WS, Miller M, Tighe AP, *et al.* Omega-3 fatty acids and coronary heart disease risk: clinical and mechanistic perspectives. *Atherosclerosis* 2008; 197(1): 12-24.

73. Wierzbicki AS. A fishy business: omega-3 fatty acids and cardiovascular disease. *Int J Clin Pract* 2008; 62(8): 1142-6.

74. Davidson MH. Mechanisms for the hypotriglyceridemic effect of marine omega-3 fatty acids. *Am J Cardiol* 2006; 98(4A): 27i-33i.

75. McKenney JM, Sica D. Role of prescription omega-3 fatty acids in the treatment of hypertriglyceridemia. *Pharmacotherapy* 2007; 27(5): 715-28.

76. Gruppo Italiano per lo Studio della Sopravvivenza nell'Infarto miocardico. Dietary supplementation with n-3 polyunsaturated fatty acids and vitamin E after myocardial infarction: results of the GISSI-Prevenzione trial. *Lancet* 1999; 354(9177): 447-55.

77. Nilsen DW, Albrektsen G, Landmark K, *et al.* Effects of a high-dose concentrate of n-3 fatty acids or corn oil introduced early after an acute myocardial infarction on serum triacylglycerol and HDL cholesterol. *Am J Clin Nutr* 2001; 74(1): 50-6.

78. Harris WS, Ginsberg HN, Arunakul N, *et al*. Safety and efficacy of Omacor in severe hypertriglyceridemia. *J Cardiovasc Risk* 1997; 4(5-6): 385-91.

79. von Schacky C. A review of omega-3 ethyl esters for cardiovascular prevention and treatment of increased blood triglyceride levels. *Vasc Health Risk Manag* 2006; 2(3): 251-62.

80. Bucher HC, Griffith LE, Guyatt GH. Systematic review on the risk and benefit of different cholesterol-lowering interventions. *Arterioscler Thromb Vasc Biol* 1999; 19(2): 187-95.

81. Bucher HC, Hengstler P, Schindler C, *et al*. N-3 polyunsaturated fatty acids in coronary heart disease: a meta-analysis of randomized controlled trials. *Am J Med* 2002; 112(4): 298-304.

82. Yokoyama M, Origasa H, Matsuzaki M, *et al*. Effects of eicosapentaenoic acid on major coronary events in hypercholesterolaemic patients (JELIS): a randomised open-label, blinded endpoint analysis. *Lancet* 2007; 369(9567): 1090-8.

83. National Institute of Health and Clinical Excellence Guideline Development Group. Myocardial Infarction: secondary prevention - Full guideline. London: Her Majesty's Stationery Office; 2007 May 23. Report No.: CG48.

84. Rauch B, Schiele R, Schneider S, *et al*. Highly purified omega-3 fatty acids for secondary prevention of sudden cardiac death after myocardial infarction - aims and methods of the OMEGA-study. *Cardiovasc Drugs Ther* 2006; 20(5): 365-75.

85. Armitage J. A Study of Cardiovascular Events iN Diabetes - A Randomized 2x2 Factorial Study of Aspirin Versus Placebo, and of Omega-3 Fatty Acid Supplementation Versus Placebo, for Primary Prevention of Cardiovascular Events in People With Diabetes. ClinicalTrials gov 2007 January 26 [cited 2008 Mar 12]; Available from: URL: http://www.clinicaltrials.gov/ct2/show/NCT00135226.

86. Mikhailidis DP, Wierzbicki AS, Daskalopoulou SS, *et al*. The use of ezetimibe in achieving low density lipoprotein lowering goals in clinical practice: position statement of a United Kingdom consensus panel. *Curr Med Res Opin* 2005; 21(6): 959-69.

87. Wierzbicki AS. Lipid-altering agents: the future. *Int J Clin Pract* 2004; 58(11): 1063-72.

88. Wierzbicki AS, Mikhailidis DP, Wray R. Drug treatment of combined hyperlipidemia. *Am J Cardiovasc Drugs* 2001; 1(5): 327-36.

89. Karas RH, Kashyap ML, Knopp RH, *et al*. Long-term safety and efficacy of a combination of niacin extended release and simvastatin in patients with dyslipidemia: the OCEANS Study. *Am J Cardiovasc Drugs* 2008; 8(2): 69-81.

90. Durrington PN, Bhatnagar D, Mackness MI, *et al*. An omega-3 polyunsaturated fatty acid concentrate administered for one year decreased triglycerides in simvastatin treated patients with coronary heart disease and persisting hypertriglyceridaemia. *Heart* 2001; 85(5): 544-8.

91. Guyton JR, Brown BG, Fazio S, *et al*. Lipid-altering efficacy and safety of ezetimibe/simvastatin coadministered with extended-release niacin in patients with type IIa or type IIb hyperlipidemia. *J Am Coll Cardiol* 2008; 51(16): 1564-72.

92. Bilz S, Wagner S, Schmitz M, *et al*. Effects of atorvastatin versus fenofibrate on apoB-100 and apoA-I kinetics in mixed hyperlipidemia. *J Lipid Res* 2004; 45(1): 174-85.

93. Watts GF, Barrett PH, Ji J, *et al*. Differential regulation of lipoprotein kinetics by atorvastatin and fenofibrate in subjects with the metabolic syndrome. *Diabetes* 2003; 52(3): 803-11.

94. Lamon-Fava S, Diffenderfer MR, Barrett PH, *et al*. Extended-release niacin alters the metabolism of plasma apolipoprotein (Apo) A-I and ApoB-containing lipoproteins. *Arterioscler Thromb Vasc Biol* 2008; 28(9): 1672-8.

95. Wierzbicki AS. Low HDL-cholesterol: Common and under-treated, but which drug to use? *Int J Clin Pract* 2006; 60(10): 1149-53.

96. Mao EQ, Tang YQ, Zhang SD. Formalized therapeutic guideline for hyperlipidemic severe acute pancreatitis. *World J Gastroenterol* 2003; 9(11): 2622-6.

97. Dominguez-Munoz JE, Malfertheiner P, Ditschuneit HH, *et al*. Hyperlipidemia in acute pancreatitis. Relationship with etiology, onset, and severity of the disease. *Int J Pancreatol* 1991; 10(3-4): 261-7.

98. Malani A, Ammar H, Mughal S. Hypertriglyceridemia. *N Engl J Med* 2008; 358(3): 310-1.

99. Monajemi H, Stroes E, Hegele RA, *et al*. Inherited lipodystrophies and the metabolic syndrome. *Clin Endocrinol* (Oxf) 2007; 67(4): 479-84.

100. Watts GF, Cameron J, Henderson A, *et al*. Lipoprotein lipase deficiency due to long-term heparinization presenting as severe hypertriglyceridaemia in pregnancy. *Postgrad Med J* 1991; 67(794): 1062-4.

101. Pschierer V, Richter WO, Schwandt P. Primary chylomicronemia in patients with severe familial hypertriglyceridemia responds to long-term treatment with (n-3) fatty acids. *J Nutr* 1995; 125(6): 1490-4.
102. Wierzbicki AS, Reynolds TM. Familial hyperchylomicronaemia. *Lancet* 1996; 348(9040): 1524-5.
103. Wierzbicki AS, Reynolds TM, Crook MA. Usefulness of orlistat in the treatment of severe hypertriglyceridemia. *Am J Cardiol* 2002; 89(2): 229-31.
104. Watts GF, Morton K, Jackson P, *et al*. Management of patients with severe hypertriglyceridaemia during pregnancy: report of two cases with familial lipoprotein lipase deficiency. *Br J Obstet Gynaecol* 1992; 99(2): 163-6.

Chapter 8

The optimal treatment of patients with familial combined hyperlipidemia

Evertine J. Abbink MD PhD, Research Physician
Jacqueline de Graaf MD PhD, Vascular Specialist
Anton F. Stalenhoef MD PhD FRCP, Professor of Medicine
Department of General Internal Medicine, Radboud University Nijmegen
Medical Centre, Nijmegen, the Netherlands

Introduction

Familial combined hyperlipidemia (FCH) was first described in 1973 by Goldstein *et al*, Rose *et al* and Nikkilä *et al* as a new inherited lipid disorder [1-3]. At present, it is the most prevalent hereditary dyslipidemia in man, with a prevalence of up to 5.7% in western society as a whole [4], of about 20% in all survivors of myocardial infarction [5] and of almost 40% in survivors of myocardial infarction at a very young age (=40 years) [6]. It is characterized by elevated plasma levels of total cholesterol (TC), triglycerides (TG) and/or apolipoprotein B (apoB) and the predominance of small dense low-density lipoprotein (sdLDL). Other characteristics of FCH are a decreased level of high-density lipoprotein cholesterol (HDL-C), abdominal obesity, insulin resistance and hypertension [4, 7-13]. Each of the characteristics may contribute to the high prevalence of coronary heart disease (CHD) in FCH patients [14-16]. The expression of the above mentioned characteristics of FCH is highly variable, not only between subjects, but also within subjects over time [17, 18]. Furthermore, FCH usually does not come to full expression until the third decade of life [19].

The elevated plasma TG levels, decreased plasma HDL-C levels, elevated blood pressure, obesity and/or elevated fasting glucose levels of FCH patients are also present in subjects with the metabolic syndrome [20-22]. This increasingly prevalent disorder in western society is one of the most important disorders underlying cardiovascular morbidity and mortality in the general population. However, although FCH shares many phenotypical features with the metabolic syndrome, important differences exist as well. First and above all, FCH is hereditary, with an evident clustering of affected subjects in certain families. Second, it has been demonstrated that in FCH (unlike in the metabolic syndrome), the abdominal obesity and insulin resistance cannot account for the observed elevated apoB levels; apoB levels are increased independently of BMI and fat distribution [23], and apoB levels and sdLDL segregate independently in FCH [24]. Because of the overlapping features with metabolic syndrome and the variability in laboratory values, FCH is often not recognized nor treated [25].

Diagnosis of FCH

Since no single specific biochemical marker exists to diagnose FCH, the diagnosis relies on accurate family history and lipid and lipoprotein measurements. Traditionally, FCH diagnosis has been based on the presence of TC and/or TG levels exceeding the 90th percentile adjusted for age and sex in a family with multiple-type hyperlipidemia and the presence of premature cardiovascular disease (CVD). However, it was shown that due to the high inter- and intra-person variability in lipid phenotype, using these criteria yields inconsistent diagnoses in 26% of the subjects [18]. Therefore, a nomogram was developed to diagnose FCH, taking into account not only age and gender adjusted percentile scores for TC and TG, but also the absolute apoB concentration, since an increased apoB stands out as the most consistent abnormality amongst FCH subjects [26] (Figure 1). According to this nomogram, subjects are defined as FCH patients when their probability of being affected is above 60%, provided that the diagnostic phenotype is also present in at least one first-degree relative and premature CVD (i.e. before the age of 60 years) is present in at least one individual in the family [6, 26]. When no percentile scores for TC and TG are available, the diagnosis of FCH can be established on an absolute apoB concentration >1200mg/L in combination with a TG concentration >1.5mmol/L (133mg/dL) [26].

Metabolic and genetic origin of FCH

Despite over 30 years of research, the exact molecular defects and pathophysiology underlying FCH are still unknown. The atherogenic lipid phenotype of FCH patients is thought to be the result of several concurrent mechanisms, of which an overproduction of very-low-density lipoprotein (VLDL) by the liver is generally regarded as the key pathophysiological defect [27-30]. Recently, the potential role of adipose tissue metabolism in the pathophysiology of FCH has been described [11, 31, 32].

When first discovered in 1973, FCH was assumed to be an autosomal dominant disorder [1]. Subsequent studies, however, learned that the inheritance of FCH is multifactorial; multiple major and modifying genes are supposed to be involved [33].

Cardiovascular risk in FCH

FCH patients have a 2- to 5-fold increased risk for CVD compared to healthy control subjects [4, 34, 35]. However, despite this marked increased overall risk, there is a considerable inter-individual variation amongst FCH patients in their tendency to develop CVD, which

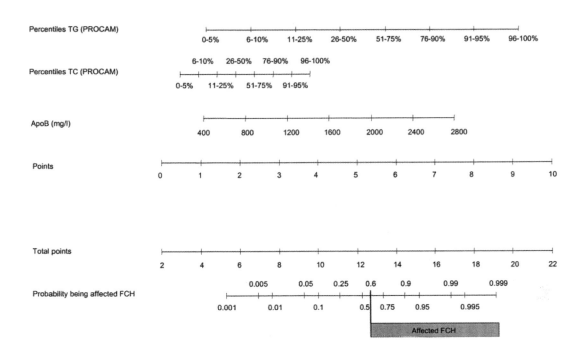

Figure 1. Nomogram to calculate probability of being affected by FCH using absolute apoB and TG-TC values adjusted for both age and gender [26]. *Reproduced with permission from Wolters Kluwer Health, © 2004.*

could be attributed to either interactions between the various risk factors present, or to variation in the duration of exposure to specific risk factors. The large inter-individual variation in the development of CVD emphasizes the need for accurate cardiovascular risk prediction for individual FCH patients. Various algorithms (i.e. Framingham, PROCAM and SCORE [36-38]) have been developed to estimate individual cardiovascular risk, and each of these algorithms can be used in FCH patients. However, calculating a 10-year risk based on CVD founded on the expression of several cardiovascular risk factors (as these algorithms do), may be inaccurate due to the highly variable phenotype in FCH. In addition, the cardiovascular risk of patients with this hereditary dyslipidemia is even larger than the risk of patients with polygenetic dyslipidemia, especially when the family history is positive for CVD at a young age. Therefore, patients who are diagnosed with FCH, which includes both the presence of dyslipidemia and the presence of premature CVD in the family, have to be treated, as recommended by the judgement of the ATP III [20]. Randomized controlled trials are lacking for familial hyperlipidemias as they are unethical to conduct considering the high risk of CVD.

FCH treatment

FCH treatment is primarily directed to correct the dyslipidemia for prevention of CVD [4, 34, 35]. The first step consists of lifestyle interventions: dietary modifications (little saturated fat and enough vegetables and fruit), weight reduction in case of obesitas, physical exercise, stop smoking and limitation of alcohol consumption [20]. These lifestyle interventions induce relatively larger decreases in TG than in LDL-cholesterol (LDL-C).

If the dyslipidemia is treated insufficiently with these interventions, drugs that lower lipids and (apo)lipoproteins should be added. Even if drug therapy is started, lifestyle changes should be continued [20]. Table 1 shows the mechanisms of action, the effects on (apo)lipoprotein levels and the most important side effects of the different types of lipid and (apo)lipoprotein-lowering agents that can be used to treat FCH patients.

Besides treatment of dyslipidemia, other cardiovascular risk factors, like hypertension, should also be treated, according to international guidelines [20].

Table 1. Mechanisms of action, effects on (apo)lipoprotein levels and most important side effects of the different types of lipid and (apo)lipoprotein-lowering agents that can be used to treat FCH patients [20].

Type of agent	Mechanism of action	Effect on (apo)lipoproteins	Most important side effects
Statin = HMG-CoA-reductase-antagonist	Inhibition of cholesterol synthesis in the liver	LDL-C ↓ (25-60%) apoB ↓ (20-25%) TG ↓ (20-40%) HDL-C ↑ (8-15%)	Tiredness Muscle ache Digestive tract symptoms Increased liver enzymes Rhabdomyolysis (seldom)
Fibrate	Stimulation of PPAR-α inducing breakdown of TG Increasing production of apoA1	TG ↓ (35-50%) HDL-C ↑ (10-25%) LDL-C ↓ (10-25%), but sometimes ↑	Digestive tract symptoms
Nicotinic acid	Not entirely known	LDL-C ↓ (5-15%) TG ↓ (15-30%) HDL-C ↑ (10-25%)	Flushing Itch
Cholesterol resorption inhibitor	Inhibition of cholesterol uptake in the intestine	LDL-C ↓ (max 20%)	Headache Digestive tract symptoms Increased liver enzymes

Treatment goals

For dyslipidemia, three different indices have been proposed as markers of atherogenic risk and adequacy of drug therapy, including LDL-C, non-HDL-C and apoB. Non-HDL-C is defined as the difference between TC and HDL-C and is a measure for cholesterol in atherogenic lipoproteins (LDL and VLDL). ApoB is an important protein on LDL and VLDL. Every LDL and VLDL particle contains one apoB molecule, so the concentration of apoB is a measure for the total amount of atherogenic lipoprotein particles.

In most guidelines, treatment is based on the concentration of LDL-C. For example, in the NCEP ATP III guidelines, LDL-C is used to evaluate the treatment of dyslipidemia [20]. In hypertriglyceridemic patients this guideline recommends non-HDL-C as a secondary goal next to LDL-C. The major reason is that in hypertriglyceridemic patients, non-HDL-C reflects risk more accurately than LDL-C as non-HDL-C is a better measure of the number of LDL-particles. sdLDL particles contain less cholesterol than larger particles and therefore LDL-C underestimates the true number of LDL-particles.

Numerous studies have shown that both apoB and non-HDL-C are superior to LDL-C as markers of cardiovascular risk [39-41] **(Ia/A)**(Table 2). In 2008, the American Diabetes Association and the American College of Cardiology Foundation incorporated apoB as a target in the guidelines for treatment of patients with cardiometabolic risk factors [42]. Recently, the American Association for Clinical Chemistry also stated that apoB is recommended as the best marker of adequacy of drug therapy [43].

The diagnosis of FCH in clinical practice is made on elevated apoB (>1200mg/L) and high TG (>1.5mmol/L). In these hypertriglyceridemic patients, treatment goals should focus on non-HDL-C or apoB, where apoB is a better reflector of sdLDL, a major characteristic of the atherogenic lipoprotein profile in FCH.

The levels of the treatment goals of LDL-C, non-HDL-C and apoB for different patient groups are summarized in Table 3.

Choice of drugs

Several clinical trials have compared statins and fibrates for the treatment of FCH. These trials reveal that statins reduce TC, LDL-C, apoB and non-HDL-C more effectively, whereas fibrates are more efficacious in lowering TG and increasing HDL-C [44-47] **(Ib/A)**. Besides those effects on lipids and lipoproteins, simvastatin and fenofibrate have comparative beneficial effects on various inflammatory markers and endothelial function [46] **(Ib/A)**. Atorvastatin is more effective in reaching lipid targets than fenofibrate [47] **(Ib/A)**. Because of their stronger LDL-C and apoB-lowering effect, statins are proposed as a first-line option in the management of FCH. In addition, statin therapy reduces cardiovascular risk by 30-40% in patients with CHD [48] **(Ib/A)**, whereas fibrates reduce the incidence of non-fatal myocardial

Table 2. Large prospective clinical trials which show that apolipoprotein B is a better marker of vascular risk than LDL cholesterol.

Study	n	Sex	Patient type
Wald et al [58]	21,520	M	Asymptomatic
The Québec Cardiovascular Study [59]	2,195	M	Asymptomatic
THROMBO [60]	1,045	M/F	Post-MI
AMORIS [61]	175,553	M/F	Asymptomatic
Northwick Park Heart Study [62]	2,508	M	Asymptomatic
Womens' Health Study [63]	15,362	F	Asymptomatic
MONICA/KORA Augsberg [64]	2,850	M/F	Asymptomatic
Casale Monferrato Study [65]	1,565	M/F	DM type 2
Québec Cardiovascular Study [66]	2,072	M	Asymptomatic
The Chinese Heart Study [67]	3,586	M/F	Asymptomatic
The Copenhagen City Heart Study [68]	9,231	M/F	Asymptomatic
Framingham Offspring Study [69]	3,322	M/F	Asymptomatic
TEKHARF Survey [70]	2,348	M/F	Asymptomatic

DM = diabetes mellitus; F= female; M = male; MI = myocardial infarction.

infarction by 24%, but have no effect on mortality [49] **(Ib/A)**. As very high triglycerides can cause acute pancreatitis, fibrate treatment should be considered when TG levels are above 10mmol/L [50].

Combination therapy of statins and fibrates has additive effects on lipids: reductions in TC, TG, LDL-C, apoB and an increase in HDL-C [45, 51-53] **(Ib/A)**. Combination of atorvastatin and fenofibrate has a beneficial effect on endothelial function and insulin sensitivity [52] **(Ib/A)**. The combination of statin and gemfibrozil increases the risk of myopathy. However, this limitation is not observed when fenofibrate, bezafibrate or ciprofibrate are coadministered with a statin [54]

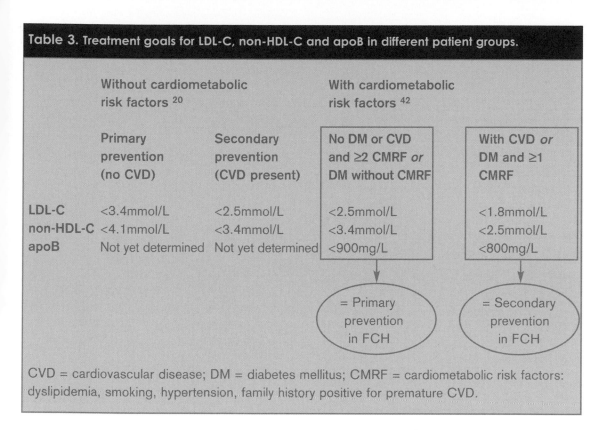

Table 3. Treatment goals for LDL-C, non-HDL-C and apoB in different patient groups.

	Without cardiometabolic risk factors [20]		With cardiometabolic risk factors [42]	
	Primary prevention (no CVD)	Secondary prevention (CVD present)	No DM or CVD and ≥2 CMRF or DM without CMRF	With CVD or DM and ≥1 CMRF
LDL-C	<3.4mmol/L	<2.5mmol/L	<2.5mmol/L	<1.8mmol/L
non-HDL-C	<4.1mmol/L	<3.4mmol/L	<3.4mmol/L	<2.5mmol/L
apoB	Not yet determined	Not yet determined	<900mg/L	<800mg/L

= Primary prevention in FCH

= Secondary prevention in FCH

CVD = cardiovascular disease; DM = diabetes mellitus; CMRF = cardiometabolic risk factors: dyslipidemia, smoking, hypertension, family history positive for premature CVD.

(Ib/A). To determine whether adding a fibrate on top of statin therapy is beneficial regarding cardiovascular risk reduction, the recent Action to Control Cardiovascular Risk in Diabetes (ACCORD) trial was conducted. However, this trial substantiated that fenofibrate on top of statins did not reduce the rate of fatal cardiovascular events, non-fatal myocardial infarction, or non-fatal stroke. Only in the subgroup of patients with elevated TG (>2.3mmol/L = 204mg/dL) and low HDL-C (<0.88mmol/L = 34mg/dL) did the addition of fenofibrate show benefit. These results do not support the general use of fibrates on top of statins in high-risk type 2 diabetes mellitus patients [55] **(Ia/A).**

A combination of the fibrate gemfibrozil and nicotinic acid offers greater improvement in detailed lipoprotein subclass distribution and apolipoprotein ratios than monotherapy [56] **(Ib/A).**

Monotherapy with ezetimibe induced LDL-C reduction, and coadministration of fenofibrate and ezetimibe had an additive effect on LDL-C [57] **(Ib/A).**

Clinical practice

In FCH patients, the first-line therapy is statins with the most important target to lower apoB (Table 2). Keep in mind that LDL-C is often not elevated in hypertriglyceridemic FCH patients, where LDL-particles are small, dense and cholesterol-depleted, but very atherogenic. Reducing apoB reflects reducing the number of LDL-particles and therefore reducing the cardiovascular risk.

At first, a low to moderate dose of statin is prescribed. If the treatment goal is not achieved after 6 weeks of treatment, the dose should be increased. If, despite statin treatment, the TG-concentration remains high (>2.3mmol/L = 204mg/dL), often in combination with low HDL-C (<0.88mmol/L = 34mg/dL), a fibrate can be added. Alternatively, nicotinic acid can be added to treat low HDL-C or hypertriglyceridemia. Ezetimibe is practically never prescribed in FCH patients. Lipids should be measured every 6 weeks and treatment should be intensified until the treatment goal is achieved [20].

Conclusions

In conclusion, the first-choice treatment of FCH patients consists of a statin, which most effectively reduces apoB, the best predictor of CVD risk. In the case of insufficient efficacy or side effects, other lipid and (apo)lipoprotein-lowering agents can be prescribed. When TG levels exeed 10mmol/L, treatment with fibrates should be considered to reduce the risk of pancreatitis.

Key points	Evidence level
◆ ApoB is a better predictor of cardiovascular risk than LDL-C and non-HDL-C, especially in hypertriglyceridemic patients.	Ia/A
◆ Statins reduce TC, LDL-C, apoB and non-HDL-C more effectively, whereas fibrates are more efficacious in lowering TG and increasing HDL-C.	Ib/A
◆ Statin therapy reduces cardiovascular risk by 30-40%.	Ib/A
◆ Fibrates reduce the incidence of non-fatal myocardial infarction by 24%, but have no effect on mortality.	Ib/A
◆ Combination therapy of statins and fibrates has additive effects on lipids: reductions in TC, TG, LDL-C, apoB and an increase in HDL-C (Ib/A). However, it has no additive impact on cardiovascular event rate compared to statin treatment alone (Ia/A). Only in the subgroup of patients with elevated TG (>2.3mmol/L = 204mg/dL) and low HDL-C (<0.88mmol/L = 34mg/dL) does the addition of fenofibrate show benefit.	Ib/A & Ia/A
◆ First-line therapy in FCH should be a statin, because of the large apoB-lowering effect and the evidence of reduction in cardiovascular risk.	Ib/A

References

1. Goldstein JL, Schrott HG, Hazzard WR, Bierman EL, Motulsky AG. Hyperlipidemia in coronary heart disease. II. Genetic analysis of lipid levels in 176 families and delineation of a new inherited disorder, combined hyperlipidemia. *J Clin Invest* 1973; 52: 1544-68.
2. Nikkilä EA, Aro A. Family study of serum lipids and lipoproteins in coronary heart-disease. *Lancet* 1973; 1: 954-9.
3. Rose HG, Kranz P, Weinstock M, Juliano J, Haft JI. Inheritance of combined hyperlipoproteinemia: evidence for a new lipoprotein phenotype. *Am J Med* 1973; 54: 148-60.
4. Hopkins PN, Heiss G, Ellison RC, Province MA, Pankow JS, Eckfeldt JH, Hunt SC. Coronary artery disease risk in familial combined hyperlipidemia and familial hypertriglyceridemia: a case-control comparison from the National Heart, Lung, and Blood Institute Family Heart Study. *Circulation* 2003; 108: 519-23.
5. Brunzell JD, Schrott HG, Motulsky AG, Bierman EL. Myocardial infarction in the familial forms of hypertriglyceridemia. *Metabolism* 1976; 25: 313-20.
6. Wiesbauer F, Blessberger H, Azar D, et al. Familial-combined hyperlipidemia in very young myocardial infarction survivors (= 40 years of age). *Eur Heart J* 2009; electronic publication ahead of print.
7. Bredie SJ, Tack CJ, Smits P, Stalenhoef AF. Nonobese patients with familial combined hyperlipidemia are insulin resistant compared with their nonaffected relatives. *Arterioscler Thromb Vasc Biol* 1997; 17: 1465-71.
8. Bredie SJ, Demacker PN, Stalenhoef AF. Metabolic and genetic aspects of familial combined hyperlipidaemia with emphasis on low-density lipoprotein heterogeneity. *Eur J Clin Invest* 1997; 27: 802-11.
9. Brunzell JD, Albers JJ, Chait A, Grundy SM, Groszek E, McDonald GB. Plasma lipoproteins in familial combined hyperlipidemia and monogenic familial hypertriglyceridemia. *J Lipid Res* 1983; 24: 147-55.
10. de Graaf J, Stalenhoef AF. Defects of lipoprotein metabolism in familial combined hyperlipidaemia. *Curr Opin Lipidol* 1998; 9: 189-96.
11. de Graaf J, Veerkamp MJ, Stalenhoef AF. Metabolic pathogenesis of familial combined hyperlipidaemia with emphasis on insulin resistance, adipose tissue metabolism and free fatty acids. *J R Soc Med* 2002; 95 (suppl 42): 46-53.
12. Hokanson JE, Austin MA, Zambon A, Brunzell JD. Plasma triglyceride and LDL heterogeneity in familial combined hyperlipidemia. *Arterioscler Thromb* 1993; 13: 427-34.
13. Keulen ET, Voors-Pette C, de Bruin TW. Familial dyslipidemic hypertension syndrome: familial combined hyperlipidemia, and the role of abdominal fat mass. *Am J Hypertens* 2001; 14: 357-63.
14. Hokanson JE, Austin MA. Plasma triglyceride level is a risk factor for cardiovascular disease independent of high-density lipoprotein cholesterol level: a meta-analysis of population-based prospective studies. *J Cardiovasc Risk* 1996; 3: 213-9.
15. Austin MA, Breslow JL, Hennekens CH, Buring JE, Willett WC, Krauss RM. Low-density lipoprotein subclass patterns and risk of myocardial infarction. *JAMA* 1988; 260: 1917-21.
16. Franceschini G, Bondioli A, Granata D, Mercuri V, Negri M, Tosi C, Sirtori CR. Reduced HDL2 levels in myocardial infarction patients without risk factors for atherosclerosis. *Atherosclerosis* 1987; 68: 213-9.
17. McNeely MJ, Edwards KL, Marcovina SM, Brunzell JD, Motulsky AG, Austin MA. Lipoprotein and apolipoprotein abnormalities in familial combined hyperlipidemia: a 20-year prospective study. *Atherosclerosis* 2001; 159: 471-81.
18. Veerkamp MJ, de Graaf J, Bredie SJ, Hendriks JC, Demacker PN, Stalenhoef AF. Diagnosis of familial combined hyperlipidemia based on lipid phenotype expression in 32 families: results of a 5-year follow-up study. *Arterioscler Thromb Vasc Biol* 2002; 22: 274-82.
19. Cortner JA, Coates PM, Liacouras CA, Jarvik GP. Familial combined hyperlipidemia in children: clinical expression, metabolic defects, and management. *J Pediatr* 1993; 123: 177-84.
20. Executive Summary of The Third Report of The National Cholesterol Education Program (NCEP) Expert Panel on Detection, Evaluation, And Treatment of High Blood Cholesterol In Adults (Adult Treatment Panel III). *JAMA* 2001; 285: 2486-97.
21. The IDF consensus worldwide definition of the metabolic syndrome. Part 1. Worldwide definition for use in clinical practice. Internet: www.idf.org. 2006.
22. Alberti KG, Zimmet P, Shaw J. Metabolic syndrome - a new world-wide definition. A Consensus Statement from the International Diabetes Federation. *Diabet Med* 2006; 23: 469-80.

23. Purnell JQ, Kahn SE, Schwartz RS, Brunzell JD. Relationship of insulin sensitivity and ApoB levels to intra-abdominal fat in subjects with familial combined hyperlipidemia. *Arterioscler Thromb Vasc Biol* 2001; 21: 567-72.

24. Jarvik GP, Brunzell JD, Austin MA, Krauss RM, Motulsky AG, Wijsman E. Genetic predictors of FCHL in four large pedigrees. Influence of ApoB level major locus predicted genotype and LDL subclass phenotype. *Arterioscler Thromb* 1994; 14: 1687-94.

25. Gaddi A, Cicero AF, Odoo FO, Poli AA, Paoletti R. Practical guidelines for familial combined hyperlipidemia diagnosis: an update. *Vasc Health Risk Manag* 2007; 3: 877-86.

26. Veerkamp MJ, de Graaf J, Hendriks JC, Demacker PN, Stalenhoef AF. Nomogram to diagnose familial combined hyperlipidemia on the basis of results of a 5-year follow-up study. *Circulation* 2004; 109: 2980-5.

27. Castro Cabezas M, Erkelens DW, Kock LA, de Bruin TW. Postprandial apolipoprotein B100 and B48 metabolism in familial combined hyperlipidaemia before and after reduction of fasting plasma triglycerides. *Eur J Clin Invest* 1994; 24: 669-78.

28. Chait A, Albers JJ, Brunzell JD. Very low density lipoprotein overproduction in genetic forms of hypertriglyceridaemia. *Eur J Clin Invest* 1980; 10: 17-22.

29. Stalenhoef AF, Demacker PN, Lutterman JA, van't Laar A. Plasma lipoproteins, apolipoproteins, and triglyceride metabolism in familial hypertriglyceridemia. *Arteriosclerosis* 1986; 6: 387-94.

30. Venkatesan S, Cullen P, Pacy P, Halliday D, Scott J. Stable isotopes show a direct relation between VLDL apoB overproduction and serum triglyceride levels and indicate a metabolically and biochemically coherent basis for familial combined hyperlipidemia. *Arterioscler Thromb* 1993; 13: 1110-8.

31. van der Vleuten GM, van Tits LJH, den Heijer M, Lemmers H, Stalenhoef AFH, de Graaf J. Decreased adiponectin levels in familial combined hyperlipidemia patients contribute to the atherogenic lipid profile. *J Lipid Res* 2005; 46: 2398-404.

32. Koenen TB, van Tits LJ, Holewijn S, Lemmers HL, den Heijer M, Stalenhoef AF, de Graaf J. Adiponectin multimer distribution in patients with familial combined hyperlipidemia. *Biochem Biophys Res Commun* 2008; 376: 164-8.

33. Suviolahti E, Lilja HE, Pajukanta P. Unraveling the complex genetics of familial combined hyperlipidemia. *Ann Med* 2006; 38: 337-51.

34. Austin MA, McKnight B, Edwards KL, *et al.* Cardiovascular disease mortality in familial forms of hypertriglyceridemia: A 20-year prospective study. *Circulation* 2000; 101: 2777-82.

35. Voors-Pette C, de Bruin TW. Excess coronary heart disease in familial combined hyperlipidemia, in relation to genetic factors and central obesity. *Atherosclerosis* 2001; 157: 481-9.

36. Assmann G, Cullen P, Schulte H. Simple scoring scheme for calculating the risk of acute coronary events based on the 10-year follow-up of the prospective cardiovascular Münster (PROCAM) study. *Circulation* 2002; 105: 310-5.

37. Wilson PW, D'Agostino RB, Levy D, Belanger AM, Silbershatz H, Kannel WB. Prediction of coronary heart disease using risk factor categories. *Circulation* 1998; 97: 1837-47.

38. Conroy RM, Pyörälä K, Fitzgerald AP, *et al.* Estimation of ten-year risk of fatal cardiovascular disease in Europe: the SCORE project. *Eur Heart J* 2003; 24: 987-1003.

39. Kastelein JJ, van der Steeg WA, Holme I, *et al.* Lipids, apolipoproteins, and their ratios in relation to cardiovascular events with statin treatment. *Circulation* 2008; 117: 3002-9.

40. Sniderman AD, Furberg CD, Keech A, Roeters van Lennep JE, Frohlich J, Jungner I, Walldius G. Apolipoproteins versus lipids as indices of coronary risk and as targets for statin treatment. *Lancet* 2003; 361: 777-80.

41. de Graaf J, Couture P, Sniderman A. A diagnostic algorithm for the atherogenic apolipoprotein B dyslipoproteinemias. *Nat Clin Pract Endocrinol Metab* 2008; 4: 608-18.

42. Brunzell JD, Davidson M, Furberg CD, *et al.* Lipoprotein management in patients with cardiometabolic risk: consensus statement from the American Diabetes Association and the American College of Cardiology Foundation. *Diabetes Care* 2008; 31: 811-22.

43. Contois JH, McConnell JP, Sethi AA, Csako G, Devaraj S, Hoefner DM, Warnick GR. Apolipoprotein B and cardiovascular disease risk: position statement from the AACC Lipoproteins and Vascular Diseases Division Working Group on Best Particles. *Clin Chem* 2009; 55: 407-19.

44. Bredie SJ, de Bruin TW, Demacker PN, Kastelein JJ, Stalenhoef AF. Comparison of gemfibrozil versus simvastatin in familial combined hyperlipidemia and effects on apolipoprotein-B-containing lipoproteins, low-density lipoprotein subfraction profile, and low-density lipoprotein oxidizability. *Am J Cardiol* 1995; 75: 348-53.

45. Zambón D, Ros E, Rodriguez-Villar C, *et al*. Randomized crossover study of gemfibrozil versus lovastatin in familial combined hyperlipidemia: additive effects of combination treatment on lipid regulation. *Metabolism* 1999; 48: 47-54.

46. Wang TD, Chen WJ, Lin JW, Cheng CC, Chen MF, Lee YT. Efficacy of fenofibrate and simvastatin on endothelial function and inflammatory markers in patients with combined hyperlipidemia: relations with baseline lipid profiles. *Atherosclerosis* 2003; 170: 315-23.

47. Arca M, Montali A, Pigna G, *et al*. Comparison of atorvastatin versus fenofibrate in reaching lipid targets and influencing biomarkers of endothelial damage in patients with familial combined hyperlipidemia. *Metabolism* 2007; 56: 1534-41.

48. Scandinavian Simvastatin Survival Study Group. Randomised trial of cholesterol lowering in 4444 patients with coronary heart disease: the Scandinavian Simvastatin Survival Study (4S). *Lancet* 1994; 344: 1383-9.

49. Keech A, Simes RJ, Barter P *et al*. Effects of long-term fenofibrate therapy on cardiovascular events in 9795 people with type 2 diabetes mellitus (the FIELD study): randomised controlled trial. *Lancet* 2005; 366: 1849-61.

50. Yadav D, Pitchumoni CS. Issues in hyperlipidemic pancreatitis. *J Clin Gastroenterol* 2003: 36: 54-62.

51. Grundy SM, Vega GL, Yuan Z, Battisti WP, Brady WE, Palmisano J. Effectiviness and tolerability of simvastatin plus fenofibrate for combined hyperlipidemia (the SAFARI trial). *Am J Cardiol* 2005; 95: 462-8.

52. Koh KK, Quon MJ, Han SH *et al*. Additive beneficial effects of fenofibrate combined with atorvastatin in the treatment of combined hyperlipidemia. *J Am Coll Cardiol* 2005; 45: 1649-53.

53. Goldberg AC, Bays HE, Ballantyne CM, *et al*. Efficacy and safety of ABT-335 (fenofibric acid) in combination with atorvastatin in patients with mixed hyperlipidemia. *Am J Cardiol* 2009; 103: 515-22.

54. Koh KK, Quon MJ, Rosenson RS, Chung WJ, Han SH. Vascular and metabolic effects of treatment of combined hyperlipidemia: focus on statins and fibrates. *Int J Cardiol* 2008; 124: 149-59.

55. The ACCORD Study Group. Effects of combination lipid therapy in Type 2 diabetes mellitus. *N Engl J Med* 2010; 362(17): 1563-74.

56. Superko HR, Garrett BC, King SB 3rd, Momary KM, Chronos NA, Wood PD. Effect of combination nicotinic acid and gemfibrozil treatment on intermediate density lipoprotein, and subclasses of low density lipoprotein and high density lipoprotein in patients with combined hyperlipidemia. *Am J Cardiol* 2009; 103: 387-92.

57. Tribble DL, Farnier M, Macdonell G, Perevozskaya I, Davies MJ, Gumbiner B, Musliner TA. Effects of fenofibrate and ezetimibe, both as monotherapy and in coadministration, on cholesterol mass within lipoprotein subfractions and low-density lipoprotein peak particle size in patients with mixed hyperlipidemia. *Metabolism* 2008; 57: 796-801.

58. Wald NJ, *et al*. Apolipoproteins and ischaemic heart disease: implications for screening. *Lancet* 1994; 343: 75-9.

59. Lamarche B, *et al*. Apolipoprotein A-I and B levels and the risk of ischemic heart disease during a five-year follow-up of men in the Québec Cardiovascular Study. *Circulation* 1996; 94: 273-8.

60. Moss AJ, *et al*. Thrombogenic factors and recurrent coronary events. *Circulation* 1999; 99: 2517-22.

61. Walldius G, *et al*. High apolipoprotein B, low apolipoprotein A-I, and improvement in the prediction of fatal myocardial infarction (AMORIS study): a prospective study. *Lancet* 2001; 358: 2026-33.

62. Talmud PJ, *et al*. Nonfasting apolipoprotein B and triglyceride levels as a useful predictor of coronary heart disease risk in middle-aged UK men. *Arterioscler Thromb Vasc Biol* 2002; 22: 1918-23.

63. Ridker PM, *et al*. Non-HDL cholesterol, apolipoproteins A-I and B100, standard lipid measures, lipid ratios, and CRP as risk factors for cardiovascular disease in women. *JAMA* 2005; 294: 326-33.

64. Meisinger C, *et al*. Prognostic value of apolipoprotein B and A-I in the prediction of myocardial infarction in middle-aged men and women: results from the MONICA/KORA Augsburg cohort study. *Eur Heart J* 2005; 26: 271-8.

65. Bruno G, *et al*. Effect of age on the association of non-high-density-lipoprotein cholesterol and apolipoprotein B with cardiovascular mortality in a Mediterranean population with type 2 diabetes: the Casale Monferrato Study. *Diabetologia* 2006; 49: 937-44.

66. St-Pierre AC, *et al*. Apolipoprotein-B, low-density lipoprotein cholesterol, and long-term risk of coronary heart disease in men. *Am J Cardiol* 2006; 97: 997-1001.

67. Chien KL, *et al*. Apolipoprotein B and non-high density lipoprotein cholesterol and the risk of coronary heart disease in Chinese. *J Lipid Res* 2007; 48: 2499-505.

68. Benn M, *et al.* Improving prediction of ischemic cardiovascular disease in the general population using apolipoprotein B: the Copenhagen City Heart Study. *Arterioscler Thromb Vasc Biol* 2007; 27: 661-70.

69. Ingelsson E, *et al.* Clinical utility of different lipid measures for prediction of coronary heart disease in men and women. *JAMA* 2007; 298: 776-85.

70. Onat A, *et al.* Serum apolipoprotein B is superior to LDL-cholesterol level in predicting incident coronary disease among Turks [Turkish]. *Anadolu Kardiyol Derg* 2007; 7: 128-33.

Chapter 9

How to manage lipid and lipoprotein disorders in children

Serena Tonstad MD PhD
Head Physician, Department of Preventive Cardiology
Oslo University Hospital Ullevål, Oslo, Norway
Professor, Clinical Nutrition, Department of Nutrition
University of Oslo, Oslo, Norway

Introduction

One of the axioms of atherosclerosis is that it is rooted in childhood. Indeed, these origins may extend to the prebirth environment and genetic antecedents. Subclinical atherosclerosis is present several decades before clinical manifestations affording ample opportunity for prevention. This said, statin therapy prevents about a third of clinical cardiovascular disease (CVD), even though treatment is started in middle age or later, and after only a few years. Could the other two thirds be prevented if treatment is started earlier? The questions of whether or when to treat children at risk of adult CVD, and which children to treat, cannot yet be answered by data linking treatment of childhood hyperlipidemia to a reduction in CVD. However, there is expert consensus that children with high risk of atherosclerosis should be identified and treated, based on rational and individualized weighing of potential risks and benefits between physician, child and family. This chapter reviews the relevant literature, supplemented by clinical observations.

Epidemiology

Prospective data from the Muscatine study [1], Bogalusa Heart Study [2, 3] and Cardiovascular Risk in Young Finns Study [4-6], as well as the autopsy-based Pathobiological Determinants of Atherosclerosis in Youth Study [7] have established independent relationships between lipid fractions measured in childhood and subsequent atherosclerosis. Lipids measured early in life have a stronger association with coronary heart disease (CHD) than later measurements [7, 8]. Prospective observational studies have shown that 1mmol/L lower serum total cholesterol is associated with ~50% lower mortality from CHD at ages 40-49 years [9]. Childhood serum cholesterol rankings tend to be maintained in adulthood, though the fate of the top 5% of the cholesterol distribution has not been studied separately [10].

The total/HDL cholesterol ratio is more than twice as informative as total cholesterol in predicting risk [9]. Non-HDL cholesterol (total minus HDL cholesterol) is another robust measure [11, 3] that encompasses all atherogenic lipid fractions and has the advantages of being measurable in the non-fasting state, and minimally affected by hypertriglyceridemia. Recently, non-HDL cholesterol levels were found to be as predictive of subclinical atherosclerosis as other lipids and lipoproteins measured early in life [3]. The apolipoprotein (apo) B/apoAI ratio measured in adolescence was recently shown to predict adult intima-media thickness (IMT) of the carotid artery [12].

While some studies have shown inconsistent relations between triglyceride concentrations and CVD, meta-analyses indicate that triglycerides are indeed independently associated with CHD and the relative risk appears to be higher in younger persons [13]. Furthermore, benefits from diet and medications are greatest in people with elevated triglyceride levels [13, 14].

Measurements and cut-off levels

For complete risk assessment a lipid profile should be measured including total, LDL and HDL cholesterol and triglycerides. LDL cholesterol can be directly measured in non-fasting serum samples, together with total and HDL cholesterol, or may be calculated using the Friedewald formula in fasting samples (LDL cholesterol = total cholesterol - HDL cholesterol - triglycerides/2.2, all in mmol/L; the formula is the same in mg/dL except that triglycerides are divided by 5). If triglycerides are >4.5mmol/L (400mg/dL) the formula cannot be used. If only total cholesterol is measured, a level >5.5mmol/L (215mg/dL) identifies high LDL cholesterol with 95% confidence [10].

Fasting lipid percentile distributions collected before the onset of the obesity epidemic are widely used for children and adolescents [15]. Cut-off levels for high-risk total and LDL cholesterol are 5.2mmol/L (200mg/dL) and 3.4mmol/L (130mg/dL), respectively. Levels of 4.4-5.1mmol/L (170-199mg/dL) for total cholesterol and 2.8-3.3mmol/L (110-129mg/dL) for LDL cholesterol are borderline. HDL cholesterol levels <0.9mmol/L (35mg/dL) are high risk and levels of 0.9-1.2mmol/L (35-45mg/dL) are borderline. The triglyceride cut-off is >1.5mmol/L (130mg/dL) and levels of 1.0-1.5mmol/L (90-129mg/dL) are borderline. These cut-offs are predictive of adult dyslipidemia [16], though for HDL cholesterol, age- and sex-specific cut-offs derived from National Health and Nutrition Examination Survey data (equivalent to a cut-off of ~1.0mmol/L; 40mg/dL) were more accurate [16]. For non-HDL cholesterol the suggested cut-off is >3.7mmol/L (144mg/dL) for high risk and 3.2-3.7mmol/L (123-143mg/dL) is borderline [17]. ApoAI and B cut-offs have also been published [17].

Risk assessment

Data on which to base CVD risk calculators for children similar to those developed for adults are not available so risk factors need to be summed and evaluated individually. In addition to lipid levels, relevant factors include blood pressure, cigarette smoking, premature CHD in first-degree relatives (before age 55 in men; before age 65 in women), obesity, fasting glucose and lack of physical activity [18]. Measurement of carotid IMT by B-mode ultrasound is a valid surrogate marker for atherosclerosis development and progression [19], and if available, provides additional risk stratification [20-22]. Endothelial dysfunction, an early manifestation of subclinical atherosclerosis, is more difficult to measure than IMT and its prognostic significance in children is not established [23].

Diagnosis of lipid disorders in children

Screening and case finding

An update of the 1998 American Academy of Pediatrics policy, mostly congruent with the 2006 American Heart Association (AHA) statement [18], recommends that children and adolescents with a positive family history of dyslipidemia or premature CVD (55 years of age for men and 65 years of age for women) be screened from the age of 2 years [24]. In addition, screening should be done in those whose family history is not known or who have other CVD risk factors, such as being overweight, obesity, hypertension, smoking or diabetes. If the lipid profile is normal testing may be repeated in 3-5 years. European recommendations are embedded in adult guidelines and likewise suggest screening children with a positive family history [25].

In contrast, the U.S. Preventive Services Task Force (USPSTF) concludes that evidence is insufficient to recommend for or against routine screening for lipid disorders below age 20 (Grade I USPSTF statement) [10]. Thus, lipid testing is not encouraged (Grade A and B recommendations), discouraged (Grade D) or given low priority (Grade C) but left to individual preference. The USPSTF found no studies that evaluated the effect of screening children on adult lipid levels or disease outcomes and pointed to the lack of evidence that clinical health benefits of cholesterol lowering apply to children.

Parental history, whether self-reported or verified, of hypercholesterolemia or CVD as a screening criterion does not seem to offer improvement over random population screening and results in many false negatives [10, 26]. However, children whose relatives have not experienced CHD are probably at lower risk and are less likely to have early manifestations of atherosclerosis than children with a positive family history [27, 28]. While family history guided screening would prevent only a very low proportion of CHD-related premature mortality [29], universal screening also has problems, as ~60% of identified high-risk adolescents would not have abnormal levels later [16]. Waiting to screen until young adulthood is an option with the caveat that young adults may be less likely to see a physician than children. Given the lack of evidence for one approach above another, a wide variety of clinical decisions between physicians and families are acceptable.

Children with genetic lipid disorders should be identified by case finding, usually when a parent or other relative is diagnosed with familial hypercholesterolemia (FH), or experiences a premature CVD event. Cascade testing (family tracing from affected patients) is cost effective [30] **(III/B)**, feasible [31] **(III/B)** and potential psychological damage does not seem to be a problem [32].

Newborns and children below 2 years

Total and LDL cholesterol increase rapidly in the first weeks of life and then gradually until age 2 years when they remain stable until puberty. Screening has poor test characteristics in newborns [33] and should be delayed until after age 2. The USPSTF found no studies that followed abnormal tests in infants from the general population by mutation analysis [10]. DNA analysis may be done if a parent has FH, the specific mutation is known and the parent wishes to know the child's status.

Children aged 2-10 years

The ability to distinguish between individuals affected and unaffected with FH based on serum cholesterol is greatest at ages 1-9 years and diminishes with increasing age [33]. Measuring serum total cholesterol detects 88% or more of cases of FH [33]. In families with known FH, testing (lipids and DNA analysis if available) children in this age group allows dietary therapy to be started at an age that is less likely to be problematic than adolescence [34].

Adolescents aged 10-18 years

At puberty, total cholesterol declines for both boys and girls, and HDL cholesterol declines for boys. Toward the end of puberty a slow increase of LDL cholesterol commences in boys, in part explaining the earlier onset of CHD in men than in women. If DNA analysis is not available, children from families with FH whose cholesterol level is low/borderline should be retested after puberty.

Work-up

The medical history should focus on any family history of CHD, potential secondary causes of lipid disorders and use of medications that affect lipids (e.g. retinoic acid derivatives, prednisone, atypical antipsychotics, anti-epileptics). Physical examination includes blood pressure, height and weight plotted on standardized growth charts, and a search for corneal arcus and tendon or skin xanthoma. Laboratory tests include glucose, thyroid-stimulating hormone, liver and renal function tests and urinalysis.

Conditions in childhood with high risk of premature atherosclerosis

AHA classification

The 2006 AHA statement selected pediatric disease settings where there is pathological or clinical evidence for manifest CHD (though not typically hyperlipidemia in some settings) and divided these into risk categories with homozygous FH, type 1 diabetes, end-stage renal disease and post-orthostatic heart transplantation in tier 1, representing the highest risk category; heterozygous FH, chronic inflammatory disease, Kawasaki disease with regressed coronary aneurysms, and type 2 diabetes in tier 2; and congenital heart disease, Kawasaki disease without detected coronary involvement and cancer treatment survivors in tier 3 [18]. In the presence of two or more other lipid abnormalities or CVD risk factors, the individual is moved to the next higher tier. For each tier, cutpoints/treatment goals are presented for body mass index (BMI), blood pressure, LDL cholesterol and fasting glucose/HbA1C.

Cholesterol-lowering medication is to be considered if after therapeutic lifestyle changes, LDL cholesterol levels remain >2.6mmol/L (100mg/dL) in tier 1, >3.4mmol/L (130mg/dL) in tier 2 and >4.1mmol/L (160mg/dL) in tier 3. The applicability of these guidelines to pediatric practice has not been tested and effectiveness, outcome measures, safety and acceptability data are lacking. However, they establish two important principles, that all classical risk factors should be addressed in children and that treatment should be based on level of risk.

Hyperlipidemic disorders

Disorders that predispose to atherosclerosis and cause hyperlipidemia are shown in Table 1. In children with genetic disorders, atherosclerosis develops earlier and therapeutic lifestyle change is frequently followed by pharmacological therapy. Statins have been shown to be effective in LDL-reduction specifically in children with FH [10] **(Ia/A)**. For children with secondary or multifactorial conditions, lifestyle intervention may be followed by lipid-lowering medication, but very little evidence is available to support this approach **(IV/C)**. The etiology of CVD in these conditions may have additional determinants. It may be noted that even in adults, e.g. postmenopausal women with hyperlipidemia, statin therapy has not consistently been associated with regression of atherosclerosis [35] and primary prevention is still controversial [36, 37].

Primary genetic lipid disorders

Familial hypercholesterolemia
FH is a well described autosomal dominant disorder caused by mutations in the LDL receptor gene. There are other genetic disorders causing the FH phenotype as well [38]. With regard to FH, LDL cholesterol is elevated before birth, contributing to accelerated atherosclerosis [17]. Carotid IMT increases several-fold faster in children with FH than in non-affected siblings, and by age 12 is clearly distinguishable from siblings' IMT [39]. LDL cholesterol is typically ≥3.5mmol/L (135mg/dL), usually ≥4.1mmol/L (160mg/dL), though lower levels (>3.1mmol/L; 120mg/dL) [40] may be identified in children carrying an LDL-receptor mutation. At least one parent should have a history of hypercholesterolemia for the diagnosis to be considered; if a parent is not available further inquiry into family history and lipid levels should be done. Only one third of children with an LDL-receptor mutation have a positive family history of premature CVD in a first-degree relative [40]. Xanthoma and corneal arcus are uncommon in children.

Table 1. Conditions in childhood that predispose to atherosclerosis or that are accompanied by secondary hyperlipidemia.

Primary lipid disorders	Chronic diseases with high prevalence of lipid disorder
Homozygous FH	Diabetes mellitus
Heterozygous FH	Organ transplant (liver, kidney, heart)
Familial defective apoB	HIV treatment
PCSK9 gain-of-function	Renal disease
Autosomal recessive hypercholesterolemia	Liver disease including intrahepatic cholestasis, biliary atresia, non-alcoholic fatty liver disease
Familial combined hyperlipidemia	Chronic inflammatory disease, e.g. SLE
Type III hyperlipoproteinemia (associated with apoE2 homozygosity)	Endocrine disease: hypothyroidism, hypopituitarism Anorexia nervosa Storage and metabolic diseases, e.g. Niemann Pick disease, Gaucher disease Lipodystrophy or lipoatrophy syndromes

DNA analysis to determine the specific LDL-receptor mutation (of which there are >1000) is helpful to confirm the diagnosis and identify other relatives with FH. Identification by gene analysis also makes it possible to identify homozygotes and introduce early appropriate treatment [41], though most homozygotes are obvious due to their extreme elevations of LDL cholesterol (>400mg/dL). Risk factors in addition to LDL cholesterol play a major role in determining risk of CVD (Table 2) [42, 43], including levels of other lipid and lipoproteins [44], and apoE4 [45] and null alleles [46].

The guidelines of the National Institute for Health and Clinical Excellence (NICE) in the United Kingdom suggest that statins licensed for the appropriate age group be considered by the age of 10 years, though earlier or later treatment may be warranted [47]. US pediatric guidelines state that statins should only be started in children <8 years in the presence of dramatic elevation of LDL cholesterol as in homozygous FH [18]. For children 8 years of age or older and no other CVD risk factors, statins may be considered at LDL cholesterol >190mg/dL despite diet; when other risk factors are present at LDL cholesterol >160mg/dL despite diet; however, it is emphasized that there is room for discretion and clinical judgment [24]. A more conservative approach is to recommend statins in children with a positive family history or substantially elevated LDL cholesterol (>190mg/dL), especially boys [43], after age 10 years [48]. Waiting until at least the start of puberty or onset of menses appears prudent [49]. Notably,

Table 2. Factors that increase risk in children with heterozygous FH.
◆ Level of LDL cholesterol
◆ Other lipid abnormality including low HDL cholesterol/elevated triglycerides, apolipoprotein (a) isoforms
◆ Male gender
◆ Null alleles
◆ Family history of CHD before age 55 in males, or before age 65 in females
◆ Other risk factors, e.g. metabolic syndrome, cigarette smoking, obesity, diabetes, hypertension

there do not seem to be psychosocial harms related to statins in children with FH; rather therapy contributes to a feeling of safety [50] **(IV/C)**.

Other genetic forms of hypercholesterolemia

Familial defective apolipoprotein B results from mutations in the apoB molecule that affects binding of LDL to its receptor [38, 51]. Clinical manifestations are similar but milder than FH [52]. Autosomal recessive hypercholesterolemia is similar to homozygous FH (but parents of index cases have normal serum cholesterol levels), though less severe and probably more responsive to medications [38]. Another mutation encodes a member of the proprotein convertase family, PCSK9, which triggers increased degradation of the LDL receptor. Rare dominant gain-of-function mutations cosegregate with hypercholesterolemia, of which one is associated with a particularly severe FH phenotype [38].

Familial combined hyperlipidemia (FCH)

This autosomal dominant disorder usually appears in adulthood but with the onset of the obesity epidemic is increasingly identified in children [53, 54]. FCH results from interactions between various gene abnormalities that affect lipid metabolism and environmental factors. There are no standardized criteria to make the diagnosis, but it should be considered in the presence of elevated LDL cholesterol, elevated triglycerides, low HDL cholesterol or combinations of these and when DNA testing does not reveal FH or related mutation. Levels of apoB are elevated reflecting the increased secretion of VLDL that is a common cause [54]. First-degree relatives may have similar or other combinations of lipid abnormalities. The Fredrickson IIB phenotype (i.e. combined hypercholesterolemia and hypertriglyceridemia) in a parent is a good predictor of expressed hyperlipidemia in children [55]. In adolescents the IIB phenotype is clearly associated with elevated IMT in adulthood [56]. Therapeutic lifestyle change is the first line of therapy. LDL cholesterol is generally lower than in FH and drug therapy can usually be postponed until late adolescence or adulthood.

Secondary hyperlipidemia in chronic disorders

Diabetes mellitus

Dyslipidemia associated with diabetes is characterized by high triglycerides and remnant particles, low HDL cholesterol, and small dense LDL particles. A wide range of prevalence of 15% to 62% has been reported in youth with type 2 diabetes [57]. Prevalence is lower in well controlled type 1 diabetes.

The American Diabetes Association (ADA) recommends lipid screening in pubertal children (>12 years) in whom diabetes has been diagnosed; for pre-pubertal children, screening is recommended only if the family history indicates risk or is unknown [58]. Retesting is recommended every 5 years thereafter if normal in patients with type 1 diabetes and every 2 years in type 2 diabetes. NICE does not recommend lipid screening for children with type 1 diabetes, stating that screening in adulthood is sufficient and that further dietary restrictions may be undesirable [59]. Measurement of non-HDL cholesterol to avoid fasting is practical [60].

While AHA guidelines placed type 1 diabetes at higher risk than type 2 [18], some experts would consider youth with type 2 diabetes at higher risk than well-controlled type 1 [60]. Many youths with type 2 diabetes have additional risk factors placing them in the AHA highest risk classification (tier 1) [18, 24]. In tier 1, statins are recommended when LDL cholesterol is >2.6mmol/L (100mg/dL) after therapeutic lifestyle change for 6 months. The ADA guidelines recommend drug therapy if LDL cholesterol is 3.4mmol/L (130mg/dL) after a 6-month trial of diet and exercise [58]. In the absence of studies demonstrating effectiveness, safety or clinical outcomes of pharmacological therapy for children with diabetes, lifestyle and glucose management should be primary.

Solid organ transplant recipients

Hypercholesterolemia is common after heart, kidney or liver transplantation and partly related to the use of cyclosporine and prednisone. To prevent transplant vasculopathy statins are routinely given to pediatric cardiac transplant patients immediately after transplantation and continued for life [18]. Pravastatin reduces lipid levels and has been tolerated well in this group [61, 62] **(Ib/A)**.

HIV treatment

As the repertoire of antiretroviral therapies and life expectancy are extended, the effect of these agents on lipids has become of concern in adults, but also in children [63]. Protease inhibitor substitution with nevirapine may improve lipid profiles [64] **(III/B)**.

Renal disease

Nephrotic syndrome or persistent proteinuria, chronic kidney failure and renal transplant are frequent causes of hyperlipidemia [65]. Small studies, primarily in transplanted children, have reported that simvastatin [66], atorvastatin [67] or pravastatin [68] seem to be safe in low doses and effective in reducing lipid levels **(Ib/A)**. It has been suggested that tacrolimus may replace cyclosporine to reduce the risk of hyperlipidemia [69].

Multifactorial dyslipidemias

Polygenetic hypercholesterolemia

In any screening program, children will be identified with hypercholesterolemia with no other lipid abnormalities or family history or findings indicating a genetic lipid disorder. Often cholesterol levels are lower upon follow-up (regression to the mean), but may increase later. Dietary treatment is recommended **(IV/C)**.

Hypertriglyceridemia

Hypertriglyceridemia in children is usually multifactorial [70]. Genetic disorders, e.g. familial combined hyperlipidemia, Fredrickson type IV familial hypertriglyceridemia, type III hyperlipoproteinemia (associated with apoE2 homozygosity) and type I familial lipoprotein lipase deficiency may underlie hypertriglyceridemia which only becomes manifest in the presence of an aggravating factor, particularly obesity or type 2 diabetes. If triglyceride levels are >1.5mmol/L (130mg/dL), lifestyle change is recommended. Dietary sugars should be restricted and a low glycemic index diet instituted [71] **(IV/C)**. If triglyceride levels are >5.6mmol/L (500mg/dL), the patient should be referred to a lipid disorder clinic. Pancreatitis or eruptive xanthoma should trigger work-up for hypertriglyceridemia.

Metabolic syndrome/obesity-related dyslipidemia

Overweight or obesity is the most prevalent cause of dyslipidemia, fuelling metabolic syndrome and increased CVD risk. The USPSTF found that childhood BMI was the second best independent predictor of adult dyslipidemia after LDL cholesterol [10]. Studies almost universally find that overweight is associated with abnormal lipids [72] and about one half of obese children have an identifiable lipid abnormality [73]. Obesity is more strongly associated with elevated triglycerides and low HDL cholesterol than hypercholesterolemia. About one fourth of obese children have metabolic syndrome and finding dyslipidemia should trigger a search for other components and treatment [74].

Children with overweight or obesity and dyslipidemia have a substantially increased risk of elevated carotid IMT [56], and the suggestion has been made to limit lipid screening in childhood to overweight or obese adolescents [56]. Weight management is the primary treatment [75], but little evidence supports its feasibility and efficacy. In a study conducted in China, obesity-related vascular dysfunction in young children was partially reversible with diet alone and particularly diet combined with exercise, with sustained improvements at 1 year in those persisting with diet plus regular exercise [76].

Non-pharmacologic management

Diet and exercise

A healthy diet has an appropriate amount of energy to promote normal growth and avoid obesity, is low in saturated and trans fat, sugar and high glycemic carbohydrates and is rich in whole grains, fruit, vegetables and dietary fibre. Recent guidelines have focused on quality more than quantity of fat [24]. The American Heart Association Step 1 diet, which recommends that total fat constitutes <30% of energy, saturated fat, <10% of energy, cholesterol, <300mg/day, and trans fat be avoided, is recommended for all high-risk pediatric patients, under the guidance of a nutritionist and with the requirement that adequate calories be provided for growth [18]. The Step 2 diet with further reduction of saturated fat to <7% of energy and of cholesterol intake to <200mg/day is recommended if LDL cholesterol is >130mg/dL (3.4mmol/L) for children with tier 2 risk and >160mg/dL (4.1mmol/L) for children with tier 3 risk [18]. In children as young as 7 months, reductions in saturated fat and cholesterol to these levels appears to be safe and does not interfere with normal growth, development and sexual maturation (Ib/A) [24]. However, the effectiveness of the diet in lowering atherogenic lipid levels in the long term has not been tested.

Studies have focused on moderate fat restriction and its effects on growth as overzealous fat restriction has been reported [77]. Though intensive dietary counselling may improve lipid levels and is safe, there is lack of evidence that dietary change is sustainable [10]. In children with FH no good quality studies of dietary therapy have been done [10]. The Dietary Intervention Study in Children, the largest study conducted in hyperlipidemic (non-FH) children, found only a 5mg/dL difference in LDL cholesterol between intervention and control groups after 1 year, which diminished to 2mg/dL by year 7 [78]. After 3 years, snack foods, desserts and pizza contributed about one third of the daily energy intake of both the intervention and control groups [79] illustrating a major barrier to healthy eating in children, namely, the abundance and accessibility of fast foods. The Finnish Special Turku Coronary Risk Factor Project found sustained effects of nutritional counselling begun in infancy on endothelial function in boys, in part due to diet-induced reductions in serum cholesterol [80], confirming the benefit of starting dietary change early as possible.

The few trials of exercise are of fair-to-poor quality and have not evaluated children with lipid disorders [10]. A meta-analysis showed that for the general population aerobic exercise does not reduce non-HDL cholesterol but improves percent body fat and aerobic capacity [81] (Ia/A). Combination diet and exercise programs have shown improvement in lipids [10] (Ia/A). Practical suggestions for implementation of diet and exercise are shown in Table 3 [82, 83].

Smoking cessation

Adolescent smokers may have a preponderance of other CVD risk factors, including increased BMI and blood pressure, low aerobic fitness, and a family history of CVD [84]. Assisting with smoking cessation is imperative, though it is not clear which programs are most successful in adolescents [85].

Other non-pharmacologic approaches

Various dietary adjuncts, e.g. soluble fibre, plant stanols and sterols and soy protein have been shown to have some effects in reducing serum lipids [10]. These studies have generally

Table 3. Dietary and physical activity recommendations to reduce CVD risk in children and adolescents.

Implementing dietary changes	Physical activity recommendations
Reduce added sugars, especially drinks and juices	60 or more minutes of physical activity daily
Use unsaturated oils in place of solid foods during food preparation	Most of the 60 or more minutes should be moderate- or vigorous-intensity aerobic activity including vigorous at least 3 days a week
Use recommended portion sizes when preparing and serving food	As part of the 60 or more minutes, muscle-strengthening activity should be included on at least 3 days of the week (playground equipment, climbing trees, playing tug-of-war)
Serve fresh, frozen and canned vegetables and fruits at every meal; be careful with added sauces and sugar	As part of the 60 or more minutes, bone-strengthening activity should be included on at least 3 days of the week (running, jumping rope, basketball, tennis, hopscotch)
Introduce and regularly serve fish as an entrée	Activities should be appropriate for age, enjoyable and offer variety
Remove the skin from poultry	
Use only lean cuts of meat and reduced-fat meat products	
Limit high calorie sauces	
Eat whole grain breads and cereals rather than refined products	
Eat more legumes (beans) and tofu in place of meat for some entrées	
Breads, breakfast cereals and prepared foods including soups may be high in salt or sugar; choose high-fibre, low-salt/low-sugar alternatives	

lasted for a few weeks, and documentation of other endpoints than lipid levels is rare. Treatment over many years would be needed to inhibit the development of atherosclerosis; however, long-term compliance is likely to be low. A recent review found that margarines and drinks containing plant sterols or stanols decrease serum cholesterol by up to 10% in individuals with FH [86] (Ia/A). Compliance with a sterol-enriched margarine for 6 months in a study of children with FH was good [87], but in some studies lipid-adjusted serum lycopene levels decreased [87]. Furthermore, stanol supplementation did not improve endothelial dysfunction despite reduction in LDL cholesterol [88].

Drug management

The main drug class to consider in children and adolescents is a statin [89]. This takes into account observations that bile acid binding resins, which were previously recommended, are difficult to administer due to unpalatability and side effects, and the wealth of evidence of effectiveness and safety of statins in adults. Treatment of children with heterozygous FH with statins for up to 2 years lowers LDL cholesterol and appears to be safe [90] (Ia/A).

Though long-term safety and clinical effects on CHD are not known due to the lack of randomized trials documenting the effects of intervention on hard clinical outcomes, statins cause regression of atherosclerotic lesions and improve endothelial function [91, 92], indicating that treatment is doing more than solely lowering blood lipids. Again, it must be emphasized that this data has only been obtained in children with a likely genetic form of hyperlipidemia, usually FH. Earlier lowering of LDL cholesterol is associated with less atherosclerosis as measured by carotid IMT, supporting the notion of starting statins early rather than late [93] (III/B). However, this evidence was solely observational.

Statins in practice

A meta-analysis found that statin therapy in children aged 8-18 years for a range of 12-104 weeks was efficacious, and safe with regard to adverse events, sexual development, and muscle or liver toxicity [90] (Ia/A). Most children in the studies were aged 10 years or older. Reductions in LDL cholesterol averaged 30%, similar to an earlier meta-analytic report [94], and more potent drugs or higher doses produced greater reductions in LDL cholesterol. There was a modest elevation in HDL cholesterol of ~4% and triglycerides were unchanged. Table 4 suggests how to start and monitor statins in children [95].

Other lipid-modifying drugs

Fibrates and nicotinic acid are effective lipid-modifying drugs, but their side effect profile suggests that they should not be used in children except in extreme circumstances [96]. Ezetimibe and colesevalam are currently being evaluated in randomized clinical trials and ezetimibe is registered for use in children in some regions. Both of these medications may be combined with statins [97].

Table 4. Starting and monitoring statins in children.

- Do a baseline evaluation including a lipid profile, glucose, TSH, creatinine, CK, ALT and AST and urinalysis

- Any approved statin registered for use in children may be used based on the preference of the physician

- If drug interactions are a concern (e.g. concomitant use of macrolide antibiotics, antifungal agents, HIV-protease inhibitors, calcium channel blockers, cyclosporine), pravastatin may be chosen

- Start with the lowest dose given once a day

- Ask the child to report all potential side effects, especially muscle stiffness, soreness, pain, or tenderness, or dark-coloured urine. Also, symptoms of hepatic dysfunction should be monitored, including fatigue, anorexia, nausea, vomiting, right upper quadrant discomfort and jaundice

- Do not prescribe statins for adolescent girls who are sexually active or may soon be sexually active without addressing the need for contraception

- Measure a lipid profile, CK, ALT and AST after 6 weeks

- Look for a 25-30% decrease in serum cholesterol level as an indicator of effective treatment

- If side effects occur, or laboratory abnormalities appear, reassess the need for the drug by weighing potential benefits and risks. Withhold the drug for at least 2 weeks before reassessing

- If the dose is changed, repeat the blood work 6 weeks later

- Monitor growth, sexual development and assess for other risk factors (smoking, overweight, blood pressure) regularly

- Once on a stable dose, the lipid profile and safety laboratory tests may be repeated every 6-12 months

Management of homozygous FH

In patients with homozygous FH, markers of atherosclerosis correlated with age at which lipid-lowering treatment was started indicating that early treatment is imperative [98]. LDL apheresis performed weekly to biweekly is the treatment of choice from the age of 6-7 years and is usually combined with statin and ezetimibe therapy [99]. Starting at age 10 or later may be too late to prevent aortic stenosis.

Growth and development of children treated with LDL apheresis appear to be normal, and the only complication is iron deficiency anemia. Apheresis may be delayed if the child responds to high-dose statin therapy (e.g. atorvastatin 40-80mg) combined with ezetimibe with a 50% reduction in LDL cholesterol. In a recent report of patients who started treatment before age 18, LDL apheresis was well tolerated and effectively lowered LDL cholesterol by 48%, though target goals were not reached [100].

Conclusions

In children and adolescents shown to have a lipid disorder, take into account age, family history, and lipid values in family members and consider secondary hyperlipidemias, in order to make a diagnosis. Diet and exercise should be optimized and stopping smoking encouraged at every visit. The use of statins is standard clinical practice for children with familial hypercholesterolemia after onset of puberty and may be indicated in other children at high risk.

Key points	Evidence level
• Identify children with genetic lipid disorders, in particular FH, through cascade testing.	III/B
• Treat high-risk children with heterozygous FH with statins if above age 10 years.	Ia/A
• Treat children with homozygous FH with LDL apheresis and lipid-lowering drugs from age 6-7.	IV/C
• Exert individualized clinical judgment regarding screening and treating of children with a family history of CVD or multiple CVD risk factors.	IV/C

References

1. Davis PH, Dawson JD, Riley WA, Lauer RM. Carotid intimal-medial thickness is related to cardiovascular risk factors measured from childhood through middle age: the Muscatine Study. *Circulation* 2001; 104: 2815-9.
2. Li S, Chen W, Srinivasan SR, Bond MG, Tang R, Urbina EM, Berenson GS. Childhood cardiovascular risk factors and carotid vascular changes in adulthood: the Bogalusa Heart Study. *JAMA* 2003; 290: 2271-6.

3.   Frontini MG, Srinivasan SR, Xu J, Tang R, Bond MG, Berenson GS. Usefulness of childhood non-high density lipoprotein cholesterol levels versus other lipoprotein measures in predicting adult subclinical atherosclerosis: The Bogalusa Heart Study. *Pediatrics* 2008; 121: 924-9.

4.   Raitakari OT, Juonala M, Kahonen M, *et al.* Cardiovascular risk factors in childhood and carotid artery intima-media thickness in adulthood: the Cardiovascular Risk in Young Finns Study. *JAMA* 2003; 290: 2777-83.

5.   Juonala M, Jarvisalo MJ, Maki-Torkko N, Kahonen M, Viikari JS, Raitakari OT. Risk factors identified in childhood and decreased carotid artery elasticity in adulthood: the Cardiovascular Risk in Young Finns Study. *Circulation* 2005; 112: 1486-93.

6.   Juonala M, Viikari JS, Rönnemaa, Marniemi J, Jula A, Loo B-M, Raitakari OT. Associations of dylipidemias from childhood to adulthood with carotid intima-media thickness, elasticity, and brachial flow-mediated dilatation in adulthood. The Cardiovascular Risk in Young Finns Study. *Arterioscler Thromb Vasc Biol* 2008; 28: 1012-7.

7.   McGill HC, McMahan A, Gidding SS. Preventing heart disease in the 21st century. Implications of the Pathobiological Determinants of Atherosclerosis in Youth (PDAY) study. *Circulation* 2008; 117: 1216-27.

8.   Klag MJ, Ford DE, Mead LA, *et al.* Serum cholesterol in young men and subsequent cardiovascular disease. *N Engl J Med* 1993; 328: 313-8.

9.   Prospective Studies Collaboration. Blood cholesterol and vascular mortality by age, sex, and blood pressure: a meta-analysis of individual data from 61 prospective studies with 55,000 vascular deaths. *Lancet* 2007; 370: 1829-39.

10. Haney EM, Huffman LH, Bougatsos C, Freeman M, Steiner RD, Nelson HD. Screening and treatment for lipid disorders in children and adolescents: systematic evidence review for the US Preventive Services Task Force. *Pediatrics* 2007; 120: e189-214.

11. Brunzell JD, Davidson M, Furberg CD, *et al.* Lipoprotein management in patients with cardiometabolic risk: consensus statement from the American Diabetes Association and the American College of Cardiology foundation. *Diabetes Care* 2008; 31: 811-22.

12. Viikari JM, Kähönen M, Solakivi T, *et al.* Childhood levels of serum apolipoproteins B and A-I predict carotid intima-media thickness and brachial endothelial function in adulthood: the Cardiovascular Risk in Young Finns Study. *J Am Coll Cardiol* 2008; 52: 293-9.

13. Criqui MH. Triglycerides and coronary heart disease revisited (again). *Ann Intern Med* 2007; 147: 425-7.

14. Ellingsen I, Hjermann I, Abdelnoor M, Hjerkinn E, Tonstad S. Dietary and antismoking advice and ischemic heart disease mortality in men with normal or high fasting triacylglycerol concentrations. A 23-y follow-up study. *Am J Clin Nutr* 2003; 78: 935-40.

15. National Cholesterol Education Program (NCEP): Highlights of the report of the Expert Panel on Blood Cholesterol Levels in Children and Adolescents. *Pediatrics* 1992; 89: 495-501.

16. Magnussen CG, Raitakari OT, Thomson R, *et al.* Utility of currently recommended pediatric dyslipidemia classifications in predicting dyslipidemia in adulthood. Evidence from the Childhood Determinants of Adults Health (CDAH) Study, Cardiovascular Risk in Young Finns study, and Bogalusa Heart Study. *Circulation* 2008; 117: 32-42.

17. Kwiterovich PO. Recognition and management of dyslipidemia in children and adolescents. *J Clin Endocrinol Metab* 2008; 93: 4200-9.

18. Kavey RE, Allada V, Daniels SR, *et al.* Cardiovascular risk reduction in high-risk pediatric patients: a scientific statement from the American Heart Association Expert Panel on Population and Prevention Science; the Councils on Cardiovascular Disease in the Young, Epidemiology and Prevention, Nutrition, Physical Activity and Metabolism, High Blood Pressure Research, Cardiovascular Nursing, and the Kidney in Heart Disease; and the Interdisciplinary Working Group on Quality of Care and Outcomes Research: endorsed by the American Academy of Pediatrics. *Circulation* 2006; 114: 2710-38.

19. De Groot E, Hovinjgh GK, Wiegman A, Duriez P, Smit AJ, Fruchart JC, Kastelein JJ. Measurement of arterial wall thickness as a surrogate marker for atherosclerosis. *Circulation* 2004; 109 (23 Suppl 1): III33-8.

20. Tonstad S, Joakimsen O, Stensland-Bugge E, Leren TP, Ose L, Russell D, Bønaa KH. Risk factors related to carotid intima-media thickness and plaque in children with familial hypercholesterolemia and control subjects. *Arterioscler Thromb Vasc Biol* 1996; 16: 984-91.

21. Slyper AH. Clinical review 168: What vascular ultrasound testing has revealed about pediatric atherogenesis, and a potential clinical role for ultrasound in pediatric risk assessment. *J Clin Endocrinol Metab* 2004; 89: 3089-95.

22. Groner JA, Joshi M, Bauer JA. Pediatric precursors of adult cardiovascular disease: noninvasive assessment of early vascular changes in children and adolescents. *Pediatrics* 2006; 118: 1683-91.

23. Tsimikas S, Witzum JL. Shifting the diagnosis and treatment of atherosclerosis to children and young adults: a new paradigm for the 21st century? *J Am Coll Cardiol* 2002; 40: 2122-4.

24. Daniels SR, Greer FR, and the Committee on Nutrition. Lipid screening and cardiovascular health in childhood. *Pediatrics* 2008; 122: 198-208.

25. De Backer G, Ambrosioni E, Borch-Johnsen K, *et al*. Third Joint Task Force of European and Other Societies on Cardiovascular Disease Prevention in Clinical Practice. European guidelines on cardiovascular disease prevention in clinical practice. *Eur Heart J* 2003; 24: 1601-10.

26. O'Loughlin J, Lauzon B, Paradis G, Hanley J, Lévy E, Delvin E, Lambert M. Usefulness of the American Academy of Pediatrics recommendations for identifying youths with hypercholesterolemia. *Pediatrics* 2004; 113: 1723-7.

27. Barra S, Gaeta G, Cuomo S, *et al*. Early increase of carotid intima-media thickness in children with parental history of premature myocardial infarction. *Heart* 2009; Jan 23 Epub ahead of print

28. de Jongh S, Lilien MR, Bakker HD, Hutten BA, Kastelein JJ, Stroes ES. Family history of cardiovascular events and endothelial dysfunction in children with familial hypercholesterolemia. *Atherosclerosis* 2002; 163: 193-7.

29. Khoury MJ, Jones K, Grosse SD. Quantifying the health benefits of genetic tests: the importance of a population perspective. *Genet Med* 2006; 8: 191-5.

30. Marks D, Wonderling D, Thorogood M, Lambert H, Humphries SE, Neil HA. Cost effectiveness analysis of different approaches of screening for familial hypercholesterolaemia. *BMJ* 2002; 324: 1303.

31. Hadfield SG, Horara S, Starr BJ *et al*. Family tracing to identify patients with familial hypercholesterolaemia: the second audit of the Department of Health Familial Hypercholesterolaemia Cascade Testing Project. *Ann Clin Biochem* 2009; 46: 24-32.

32. van Maarle MC, Stouthard MEA, Bonsel GJ. Quality of life in a family based cascade screening programme for familial hypercholesterolemia: a longitudinal study among participants. *J Med Genet* 2003; 40: e3.

33. Wald DS, Betwick JP, Wald NJ. Child-parent screening for familial hypercholesterolaemia: screening strategy based on a meta-analysis. *BMJ* 2007; 335: 599-607.

34. Tonstad S. Choices for treatment of hyperlipidaemia. *J Inherit Metab Dis* 2003; 26: 289-98.

35. Stein EA. Additional lipid lowering trials using surrogate measurements of atherosclerosis by carotid intima-media thickness. *J Am Coll Cardiol* 2008; 52: 2206-9.

36. Peterson ED, Wang TY. The great debate of 2008 - how low to go in preventive cardiology? *JAMA* 2008; 299: 1718-20.

37. Rashid S, Francis GA. Statins and primary prevention: is all the evidence in? *Can J Cardiol* 2008; 24: 301-3.

38. Rahalkar AR, Hegele RA. Monogenic pediatric dyslipidemias: classification, genetics and clinical spectrum. *Mol Genet Metab* 2008; 93: 282-94.

39. Wiegman A, Groot E, Hutten BA, *et al*. Arterial intima-media thickness in children heterozygous for familial hypercholesterolemia. *Lancet* 2004; 363: 369-70.

40. Wiegman A, Rodenburg J, de Jongh S, Defesche JC, Bakker HD, Kastelein JJ, Sijbrands EJ. Family history and cardiovascular risk in familial hypercholesterolemia: data in more than 1000 children. *Circulation* 2003; 107: 1473-8.

41. Kubalska J, Chmara M, Limon J, *et al*. Clinical course of homozygous familial hypercholesterolemia during childhood: report of 4 unrelated patients with homozygous or compound heterozygous mutations in the LDLR gene. *J Appl Genet* 2008; 49: 109-13.

42. Jansen AC, van Aalst-Cohen ES, Tanck MW, *et al*. The contribution of classical risk factors to cardiovascular disease in familial hypercholesterolaemia: data in 2400 patients. *J Intern Med* 2004; 256: 482-90.

43. Sijbrands EJ, Westerndorp RG, Paola Lombardi M Havekes LM, Frants RR, Kastelein JJ, Smelt AH. Additional risk factors influence excess mortality in heterozygous familial hypercholesterolaemia. *Atherosclerosis* 2000; 149: 421-5.

44. van der Graaf A, Rodenburg J, Vissers MN, *et al*. Atherogenic lipoprotein particle size and concentrations and the effect of pravastatin in children with familial hypercholesterolemia. *J Pediatr* 2008; 152: 873-8.

45. Wiegman A, Sijbrands EJ, Rodenburg J, Defesche JC, de Jongh S, Bakker HD, Kastelein JJ. The apolipoprotein epsilon4 allele confers additional risk in children with familial hypercholesterolemia. *Pediatr Res* 2003; 53: 1008-12.

46. Koeijvoets KC, Rodenburg J, Hutten BA, Wiegman A, Kastelein JJ, Sijbrands EJ. Low-density lipoprotein receptor genotype and response to pravastatin in children with familial hypercholesterolemia: substudy of an intima-media thickness trial. *Circulation* 2005; 112: 3168-73.

47. Wierzbicki AS, Humphries SE, Jinhas R, on behalf of the Guideline Development Group. Familial hypercholesterolemia: summary of NICE guidance. *BMJ* 2008; 337: 509-10.

48. Tonstad S. A rational approach to treating hypercholesterolaemia in children. Weighing the risks and benefits. *Drug Safety* 1997; 16: 330-41.

49. Stein EA. Statins and children. Whom do we treat and when? *Circulation* 2007; 116: 594-5.

50. De Jongh S, Kerckhoffs MC, Grootenhuis MA, Bakker HD, Heymans HS, Last BF. Quality of life, anxiety and concerns among statin-treated children with familial hypercholesterolemia and their parents. *Acta Paediatr* 2003; 92: 1096-101.

51. Soutar AK, Naoumova RP. Mechanisms of disease: genetic causes of familial hypercholesterolemia. *Nat Clin Pract Cardiovasc Med* 2007; 4: 214-25.

52. Pimstone SN, Defesche JC, Clee SM, Bakker HD, Hayden MR, Kastelein JJ. Differences in the phenotype between children with familial defective apolipoprotein B-100 and familial hypercholesterolemia. *Arterioscler Thromb Vasc Biol* 1997; 17: 826-33.

53. Kuromori Y, Okada T, Iwata F, Hara M, Noto N, Harada K. Familial combined hyperlipidemia (FCHL) in children: the significance of early development of hyperapoB lipoproteinemia, obesity and aging. *J Atheroscler Thromb* 2002; 9: 314-20.

54. ter Avest E, Sniderman AD, Bredie SJ, Wiegman A, Stalenhoef AF, de Graaf J. Effect of aging and obesity on the expression of dyslipidaemia in children from families with familial combined hyperlipidaemia. *Clin Sci* 2007; 112: 131-9.

55. Lapinleimu J, Nuotio IO, Lapinleimu H, Simell OG, Rask-Nissila L, Viikari JS. Recognition of familial dyslipidemias in 5-year-old children using the lipid phenotypes of parents. The STRIP project. *Atherosclerosis* 2002; 160: 417-23.

56. Magnussen CG, Venn A, Thomson R, *et al.* The association of pediatric low- and high-density lipoprotein cholesterol dyslipidemia classifications and change in dyslipidemia status with carotid intima-media thickness in adulthood. *J Am Coll Cardiol* 2009; 53: 860-9.

57. Pinhas-Hamiel O, Zeiler P. Acute and chronic complications of type 2 diabetes mellitus in children and adolescents. *Lancet* 2007; 369: 1823-31.

58. American Diabetes Association. Standards of medical care in diabetes. *Diabetes Care* 2005. 28 (suppl 1): S4-36.

59. NICE. Guidelines for the diagnosis and management of type 1 diabetes in children and young adults. National Institute of Health and Clinical Excellence, July 2004.

60. Maahs DM, Wadwa RP, Bishop F, Daniels SR, Rewers M, Klingensmith GJ. Dyslipidemia in youth with diabetes: to treat or not to treat? *J Pediatr* 2008; 153: 458-65.

61. Seipelt IM, Crawford SE, Rodgers S, Backer C, Mavroudis C, Seipelt RG, Pahl E. Hypercholesterolemia is common after pediatric heart transplantation: initial experience with pravastatin. *J Heart Lung Transplant* 2004; 23: 317-22.

62. Penson MG, Fricker FJ, Thompson JR. Safety and efficacy of pravastatin therapy for the prevention of hyperlipidemia in pediatric and adolescent cardiac transplant recipients. *J Heart Lung Transplant* 2001; 20: 611-8.

63. Tassiopoulos K, Williams PL, Seage GR 3rd, Crain M, Oleske J, Farley J; International Maternal Pediatric Adolescent AIDS clinical Trials 219C Team. Association of hypercholesterolemia incidence with antiretroviral treatment, including protease inhibitors, among perinatally HIV-infected children. *J Acquir Immune Defic Syndr* 2008; 47: 607-14.

64. Gonzalez-Tome MI, Amador JT, Peña MJ, Gomez ML, Conejo PR, Fontelos PM. Outcome of protease inhibitor substitution with nevirapine in HIV-1 infected children. *BMC Infect Dis* 2008; 8: 144.

65. Lechner BL, Bockenhauer D, Iragorri S, Kennedy TL, Siegel NJ. The risk of cardiovascular disease in adults who have had childhood nephritic syndrome. *Pediatr Nephrol* 2004; 19: 744-8.

66. Garcia-de-la-Puente S, Arredondo-Garia J, Gutiérrez-Castrellón P, Bojorquez-Ochoa A, Reyna Maya E, Del Pilar Pérez-Martinez M. Efficacy of simvastatin in children with hyperlipidemia secondary to kidney disorders. *Pediatr Nephrol* 2009; Feb 24: Epub ahead of print.

67. Argent E, Kainer G, Aitken M, Rosenberg AR, Mackie FE. Atorvastatin treatment for hyperlipidemia in pediatric renal transplant recipients. *Pediatr Transplant* 2003; 7: 38-42.

68. Butani L. Prospective monitoring of lipid profiles in children receiving pravastatin preemptively after renal transplantation. *Pediatr Transplant* 2005; 9: 746-53.

69. Silverstein DM. Indications and outcome of treatment of hyperlipidemia in pediatric allograft recipients. *Pediatr Transplant* 2003; 7: 7-10.

70. Manhliot C, Larsson P, Gurofsky RC, *et al.* Spectrum and management of hypertriglyceridemia among children in clinical practice. *Pediatrics* 2009; 123: 458-65.

71. Sondike SB, Kay GA, Emmett MK. Weight loss regimens that control for carbohydrate quality or quantity: a review. *Pediatric Diabetes* 2008; 9 (Part II): 33-45.

72. Freedman DS, Dietz WH, Srinivasan SR, *et al.* The relation of overweight to cardiovascular risk factors among children and adolescents: the Bogalusa Heart Study. *Pediatrics* 1999; 103: 1175-82.

73. Korsten-Reck U, Kromeyer-Hauschild K, Korsten K, Baumstark MW, Dickhuth H-H, Berg A. Frequency of secondary dyslipidemia in obese children. *Vascular Health Risk Management* 2008; 4: 1089-94.

74. Steinberger J, Daniels SR, Eckel RH, *et al.* Progress and challenges in metabolic syndrome in children and adolescents: a scientific statement from the American Heart Association Atherosclerosis, Hypertension, and Obesity in the Young Committee of the Council on Cardiovascular Disease in the Young; Council on Cardiovascular Nursing; and Council on Nutrition, Physical Activity, and Metabolism. *Circulation* 2009; 119: 628-47.

75. Spear BA, Barlow SE, Ervin C, Ludwig DS, Saelens BE, Schetzina KE, Taveras EM. Recommendations for treatment of children and adolescent overweight and obesity. *Pediatrics* 2007; 120 Suppl 4; S254-88.

76. Koo KS, Chook P, Yu CW, *et al.* Effects of diet and exercise on obesity-related vascular dysfunction in children. *Circulation* 2004; 109: 1981-6.

77. Kaistha A, Deckelbaum RJ, Starc TJ, Couch SC. Overrestriction of dietary fat intake before formal nutritional counseling in children with hyperlipidemia. *Arch Pediatr Adolesc Med* 2001; 155: 1225-30.

78. Obarzanek E, Kimm SY, Barton BA, *et al.* Long-term safety and efficacy of a cholesterol-lowering diet in childen with elevated low-density lipoprotein cholesterol: seven-year results of the Dietary Intervention Study in Children (DISC). *Pediatrics* 2001; 107: 256-64.

79. Van Horn L, Obarzanek E, Friedman LA, Gernhofer N, Barton B. Children's adaptations to a fat-reduced diet: the Dietary Intervention Study in Children (DISC). *Pediatrics* 2005; 115: 1723-33.

80. Raitakari OT, Ronnemaa T, Jarvisalo MJ, *et al.* Endothelial function in healthy 11-year-old children after dietary intervention with onset in infancy: the Special Turku Coronary Risk Factor Intervention Project for children (STRIP). *Circulation* 2005; 112: 3786-94.

81. Kelley GA. Kelley KS. Effects of aerobic exercise on non-high-density lipoprotein cholesterol in children and adolescents: a meta-analysis of randomized controlled trials. *Prog Cardiovasc Nurs* 2008; 23: 128-32.

82. Gidding SS, Dennison BA, Birch LL *et al.* Dietary recommendations for children and adolescents. A guide for practitioners. Consensus statement from the American Heart Association. *Circulation* 2005; 112: 2061-75.

83. 2008 Physical Activity Guidelines for Americans Summary. Accessed at http://www.health.gov/PAGuidelines/ on March 24, 2009.

84. Flouris AD, Faught BE, Klentrou P. Cardiovascular disease risk in adolescent smokers: evidence of a 'smoker lifestyle'. *J Child Health Care* 2008; 12: 221-31.

85. Grimshaw GM, Stanton A. Tobacco cessation interventions for young people. *Cochrane Database Syst Rev* 2006; CD003289.

86. Moruisi K, Oosthuizen W, Opperman AM. Phytosterols/stanols lower cholesterol concentrations in familial hypercholesterolemic subjects: a systematic review with meta-analysis. *J Am Coll Nutr* 2006; 25: 41-8.

87. Amundsen AL, Ntanios F, Put N, Ose L. Long-term compliance and changes in plasma lipids, plant sterols and carotenoids in children and parents with FH consuming plant sterol ester-enriched spread. *Eur J Clin Nutr* 2004; 58: 1612-20.

88. Jakulj L, Vissers MN, Rodenburg J, Wiegman A, Trip MD, Kastelein JJ. Plant stanols do not restore endothelial function in pre-pubertal children with familial hypercholesterolemia despite reduction of low-density lipoprotein cholesterol levels. *J Pediatr* 2006; 148: 495-500.

89. McCrindle BW, Urbina EM, Dennison BA, *et al.* Drug therapy for high-risk lipid abnormalities in children and adolescents: a scientific statement from the American Heart Association Atherosclerosis, Hypertension, and Obesity in Youth Committee, Council of Cardiovascular Disease in the Young with the Council on Cardiovascular Nursing. *Circulation* 2007; 115: 1948-67.

90. Avis HJ, Vissers MN, Stein EA, Wijburg FA, Trip MD, Kastelein JJP, Hutten GA. A systematic review and meta-analysis of statin therapy in children with familial hypercholesterolemia. *Arterioscler Thromb Vasc Biol* 2007; 27: 1803-10.

91. De Jongh S, Lilien MR, op't Roodt J, Stroes ES, Bakker HD, Katelein JJ. Early statin therapy restores endothelial function in children with familial hypercholesterolemia. *J Am Coll Cardiol* 2002; 40: 2117-21.

92. Wiegman A, Hutten BA, de Groot E, *et al*. Efficacy and safety of statin therapy in children with familial hypercholesterolemia: a randomized controlled trial. *JAMA* 2004; 292: 331-7.

93. Rodenburg J, Vissers MN, Wiegman A, *et al*. Statin treatment in children with familial hypercholesterolemia. The younger, the better. *Circulation* 2007; 116: 664-8.

94. Arambepola C, Farmer AJ, Perera R, Heil HAW. Statin treatment for children and adolescents with heterozygous familial hypercholesterolaemia. A systematic review and meta-analysis. *Atherosclerosis* 2007; 195: 339-47.

95. McCrindle BW. Hyperlipidemia in children. *Thromb Res* 2006; 118: 49-58.

96. Rodenburg J, Vissers MN, Daniels SR, Wiegman A, Kastelein JJ. Lipid-lowering medications. *Pediatr Endocrinol Rev* 2004; 2 Suppl 1: 171-80.

97. van der Graaf A, Cuffie-Jackson C, Vissers MN, *et al*. Efficacy and safety of coadministration of ezetimibe and simvastatin in adolescents with heterozygous familial hypercholesterolemia. *J Am Coll Cardiol* 2008; 52: 1421-9.

98. Kolansky DM, Cuchel M, Clark BJ, *et al*. Longitudinal evaluation and assessment of cardiovascular disease in patients with homozygous familial hypercholesterolemia. *Am J Cardiol* 2008; 102: 1438-43.

99. Gilbert GR, Heart UK LDL apheresis Working Group. Recommendations for the use of LDL apheresis. *Atherosclerosis* 2008; 198: 247-55.

100. Hudgins LC, Bleinman B, Scheuer A, White S, Gordon BR. Long-term safety and efficacy of low-density lipoprotein apheresis in childhood for homozygous familial hypercholesterolemia. *Am J Cardiol* 2008; 102: 1199-204.

Chapter 10

Contribution of the atherogenic dyslipidemic phenotype to the increased cardiovascular disease risk of the metabolic syndrome and diabetes mellitus

Benoit J. Arsenault PhD, Researcher
Jean-Pierre Després PhD FAHA, Director of Research, Cardiology
Centre de Recherche de l'Institut Universitaire de
Cardiologie et de Pneumologie de Québec, Canada

Introduction

The discovery of insulin in the 1920s has transformed diabetes, an initially lethal metabolic disease, into a condition which, when properly managed, no longer has a major impact on life expectancy and quality. Later on, a distinction was made when investigators realized that the hyperglycemic state of diabetes could result from a lack of insulin secretion (type 1 diabetes) or from resistance to its effects (type 2 diabetes) [1] **(IV/C)**. Until recently, type 2 diabetes was considered as a relatively mild metabolic condition associated with ageing without any severe consequences on global population health. However, as a result of poor nutritional habits and sedentary lifestyle, there has been a sharp increase in the worldwide prevalence of type 2 diabetes. According to the World Health Organization, more than 180 million people have diabetes and conservative estimates suggest that this number will double over the next 20 years [2] **(IV/C)**. Diabetes mellitus is now considered as one of the major contemporary causes of premature mortality and morbidity in both developed and developing countries. In several regions of the world, diabetes is the leading cause of microvascular diseases such as renal failure, blindness and lower limb amputation [3]. As approximately half of people with diabetes will die from cardiovascular disease (CVD), it is also now one of the leading causes of death. Several studies have suggested that patients with diabetes mellitus without any CVD history carry the same risk of having a myocardial infarction than patients without diabetes mellitus who had previously suffered a myocardial infarction (Figure 1) [4, 5] **(IIa/B)**. Given the alarming rates of diabetes and its harmful consequences on cardiovascular mortality and morbidity, understanding the molecular basis of this metabolic disease and its relationship with CVD are topics of considerable clinical interest with important public health implications.

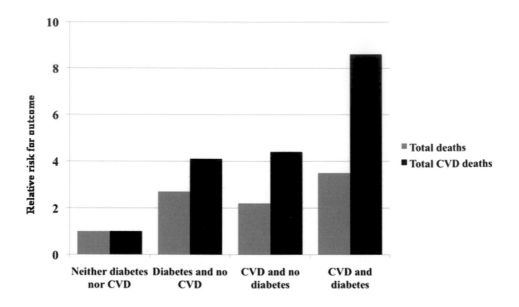

Figure 1. Hazard ratio for total and cardiovascular mortality over a follow-up of 24 years among men of the Québec Cardiovascular study classified on the basis of baseline clinical status (with vs. without CVD and with vs. without diabetes). *Reproduced with permission [5]. This work is protected by copyright and the making of this copy was with the permission of Access Copyright. Any alteration of its content or further copying in any form whatsoever is strictly prohibited unless otherwise permitted by law. © 2009 Canadian Medical Association.*

Several risk factors for type 2 diabetes mellitus have been identified. They include non-modifiable risk factors such as ageing, ethnicity, family history of diabetes and intra-uterine environment. Although these risk factors may account to a certain extent for the increased diabetes mellitus rates, it is now well accepted that the rapid increase in the prevalence of obesity that is witnessed in almost every region of the world plays a major role in the increasing prevalence of type 2 diabetes. In fact, more than 80% of patients with type 2 diabetes are obese. Obesity, and particularly abdominal obesity, is a major risk factor for diabetes mellitus [6, 7]. There are several pathophysiological links between abdominal obesity and diabetes mellitus including insulin resistance, inflammation, dyslipidemia, ectopic fat deposition, hypertension, etc. Over many decades, many investigators have attempted to put a nametag on the 'prediabetic' condition. Although it is not our objective to review the history of the conceptual definition that led to the concept of metabolic syndrome (a constellation of CVD risk factors associated with insulin resistance, dyslipidemia, hypertension and abdominal obesity), we will discuss the pathophysiology and management of the diabetic or atherogenic dyslipidemia, a typical dyslipidemic phenotype that almost always coexists with visceral obesity/ectopic fat, insulin resistance and features of the metabolic syndrome.

Visceral adipose tissue/ectopic fat: the epicenter of the type 2 diabetes pandemic

Compared to Europids, South Asians develop abdominal obesity earlier in their lives and are more susceptible to the vascular consequences of obesity, even with a lower amount of total body fat [8]. In a recent attempt to identify the biological factors that might predispose South Asians to these adverse consequences, Sniderman and colleagues [9] have suggested that lipid overload and overflow from a metabolically inert and functional superficial subcutaneous adipose tissue to other compartments, mainly visceral adipose tissue and other organs such as the liver, skeletal muscles, the heart and even the pancreas might account to a very significant extent for these differences among ethnicities. Although this might explain why South Asians are more susceptible to develop diabetes mellitus, based on this hypothesis, each and every individual who carry a certain amount of visceral fat, independent from ethnicity, is at risk for diabetes mellitus. Figure 2 shows the temporal relationship and the links between visceral fat accumulation and the diabetes-driven CVD risk.

There is now compelling evidence suggesting that, as opposed to superficial subcutaneous fat accumulation located in the abdomen, around the thighs or the legs, visceral or intra-abdominal adipose tissue is closely associated with features of insulin resistance and the metabolic syndrome [10]. This heterogeneity among different fat

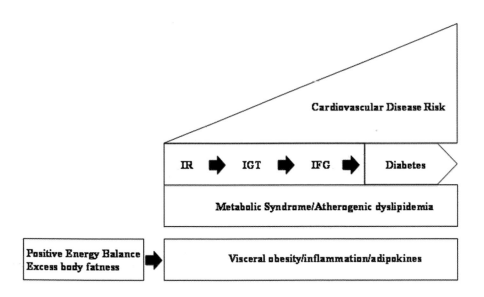

Figure 2. Relationship between visceral fat accumulation and associated metabolic consequences and the diabetes-driven CVD risk. IR = insulin resistance; IGT = impaired glucose tolerance; IFG = impaired fasting glucose. *Reproduced with permission from Rader DJ. Effect of insulin resistance, dyslipidemia, and intra-abdominal adiposity on the development of cardiovascular disease and diabetes mellitus. The American Journal of Medicine 2007; 120(3): 1. © 2007, Elsevier Limited.*

compartments is most likely to be attributable to the biology and the local environment of the visceral adipocyte. It is well accepted that the most important function of adipose tissue, independent from its anatomical location, is to store excess energy. This process is mediated by the lipoprotein lipase (LPL), a central enzyme in lipoprotein-lipid metabolism. Its main function is to hydrolyze chylomicrons and very-low-density lipoproteins (VLDL) or triglyceride-rich lipoproteins [11]. Upon hydrolysis, triglycerides are stored inside adipocytes into large vacuoles. Under homeostatic conditions, insulin concentrations are increased during the post-prandial state. Insulin is of primary importance to stimulate glucose uptake by most of the organs of the human body including adipose tissue. Another important action of insulin is to stimulate the expression of LPL. However, a local insulin resistance state within the visceral fat depot is known to alter insulin-mediated LPL expression/activity. As LPL is considered the rate-limiting enzyme for triglyceride storage in adipose tissue, downregulation of LPL promotes delayed post-prandial lipid clearance and, therefore, increases post-prandial lipemia, an important risk factor for CVD [12]. Similarly, apolipoprotein CIII (apoCIII) also contributes to the link between insulin resistance and dyslipidemia. ApoCIII has been shown to inhibit the LDL receptor-mediated uptake of remnant lipoproteins and to be a potent inhibitor of LPL. Evidence suggested that apoCIII genetic variants such as the apoCIII SstI polymorphism could modulate the magnitude of the dyslipidemic state in abdominally obese individuals [13]. As the hepatic production of apoCIII is increased in insulin resistance, the catabolism of triglyceride-rich lipoproteins is significantly altered, thereby contributing to the increased plasma levels of remnant-like particles [14].

Meanwhile, as opposed to subcutaneous adipocytes, visceral adipocytes have an increased density in β2- and β3-adrenoreceptors [15]. As a result, adipocytes located in the visceral depots have an increased susceptibility to catecholamine-induced lipolysis, i.e. the hydrolysis of stored triglycerides into free fatty acids (FFA) and glycerol. This process is mediated by the hormone-sensitive lipase (HSL), which, upon activation, promotes lipolysis. The end products of lipolysis are then secreted into the bloodstream. These FFA are drained out from visceral adipocytes by the portal vein, which carries adipose tissue-derived FFA up to the liver. The simultaneous effect of LPL downregulation and the impaired insulin action on HSL inhibition in people who are insulin resistant is an important cause of the diabetic dyslipidemia that will be discussed in the next section.

Although the above-mentioned dysregulation of fatty acid storage and enhanced lipolysis model explains to a great extent the close association between 'sick' visceral adipose tissue and dyslipidemia, one must not disregard the primary importance of adipose tissue macrophage polarization and the associated adipokine secretion hypothesis [16]. It was not until 15 years ago that the scientific and medical communities came to appreciate one of the most important and fascinating biological aspects of adipose tissue: its 'endocrine' activity. Both visceral and subcutaneous fat depots secrete several adipokines that may impact numerous biological systems of the human body such as glucose-insulin homeostasis, lipoprotein-lipid metabolism, the immune response, thrombosis and the regulation of blood pressure. This has led several investigators to suggest that adipose tissue is at the center of an important cross-talk that includes several other organs such as the liver, skeletal muscles, the heart, the pancreas and the brain. More than 15 years ago, leptin was the first ever-identified adipokine [17]. Leptin secretion by adipocytes increases as a function of total fat accumulation. Although its main function is to act centrally where it influences food intake and the regulation of body weight, leptin may also reach the liver and downregulate the lipogenic transcription factor sterol regulatory element binding-protein (SREBP)-1c and activate 5' adenosine monophosphate-activated protein (AMP)-kinase, thereby increasing fatty acid oxidation and limiting liver fat accumulation [18]. However, as adipose tissue mass expands, a state of leptin resistance slowly develops, which may lead to increased liver fat accumulation. Some have proposed that leptin resistance is an early step in the development of the metabolic syndrome [19]. In addition, the relatively high concentrations of leptin found in the obese are also responsible for an increased macrophage and T-cell infiltration not only within the visceral adipose depot, but also within the arterial wall where it directly promotes atherosclerosis [20]. The role of leptin as an important immune regulator is also supported by the role of this adipokine in promoting the release of several other cytokines such as tumor necrosis factor-α (TNF-α) and interleukin-6 (IL-6) [21]. It has also been shown that several cell populations located within the visceral adipose tissue contribute to the production of these cytokines, including fat cells themselves, but also macrophages residing within visceral adipose tissue [22].

Although it is beyond the scope of this chapter to discuss the numerous effects of these inflammatory cytokines on the vasculature, there is increasing evidence suggesting that these adipokines modulate the release of FFA by visceral adipocytes and may substantially contribute to the atherogenic dyslipidemia of insulin resistance. On top of regulating several inflammatory processes, TNF-α plays several key roles within the adipose tissue and is involved at numerous stages of the local insulin resistance state. First, TNF-α can slow the differentiation process of pre-adipocytes into mature adipocytes by inhibiting the nuclear transcription factor CCAAT enhancer binding protein (C/EBP)-β as well as the peroxisome-proliferator activated receptor (PPAR)-γ (Figure 3). Therefore, by inhibiting adipocyte maturation and differentiation on one hand, and by inducing apoptosis of adipocytes, TNF-α favours adipocyte hypertrophy [23]. As a consequence, since they can no longer replicate, visceral adipocytes must keep up with triglyceride storage by increasing their size, which makes them resistant to the local effects of insulin. This is believed to be one of the most important mechanisms linking inflammation and lipolysis. Moreover, it has been shown that TNF-α itself can increase the expression of IL-6 by visceral adipocytes [24]. Similar to TNF-α, IL-6 has several autocrine and paracrine roles and this adipokine is thought to promote insulin resistance as well as the development of atherosclerosis. IL-6 is an important regulator of the hepatic systemic inflammatory response [25]. It has been shown that IL-6 would be the most important hormonal factor contributing to the hepatic expression of acute phase proteins such as serum amyloid-A (SAA) and C-reactive protein (CRP) as well as prothrombotic factors such as fibrinogen [26-28].

Not all adipose tissue-derived hormones are detrimental for cardiovascular health. It has been shown that plasma levels of adiponectin are decreased in viscerally obese men, a phenomenon likely to be attributable to adipocyte hypertrophy and local inflammation [29]. Adiponectin, unlike the above-mentioned adipokines, has anti-inflammatory effects and prevents the development of insulin resistance. A reduction in plasma adiponectin concentrations may have a negative impact on the development of atherosclerosis via several mechanisms that have been previously reviewed [30, 31]. Adiponectin is also thought to play a

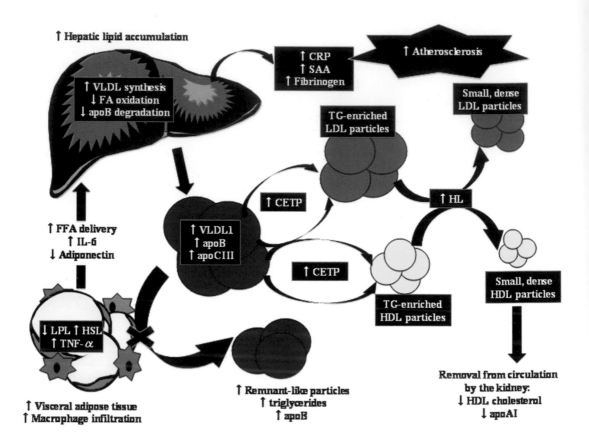

↑ Hepatic lipid accumulation

↑ VLDL synthesis
↓ FA oxidation
↓ apoB degradation

↑ CRP
↑ SAA
↑ Fibrinogen

↑ Atherosclerosis

Small, dense
LDL particles

TG-enriched
LDL particles

↑ CETP

↑ HL

↑ FFA delivery
↑ IL-6
↓ Adiponectin

↑ VLDL1
↑ apoB
↑ apoCIII

↑ CETP

↓ LPL ↑ HSL
↑ TNF-α

Small, dense
HDL particles

TG-enriched
HDL particles

Removal from circulation
by the kidney:
↓ HDL cholesterol
↓ apoAI

↑ Visceral adipose tissue
↑ Macrophage infiltration

↑ Remnant-like particles
↑ triglycerides
↑ apoB

Figure 3. Lipoprotein-lipid metabolism under the influence of visceral obesity and ectopic fat deposition. LPL = lipoprotein lipase; HSL = hormone-sensitive lipase; TNF-α = tumor necrosis factor-α; IL-6 = interleukin-6; FFA = free fatty acids; FA = fatty acids; VLDL = very-low-density lipoprotein; LDL = low-density lipoprotein; HDL = high-density lipoprotein; apoB = apolipoprotein B; apoAI = apolipoprotein AI; apoCIII = apolipoprotein CIII; TG = triglycerides; CETP = cholesteryl ester transfer protein; HL = hepatic lipase; CRP = C-reactive protein; SAA = serum amyloid-A.

direct role in lipoprotein-lipid metabolism. Low adiponectin concentrations are associated with increased levels of both liver fat and visceral adipose tissue and may thus represent a fairly good marker of poor lipid handling by peripheral tissues [32]. In the liver, adiponectin decreases gluconeogenesis and increases fatty acid oxidation (via AMP-kinase) and, therefore, decreases the production of triglyceride-enriched VLDL particles.

In summary, visceral adipose tissue has a fundamental role to play in the etiology of insulin resistance and metabolic syndrome. Because it is plunged in an insulin resistant and pro-inflammatory milieu, visceral adipose tissue cannot maintain its biological function of triglyceride storage. A large visceral adipose tissue depot is therefore a 'sick' type of adipose tissue that closely correlates with accumulation of fat into other tissues such as the liver, the skeletal muscle, the pancreas and the heart. The following sections will focus on the clinical manifestations associated with ectopic fat deposition (i.e. metabolic syndrome) and on the management of the often underdiagnosed CVD risk factors associated with visceral obesity.

Metabolic origins of the diabetic dyslipidemic state

Many patients with diabetes mellitus carry a dyslipidemic phenotype which includes high triglyceride and low HDL cholesterol levels, with a preponderance of small, dense LDL particles; such condition often being referred to as the atherogenic lipid triad [33, 34]. It is important to highlight that, except for individuals with specific genetic diseases, these metabolic alterations are not found in isolation and rather tend to cluster, especially among sedentary individuals who are viscerally obese. The lipid triad is also highly prevalent in individuals without diabetes mellitus but who are nevertheless characterized by excessive accumulation of visceral adipose tissue/ectopic fat.

The consequences of the hyperlipolytic activity of visceral adipocytes, combined with their relative reduced ability to efficiently catabolize triglyceride-rich lipoproteins, lead to increased FFA concentrations which are transported to the liver, thereby contributing to increased lipid deposition in the liver and overproduction and increased secretion of apolipoprotein-B (apoB) containing very-low-density lipoproteins (VLDL). As a consequence, plasma triglyceride and apoB concentrations are often elevated in individuals who are insulin resistant or diabetic, with major consequences on LDL integrity. Hypertriglyceridemia is an important marker of CVD risk. In a meta-analysis that included 262,525 participants of whom 10,158 were coronary artery disease (CAD) cases that were drawn from 29 prospective studies, after adjusting for age, sex, smoking, blood pressure and LDL cholesterol, the odds ratio for future CAD was 1.72 (95% CI, 1.56-1.90) for participants of the top triglyceride tertile compared to the bottom tertile [35] (Ia/A). Similarly, post hoc analyses conducted in the PROVE-IT TIMI 22 trial have shown that patients with prior acute coronary syndrome who achieved low triglyceride levels (<150mg/dL) upon statin treatment were at lower risk of recurrent CHD events, thereby underlining the importance of achieving low triglyceride concentrations on top of low LDL cholesterol levels [36] (Ib/A). Triglyceride levels are correlated with other parameters of the lipoprotein-lipid profile such as non-HDL cholesterol levels, apoB levels and LDL particle size, but not with plasma LDL concentrations (Figure 4). Although hypertriglyceridemia does not impact LDL cholesterol concentration *per se*, the hypertriglyceridemic state associated with insulin resistance significantly alters the physicochemical properties of LDL particles. Indeed, it is now well recognized that mean LDL particle size is reduced in patients with type 2 diabetes and studies have shown that visceral adiposity is an important factor to explain the high prevalence of the small LDL phenotype in patients with type 2 diabetes [37, 38]. However, independently of the glycemic status, LDL particle size correlates well with triglycerides, HDL cholesterol levels and the total to HDL cholesterol ratio, which suggests that this atherogenic phenotype can be observed among individuals who have visceral obesity and high triglycerides, even if they are not diabetic [39]. Based on this evidence, assessing LDL quality on top of LDL cholesterol levels is of primary

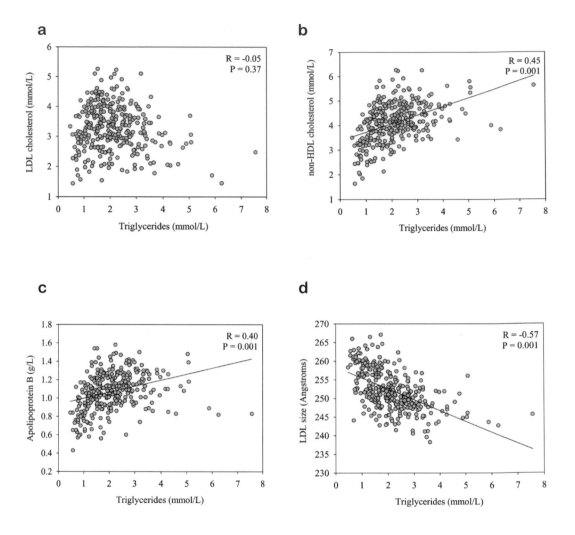

Figure 4. The relationship between plasma triglyceride levels and (a) LDL cholesterol levels, (b) non-HDL cholesterol levels, (c) apolipoprotein B levels, (d) LDL particle size, in a sample of 320 healthy men without diabetes.

importance for the optimal assessment and management of lipid disorders in diabetes mellitus. In this regard, as each LDL particle contains one molecule of apoB, the measurement of apoB could provide valuable information in the evaluation of the number of circulating LDL particles in clinical settings [40]. Plasma apoB levels could therefore represent an inexpensive and very useful marker of both LDL quantity and quality [41].

It is also well recognized that plasma levels of HDL cholesterol are reduced in patients with diabetes mellitus. Reduction of plasma HDL cholesterol levels in insulin resistant and diabetic patients are most likely to be attributable to the increased catabolism of HDL via apolipoprotein AI (apoAI), the most important core surface protein of HDLs [42, 43]. On top of HDL cholesterol levels, mean HDL particle size is also reduced in insulin resistant individuals [44]. Reduction in HDL size is known to be a consequence of the increased hepatic lipase (HL) activity, which alters HDL size, especially in the presence of hypertriglyceridemia. Upon these biological circumstances, small HDL particles are rapidly removed from the circulation by the kidney, which further contribute to reduce HDL cholesterol levels [45].

The cholesteryl ester transfer protein (CETP) is another enzyme involved in the remodelling of lipoprotein particles. The main biological role of CETP is to transfer cholesteryl esters from HDL particles into apoB-containing lipoproteins in exchange for triglycerides, thus making HDL particles smaller, denser and more prone to hydrolysis by HL [46]. Increased CETP and triglyceride concentrations have been shown to be associated with increased plasma cholesteryl ester transfer; such a process being also correlated with carotid intima-media thickness in patients with and without diabetes mellitus [47] **(IIa/B)**. A prospective study has also shown that CETP concentrations are associated with incident coronary artery disease, especially in participants who showed elevated triglyceride concentrations [48] **(IIa/B)**. Meanwhile, a recent meta-analysis has reported that well described genetic variants of the *CETP* gene are associated with a reduced CETP activity and with a reduced CVD risk that was most likely attributable to the increased HDL cholesterol levels found in carriers of the favourable genotype [49] **(Ia/A)**. Figure 3 summarizes the pathobiological pathways linking excess visceral adipose tissue and liver fat accumulation with the atherogenic dyslipidemia of insulin resistance.

Management of the atherogenic dyslipidemia of insulin resistance

Conventional lipid-lowering therapy

In patients with diabetes mellitus, intensive glycemic control is at the cornerstone of management of microvascular risk. However, recent trials have shown that intensive therapy targeting glycemic control does not significantly reduce the risk of major cardiovascular events and could even increase mortality under some circumstances [50-52] **(Ia/A)**. Therefore, in order to reduce the macrovascular complications of diabetes mellitus, targeting other risk factors such as lipids is of primary importance. As a significant proportion of individuals with impaired glucose tolerance are on their way to developing full-blown diabetes mellitus, the optimal management of lipids could also be important in prediabetic individuals. Several studies have tested the effects of HMG-CoA inhibitors or statins, in patients with diabetes mellitus. The first clinical outcome trial to measure the efficacy of statin therapy in patients with diabetes (who were also characterized by the presence of another CVD risk factor) was CARDS (Collaborative Atorvastatin Diabetes Study). The CARDS investigators reported a 37% decrease in the incidence of major cardiovascular events in patients treated with atorvastatin over a 3.9-year follow-up [53] **(Ia/A)**. In a similar study conducted among patients at lower global CVD risk, the ASPEN (Atorvastatin Study for Prevention of Coronary Heart Disease Endpoints in Non-Insulin-Dependant Diabetes Mellitus) found a similar risk reduction (approximately 10%) in patients treated with atorvastatin 10mg [54] **(Ia/A)**. In another study performed among patients with diabetes mellitus with high triglyceride levels, both low-dose and high-dose statin therapy induced important changes in triglyceride levels [55] (Ia/A). Outcome studies are needed to investigate whether statin therapy would reduce CVD risk in these diabetic patients with high triglyceride levels. A recent meta-analysis using data from 18,686 patients with diabetes in 14 randomized prospective trials nevertheless confirmed the benefits of statin therapy in these patients [56] (Ia/A). This study showed that statin therapy was associated with a 21-25% decreased risk in various cardiovascular outcomes per 1mmol/L reduction in LDL cholesterol while reporting a 9% decreased risk in all-cause mortality. The results of the meta-analysis of the Cholesterol Treatment Trialists' Collaborators reported that even in patients who achieved targeted LDL cholesterol levels, the presence of low HDL cholesterol and/or elevated triglyceride concentrations remained predictive of an increased CVD risk. In addition, a recently published post hoc analysis of the Treating to New Targets (TNT) trial has shown that in patients with documented coronary heart disease with or without diabetes, patients with the metabolic syndrome had a more beneficial impact of high-dose statin therapy (atorvastatin 80mg) compared to those without the metabolic syndrome [57] (Ia/A). Also, this study showed that the magnitude of risk reduction observed with high-dose statin therapy was positively associated with the number of metabolic syndrome components as patients with all five components of the metabolic syndrome treated with high-dose statin had a higher risk reduction than those treated with low-dose statin (atorvastatin 10mg).

As previously stated, LDL cholesterol concentrations are not always elevated in the atherogenic dyslipidemia of insulin resistance. Therefore, pharmacological agents targeting other components of the lipoprotein-lipid profile such as the lipid triad might be effective to lower macrovascular risk in insulin resistant individuals. In that regard, fibric acid derivatives, or fibrates, have been shown to improve several markers of the lipoprotein profile through the hepatic activation of PPAR-α. Fibrates are known to reduce the secretion of VLDL particles as well as apoCIII by the liver. PPAR-α activation also increases plasma apoAI levels, and increases LPL activity in the adipose tissue. Such changes contribute to improve the catabolism of triglyceride-rich lipoproteins, leading to a shift in the size and density of LDL particles towards larger and more buoyant cholesteryl ester-rich LDL particles [58, 59]. Several studies described below have shown that despite having a moderate effect on plasma LDL cholesterol levels, fibrates induce 20-50% decreases in triglyceride levels while increasing HDL cholesterol by 10-35%. Because of these favourable impacts on the lipid triad, the efficiency of fibrates has been tested in large multicenter randomized trials. For instance, in the Veterans Affairs High-Density Lipoprotein Intervention Trial (VA-HIT) [60] (Ia/A), which tested the efficacy of gemfibrozil for the secondary prevention of coronary heart disease in men with low HDL levels, a significant reduction in the risk of major cardiovascular events in patients with coronary disease was observed. Another trial specifically designed to assess the potential contribution of another fibrate, fenofibrate, in patients with type 2 diabetes, the Fenofibrate Intervention and Event Lowering in Diabetes (FIELD) study, failed to report a lowering of CHD events with fenofibrate in this large population of patients with diabetes mellitus [61] (Ia/A). However, post hoc analyses conducted in the FIELD study population and in other fibrate trials have suggested that the cardiovascular benefits of fibrate therapy may be limited to patients with either insulin resistance or to those with the metabolic syndrome [62-64]. Thus, these observations suggest that fibrate therapy is not suitable for every diabetic patient.

In fact, the recent Action to Control Cardiovascular Risk in Diabetes (ACCORD) trial substantiated that fenofibrate on top of statins did not reduce the rate of fatal cardiovascular events, non-fatal myocardial infarction, or non-fatal stroke. These results do not support the routine use of fibrates on top of statins in high-risk type 2 diabetes mellitus patients, especially in those with triglyceride and HDL levels in the normal range [65] **(Ia/A)**.

PPAR-γ agonists or thiazolidinediones (TZD) are often used in patients with diabetes mellitus and/or impaired glucose tolerance. Over the past few years, studies have shown that treatment with either pioglitazone or rosiglitazone, two commonly used TZDs, improved several indices of insulin resistance as well as other features of the cardiometabolic risk profile. For instance, the Pioglitazone Effect on Regression of Intravascular Sonographic Coronary Obstruction Prospective Evaluation (PERISCOPE) trial as well as the Carotid Intima-Media Thickness in Atherosclerosis Using Pioglitazone (CHICAGO) trial have shown that pioglitazone may slow the progression of atherosclerosis in patients with CHD and diabetes [66, 67] **(Ia/A)**. It has also been suggested that the beneficial impact of pioglitazone on carotid intima-media thickness (cIMT) was largely attributable to the impact of pioglitazone on specific features of the cardiometabolic risk profile such as plasma HDL cholesterol levels [68]. Similarly, rosiglitazone treatment has been shown to reduce the incidence of diabetes in patients with impaired glucose tolerance. For instance, in the Diabetes Reduction Assessment with Ramipril and Rosiglitazone Medication (DREAM) trial, which included 5269 participants with impaired glucose tolerance, the incidence of diabetes was reduced by 60% in participants treated with rosiglitazone 8mg/day compared to those treated with placebo [69] **(Ia/A)**. In this trial, rosiglitazone also induced a moderate reduction of cIMT [70]. Moreover, despite causing significant weight gain, TZDs have been shown to improve plasma levels of several cardiometabolic risk markers such as triglycerides, HDL cholesterol, C-reactive protein, adiponectin and circulating free-fatty acids [67, 68] **(IIa/B)**. Kim and colleagues [71] **(IIa/B)** tested the effect of rosiglitazone (4mg/day) on body fat distribution in 173 patients with diabetes mellitus. They found that although treatment with rosiglitazone induced weight gain (approximately 0.8kg), it did not increase the amount of atherogenic visceral fat. Rather, treatment with rosiglitazone significantly increased the amount of subcutaneous fat mass, which was found to be an independent predictor of changes in fasting glucose. These results suggest that, by increasing subcutaneous fat mass, TZDs create a 'metabolic sink' that could store excess energy and protect peripheral organs from lipid deposition. Although TZDs may be helpful to treat patients with insulin resistance and associated dyslipidemia, the impact of this class of drug on body weight and its potential harmful effects on cardiovascular risk warrant prudency. Indeed, an early meta-analysis of randomized controlled trials that have studied the relationship between rosiglitazone treatment and the incidence of CVD had reported that this drug may potentially increase CVD risk [72] **(Ia/A)**. However, recently published randomized controlled trials such as the Diabetes Outcome Progression trial (ADOPT) confirmed that despite causing weight gain, rosiglitazone did not increase the risk of major cardiovascular events [73] **(Ia/A)**. In this regard, the Rosiglitazone Evaluated for Cardiac Outcomes and Regulation of Glycaemia in Diabetes (RECORD) study reported that rosiglitazone treatment may increase the risk of heart failure, but does not appear to increase cardiovascular morbidity in patients with type 2 diabetes [74] **(Ia/A)**. Thus, although there is robust evidence that TZDs can prevent or at least delay the development of type 2 diabetes and improve glycemic control and several CVD risk factors in patients with type 2 diabetes, the relevance of this class of drugs to the management of CVD remains debated.

Finally, other therapeutic options may be useful in the treatment of atherogenic dyslipidemia such as nicotinic acid, bile acid sequestrants, ezetimibe, dual PPAR-α and PPAR-γ agonists, CETP inhibitors or omega-3 fatty acids [75].

Visceral obesity/ectopic fat: a new therapeutic target for management of CVD risk in patients with type 2 diabetes/metabolic syndrome?

As previously stated, more than 80% of patients with diabetes are either obese and/or have the metabolic syndrome. As diabetes and its associated dyslipidemic state largely result from an excess of visceral adipose tissue/ectopic fat, targeting visceral obesity via lifestyle modification therapy should remain at the forefront of lipid management not only in patients with diabetes mellitus, but also in all individuals with atherogenic dyslipidemia of insulin resistance. Evidence supporting the use of lifestyle therapy in the prevention of diabetes mellitus came from only a few studies. Among them, the Diabetes Prevention Program (DPP) randomly assigned 3234 participants with impaired glucose tolerance to either a placebo with standard lifestyle recommendations, to the antihyperglycemic agent, metformin, with standard lifestyle recommendations or to a lifestyle-modifying program aiming at promoting and maintaining a 7% body weight reduction [76] (Ia/A). During the 3.2-year follow-up, diabetes incidence was reduced by 58% and by 31% in the lifestyle and metformin groups, respectively, as compared to the placebo arm. Importantly, compared to the metformin group, a larger proportion of subjects of the lifestyle group had normal post-load glucose values at the end of the follow-up. A secondary analysis of the DPP showed that visceral fat, but not subcutaneous fat predicted the onset of diabetes mellitus in the placebo and in the lifestyle groups, most likely because metformin reduces the incidence of diabetes without influencing body composition [77] (Ib/A). An additional post hoc analysis from the DPP revealed that the lifestyle modification program reduced the incidence of the metabolic syndrome by 45% in participants who did not have it at baseline [78] (Ia/A). Accordingly, another study found that even without weight loss, exercise training could promote an important loss of visceral fat [79]. In fact, a meta-analysis reported the existence of a dose response relationship between endurance exercise training and visceral fat reduction [80] (Ia/A). Meanwhile, several studies have shown that the relationship between physical activity and/or abdominal obesity and CVD risk are to a very significant extent explained by underlying abnormalities such as inflammation, dyslipidemia and blood pressure [81, 82]. Meanwhile, although studies have shown that visceral adiposity is more closely associated with a deteriorated cardiometabolic risk profile than cardiorespiratory fitness [83, 84] (III/B), cardiorespiratory fitness is an independent and important risk factor for CVD and overall mortality [85, 86]. A recent meta-analysis conducted on the topic concluded that cardiorespiratory fitness is at least as strongly associated with CVD risk than other established risk factors such as blood pressure, waist circumference, triglyceridemia or glycemia [87] (Ia/A). Based on these observations, prevention strategies for diabetes mellitus and CVD must also consider increasing daily energy expenditure via regular exercise and decreasing energy intake to prevent the accumulation of body fat mass. Unfortunately, long-term adherence to such lifestyle modifications has been reported to be poor and even after successful weight loss, weight regain is often inevitable [88].

Given the poor success rates of lifestyle modification approaches, obese individuals, particularly massively obese individuals are often advised to undergo bariatric surgery. Such intervention has been shown to induce dramatic weight loss and prevent the onset of diabetes mellitus [89] **(IIa/B)**. Bariatric surgery could even cause remission of diabetes mellitus in some massively obese patients [90]. At the tissue level, such an intervention improves the ability of fat tissue to store lipids as well as its insulin sensitivity and reduces macrophage infiltration [91]. However, such intervention was limited to massively obese patients but the spectacular metabolic improvements observed in more moderately obese patients with type 2 diabetes have opened a debate on the large-scale use of bariatric surgery for the management of type 2 diabetes [92]. At the time being, bariatric surgery should be considered as a proof of concept approach to prove the hypothesis that targeting visceral obesity and excess ectopic fat accumulation should be our number one priority to treat the atherogenic dyslipidemia of insulin resistance and even prevent diabetes mellitus onset in high-risk individuals.

Conclusions

Abdominal obesity is ubiquitous in people with insulin resistance and/or diabetes mellitus. These patients have a dysfunctional adipose organ which fails to efficiently store excess energy and rather secretes numerous 'hormones' that alter several biological processes including insulin-mediated glucose uptake in peripheral organs, thereby increasing the risk of diabetes mellitus. Visceral and ectopic fat accumulation is also associated with low-grade inflammation, hypertension and a typical dyslipidemic state that is characterized by high triglyceride and low HDL cholesterol levels as well as by the presence of small LDL and HDL particles, even if LDL cholesterol levels are often 'on target' with statin therapy in these individuals. Targeting visceral adipose tissue/ectopic fat, e.g. the source of this atherogenic dyslipidemia, should be an important therapeutic objective. Visceral adipose tissue and ectopic fat are modifiable CVD/diabetes risk factors that need to be targeted via lifestyle therapy. Aggressive public health policies should be conducted to facilitate the adoption of healthy behaviors at the population level all over the world.

Key points	Evidence level
◆ Individuals with type 2 diabetes mellitus and/or the metabolic syndrome are often characterized by ectopic fat deposition including high levels of intra-abdominal (visceral) adipose tissue.	III/B
◆ Although excess visceral adiposity does not predict increased plasma LDL cholesterol levels, individuals with visceral obesity are very likely to be characterized by the lipid triad, e.g. the combination of elevated triglyceride concentrations, low HDL cholesterol levels and an increased preponderance of small, dense LDL particles.	III/B
◆ Although achieving optimal glucose control is of primary importance in the management of type 2 diabetes, intensive therapy targeting glycemic control does not significantly reduce the risk of major cardiovascular events and could even increase mortality under some circumstances.	Ia/A
◆ Although the vast majority of individuals with type 2 diabetes are treated with statins, results of recent studies have suggested that statin treatment is particularly effective in patients with a deteriorated cardiometabolic risk profile such as those with the atherogenic lipid triad or those with the metabolic syndrome, independently from diabetes status.	Ia/A
◆ Whereas fibrates can be helpful in the management of lipid disorders in patients with the metabolic syndrome or in patients with type 2 diabetes, there is no additive value on cardiovascular event rate compared to statin treatment alone in patients without dyslipidemia.	Ia/A
◆ PPAR-γ agonists, or thiazolidinediones, are insulin sensitizers that are particularly effective in patients with type 2 diabetes characterized by an increased visceral adipose tissue accumulation. Although this class of drugs improves glycemic control and several cardiometabolic risk markers, their contribution to the management of cardiovascular disease risk remains uncertain.	IV/C
◆ Thiazolidinediones may reduce the risk of type 2 diabetes or at least retard its development in individuals with impaired fasting glucose. However, questions have been raised regarding the detrimental side effects of thiazolidinediones, particularly in patients with heart failure.	Ia/A
◆ Improving nutritional and physical activity/exercise habits should be promoted by all means to reduce CVD and diabetes risk in people with the metabolic syndrome.	Ia/A
◆ When lifestyle therapy is not effective, bariatric surgery might be helpful in the management of severely obese patients. Such intervention has been shown to induce dramatic weight loss and prevent the onset of type 2 diabetes. Bariatric surgery could even cause remission of diabetes mellitus in some massively obese patients.	IIa/B

References

1. Report of the Expert Committee on the Diagnosis and Classification of Diabetes Mellitus. *Diabetes Care* 1997; 20(7): 1183-97.
2. http://www.who.int/mediacentre/factsheets/fs312/en/index.html. Accessed 8 May, 2009.
3. Orasanu G, Plutzky J. The pathologic continuum of diabetic vascular disease. *J Am Coll Cardiol* 2009; 53(5 Suppl): S35-42.
4. Haffner SM, Lehto S, Ronnemaa T, Pyorala K, Laakso M. Mortality from coronary heart disease in subjects with type 2 diabetes and in nondiabetic subjects with and without prior myocardial infarction. *N Engl J Med* 1998; 339(4): 229-34.
5. Dagenais GR, St-Pierre A, Gilbert P, Lamarche B, Després JP, Bernard PM, et al. Comparison of prognosis for men with type 2 diabetes mellitus and men with cardiovascular disease. *CMAJ* 2009; 180(1): 40-7.
6. Ohlson LO, Larsson B, Svardsudd K, Welin L, Eriksson H, Wilhelmsen L, et al. The influence of body fat distribution on the incidence of diabetes mellitus. 13.5 years of follow-up of the participants in the study of men born in 1913. *Diabetes* 1985; 34(10): 1055-8.
7. Balkau B, Deanfield JE, Després JP, Bassand JP, Fox KA, Smith SC, Jr., et al. International Day for the Evaluation of Abdominal Obesity (IDEA): a study of waist circumference, cardiovascular disease, and diabetes mellitus in 168,000 primary care patients in 63 countries. *Circulation* 2007; 116(17): 1942-51.
8. Appropriate body-mass index for Asian populations and its implications for policy and intervention strategies. *Lancet* 2004; 363(9403): 157-63.
9. Sniderman AD, Bhopal R, Prabhakaran D, Sarrafzadegan N, Tchernof A. Why might South Asians be so susceptible to central obesity and its atherogenic consequences? The adipose tissue overflow hypothesis. *Int J Epidemiol* 2007; 36(1): 220-5.
10. Carr DB, Utzschneider KM, Hull RL, Kodama K, Retzlaff BM, Brunzell JD, et al. Intra-abdominal fat is a major determinant of the National Cholesterol Education Program Adult Treatment Panel III criteria for the metabolic syndrome. *Diabetes* 2004; 53(8): 2087-94.
11. Eckel RH. Lipoprotein lipase. A multifunctional enzyme relevant to common metabolic diseases. *N Engl J Med* 1989; 320(16): 1060-8.
12. Nordestgaard BG, Benn M, Schnohr P, Tybjaerg-Hansen A. Nonfasting triglycerides and risk of myocardial infarction, ischemic heart disease, and death in men and women. *JAMA* 2007; 298(3): 299-308.
13. Couillard C, Vohl MC, Engert JC, Lemieux I, Houde A, Alméras N, et al. Effect of apoC-III gene polymorphisms on the lipoprotein-lipid profile of viscerally obese men. *J Lipid Res* 2003; 44(5): 986-93.
14. Chan DC, Nguyen MN, Watts GF, Barrett PH. Plasma apolipoprotein C-III transport in centrally obese men: associations with very low-density lipoprotein apolipoprotein B and high-density lipoprotein apolipoprotein A-I metabolism. *J Clin Endocrinol Metab* 2008; 93(2): 557-64.
15. Mauriège P, Galitzky J, Berlan M, Lafontan M. Heterogeneous distribution of beta and alpha-2 adrenoceptor binding sites in human fat cells from various fat deposits: functional consequences. *Eur J Clin Invest* 1987; 17(2): 156-65.
16. Berg AH, Scherer PE. Adipose tissue, inflammation, and cardiovascular disease. *Circ Res* 2005; 96(9): 939-49.
17. Zhang Y, Proenca R, Maffei M, Barone M, Leopold L, Friedman JM. Positional cloning of the mouse obese gene and its human homologue. *Nature* 1994; 372(6505): 425-32.
18. Muller-Wieland D, Kotzka J. SREBP-1: gene regulatory key to syndrome X? *Ann N Y Acad Sci* 2002; 967: 19-27.
19. Unger RH. Lipid overload and overflow: metabolic trauma and the metabolic syndrome. *Trends Endocrinol Metab* 2003; 14(9): 398-403.
20. Schafer K, Halle M, Goeschen C, Dellas C, Pynn M, Loskutoff DJ, et al. Leptin promotes vascular remodeling and neointimal growth in mice. *Arterioscler Thromb Vasc Biol* 2004; 24(1): 112-7.
21. Zarkesh-Esfahani H, Pockley G, Metcalfe RA, Bidlingmaier M, Wu Z, Ajami A, et al. High-dose leptin activates human leukocytes via receptor expression on monocytes. *J Immunol* 2001; 167(8): 4593-9.
22. Fain JN. Release of interleukins and other inflammatory cytokines by human adipose tissue is enhanced in obesity and primarily due to the nonfat cells. *Vitam Horm* 2006; 74: 443-77.
23. Prins JB, Niesler CU, Winterford CM, Bright NA, Siddle K, O'Rahilly S, et al. Tumor necrosis factor-alpha induces apoptosis of human adipose cells. *Diabetes* 1997; 46(12): 1939-44.

24. Kern PA, Ranganathan S, Li C, Wood L, Ranganathan G. Adipose tissue tumor necrosis factor and interleukin-6 expression in human obesity and insulin resistance. *Am J Physiol Endocrinol Metab* 2001; 280(5): E745-51.

25. Yudkin JS, Kumari M, Humphries SE, Mohamed-Ali V. Inflammation, obesity, stress and coronary heart disease: is interleukin-6 the link? *Atherosclerosis* 2000; 148(2): 209-14.

26. O'Brien KD, Chait A. Serum amyloid A: the 'other' inflammatory protein. *Curr Atheroscler Rep* 2006; 8(1): 62-8.

27. Arnaud C, Burger F, Steffens S, Veillard NR, Nguyen TH, Trono D, *et al*. Statins reduce interleukin-6-induced C-reactive protein in human hepatocytes: new evidence for direct antiinflammatory effects of statins. *Arterioscler Thromb Vasc Biol* 2005; 25(6): 1231-6.

28. Juhan-Vague I, Morange PE, Alessi MC. The insulin resistance syndrome: implications for thrombosis and cardiovascular disease. *Pathophysiol Haemost Thromb* 2002; 32(5-6): 269-73.

29. Côté M, Mauriège P, Bergeron J, Alméras N, Tremblay A, Lemieux I, *et al*. Adiponectinemia in visceral obesity: impact on glucose tolerance and plasma lipoprotein and lipid levels in men. *J Clin Endocrinol Metab* 2005; 90(3): 1434-9.

30. Okamoto Y, Kihara S, Funahashi T, Matsuzawa Y, Libby P. Adiponectin: a key adipocytokine in metabolic syndrome. *Clin Sci* (Lond). 2006; 110(3): 267-78.

31. Kadowaki T, Yamauchi T, Kubota N, Hara K, Ueki K, Tobe K. Adiponectin and adiponectin receptors in insulin resistance, diabetes, and the metabolic syndrome. *J Clin Invest* 2006; 116(7): 1784-92.

32. Matikainen N, Manttari S, Westerbacka J, Vehkavaara S, Lundbom N, Yki-Jarvinen H, *et al*. Postprandial lipemia associates with liver fat content. *J Clin Endocrinol Metab* 2007; 92(8): 3052-9.

33. Nesto RW. Beyond low-density lipoprotein: addressing the atherogenic lipid triad in type 2 diabetes mellitus and the metabolic syndrome. *Am J Cardiovasc Drugs* 2005; 5(6): 379-87.

34. Rizzo M, Berneis K. Lipid triad or atherogenic lipoprotein phenotype: a role in cardiovascular prevention? *J Atheroscler Thromb* 2005; 12(5): 237-9.

35. Sarwar N, Danesh J, Eiriksdottir G, Sigurdsson G, Wareham N, Bingham S, *et al*. Triglycerides and the risk of coronary heart disease: 10,158 incident cases among 262,525 participants in 29 Western prospective studies. *Circulation* 2007; 115(4): 450-8.

36. Miller M, Cannon CP, Murphy SA, Qin J, Ray KK, Braunwald E. Impact of triglyceride levels beyond low-density lipoprotein cholesterol after acute coronary syndrome in the PROVE IT-TIMI 22 trial. *J Am Coll Cardiol* 2008; 51(7): 724-30.

37. Tchernof A, Lamarche B, Prud'Homme D, Nadeau A, Moorjani S, Labrie F, *et al*. The dense LDL phenotype. Association with plasma lipoprotein levels, visceral obesity, and hyperinsulinemia in men. *Diabetes Care* 1996; 19(6): 629-37.

38. Sam S, Haffner S, Davidson MH, D'Agostino RB, Sr., Feinstein S, Kondos G, *et al*. Relationship of abdominal visceral and subcutaneous adipose tissue with lipoprotein particle number and size in type 2 diabetes. *Diabetes* 2008; 57(8): 2022-7.

39. Després JP. Cardiovascular disease under the influence of excess visceral fat. *Critical Pathways in Cardiology* 2007; 6(2): 51-9.

40. Sniderman AD. Applying apoB to the diagnosis and therapy of the atherogenic dyslipoproteinemias: a clinical diagnostic algorithm. *Curr Opin Lipidol* 2004; 15(4): 433-8.

41. Walldius G, Jungner I. Is there a better marker of cardiovascular risk than LDL cholesterol? Apolipoproteins B and A-I - new risk factors and targets for therapy. *Nutr Metab Cardiovasc Dis* 2007; 17(8): 565-71.

42. Lewis GF, Rader DJ. New insights into the regulation of HDL metabolism and reverse cholesterol transport. *Circ Res* 2005; 96(12): 1221-32.

43. Arsenault BJ, Lemieux I, Despres JP, Gagnon P, Wareham NJ, Stroes ES, *et al*. HDL particle size and the risk of coronary heart disease in apparently healthy men and women: The EPIC-Norfolk prospective population study. *Atherosclerosis* 2009; 206(1): 276-81.

44. Pascot A, Lemieux I, Prud'homme D, Tremblay A, Nadeau A, Couillard C, *et al*. Reduced HDL particle size as an additional feature of the atherogenic dyslipidemia of abdominal obesity. *J Lipid Res* 2001; 42(12): 2007-14.

45. Rashid S, Barrett PH, Uffelman KD, Watanabe T, Adeli K, Lewis GF. Lipolytically modified triglyceride-enriched HDLs are rapidly cleared from the circulation. *Arterioscler Thromb Vasc Biol* 2002; 22(3): 483-7.

46. Tan KC, Cooper MB, Ling KL, Griffin BA, Freeman DJ, Packard CJ, *et al*. Fasting and postprandial determinants for the occurrence of small dense LDL species in non-insulin-dependent diabetic patients with

and without hypertriglyceridaemia: the involvement of insulin, insulin precursor species and insulin resistance. *Atherosclerosis* 1995; 113(2): 273-87.

47. de Vries R, Perton FG, Dallinga-Thie GM, van Roon AM, Wolffenbuttel BH, van Tol A, *et al.* Plasma cholesteryl ester transfer is a determinant of intima-media thickness in type 2 diabetic and nondiabetic subjects: role of CETP and triglycerides. *Diabetes* 2005; 54(12): 3554-9.

48. Boekholdt SM, Kuivenhoven JA, Wareham NJ, Peters RJ, Jukema JW, Luben R, *et al.* Plasma levels of cholesteryl ester transfer protein and the risk of future coronary artery disease in apparently healthy men and women: the prospective EPIC (European Prospective Investigation into Cancer and nutrition) - Norfolk population study. *Circulation* 2004; 110(11): 1418-23.

49. Thompson A, Di Angelantonio E, Sarwar N, Erqou S, Saleheen D, Dullaart RP, *et al.* Association of cholesteryl ester transfer protein genotypes with CETP mass and activity, lipid levels, and coronary risk. *JAMA* 2008; 299(23): 2777-88.

50. UK Prospective Diabetes Study (UKPDS) Group. Intensive blood-glucose control with sulphonylureas or insulin compared with conventional treatment and risk of complications in patients with type 2 diabetes (UKPDS 33). *Lancet* 1998; 352(9131): 837-53.

51. Gerstein HC, Miller ME, Byington RP, Goff DC, Jr., Bigger JT, Buse JB, *et al.* Effects of intensive glucose lowering in type 2 diabetes. *N Engl J Med* 2008; 358(24): 2545-59.

52. Patel A, MacMahon S, Chalmers J, Neal B, Billot L, Woodward M, *et al.* Intensive blood glucose control and vascular outcomes in patients with type 2 diabetes. *N Engl J Med* 2008; 358(24): 2560-72.

53. Colhoun HM, Betteridge DJ, Durrington PN, Hitman GA, Neil HA, Livingstone SJ, *et al.* Primary prevention of cardiovascular disease with atorvastatin in type 2 diabetes in the Collaborative Atorvastatin Diabetes Study (CARDS): multicentre randomised placebo-controlled trial. *Lancet* 2004; 364(9435): 685-96.

54. Knopp RH, d'Emden M, Smilde JG, Pocock SJ. Efficacy and safety of atorvastatin in the prevention of cardiovascular end points in subjects with type 2 diabetes: the Atorvastatin Study for Prevention of Coronary Heart Disease Endpoints in non-insulin-dependent diabetes mellitus (ASPEN). *Diabetes Care* 2006; 29(7): 1478-85.

55. Diabetes Atorvastin Lipid Intervention (DALI) Study Group. The effect of aggressive versus standard lipid lowering by atorvastatin on diabetic dyslipidemia: the DALI study: a double-blind, randomized, placebo-controlled trial in patients with type 2 diabetes and diabetic dyslipidemia. *Diabetes Care* 2001; 24(8): 1335-41.

56. Kearney PM, Blackwell L, Collins R, Keech A, Simes J, Peto R, *et al.* Efficacy of cholesterol-lowering therapy in 18,686 people with diabetes in 14 randomised trials of statins: a meta-analysis. *Lancet* 2008; 371(9607): 117-25.

57. Deedwania P, Barter P, Carmena R, Fruchart JC, Grundy SM, Haffner S, *et al.* Reduction of low-density lipoprotein cholesterol in patients with coronary heart disease and metabolic syndrome: analysis of the Treating to New Targets study. *Lancet* 2006; 368(9539): 919-28.

58. Lemieux I, Salomon H, Després JP. Contribution of apo CIII reduction to the greater effect of 12-week micronized fenofibrate than atorvastatin therapy on triglyceride levels and LDL size in dyslipidemic patients. *Ann Med* 2003; 35(6): 442-8.

59. Fruchart JC, Staels B, Duriez P. PPARS, metabolic disease and atherosclerosis. *Pharmacol Res* 2001; 44(5): 345-52.

60. Rubins HB, Robins SJ, Collins D, Fye CL, Anderson JW, Elam MB, *et al.* Gemfibrozil for the secondary prevention of coronary heart disease in men with low levels of high-density lipoprotein cholesterol. Veterans Affairs High-Density Lipoprotein Cholesterol Intervention Trial Study Group. *N Engl J Med* 1999; 341(6): 410-8.

61. Keech A, Simes RJ, Barter P, Best J, Scott R, Taskinen MR, *et al.* Effects of long-term fenofibrate therapy on cardiovascular events in 9795 people with type 2 diabetes mellitus (the FIELD study): randomised controlled trial. *Lancet* 2005; 366(9500): 1849-61.

62. Tenenbaum A, Motro M, Fisman EZ, Tanne D, Boyko V, Behar S. Bezafibrate for the secondary prevention of myocardial infarction in patients with metabolic syndrome. *Arch Intern Med* 2005; 165(10): 1154-60.

63. Scott R, O'Brien R, Fulcher G, Pardy C, D'Emden M, Tse D, *et al.* Effects of fenofibrate treatment on cardiovascular disease risk in 9,795 individuals with type 2 diabetes and various components of the metabolic syndrome: the Fenofibrate Intervention and Event Lowering in Diabetes (FIELD) study. *Diabetes Care* 2009; 32(3): 493-8.

64. Robins SJ, Rubins HB, Faas FH, Schaefer EJ, Elam MB, Anderson JW, *et al.* Insulin resistance and cardiovascular events with low HDL cholesterol: the Veterans Affairs HDL Intervention Trial (VA-HIT). *Diabetes Care* 2003; 26(5): 1513-7.

65. The ACCORD Study Group. Effects of combination lipid therapy in Type 2 diabetes mellitus. *N Engl J Med* 2010; 362(17): 1563-74.

66. Mazzone T, Meyer PM, Feinstein SB, Davidson MH, Kondos GT, D'Agostino RB, Sr., *et al.* Effect of pioglitazone compared with glimepiride on carotid intima-media thickness in type 2 diabetes: a randomized trial. *JAMA* 2006; 296(21): 2572-81.

67. Nissen SE, Nicholls SJ, Wolski K, Nesto R, Kupfer S, Perez A, *et al.* Comparison of pioglitazone vs glimepiride on progression of coronary atherosclerosis in patients with type 2 diabetes: the PERISCOPE randomized controlled trial. *JAMA* 2008; 299(13): 1561-73.

68. Davidson M, Meyer PM, Haffner S, Feinstein S, D'Agostino R, Sr., Kondos GT, *et al.* Increased high-density lipoprotein cholesterol predicts the pioglitazone-mediated reduction of carotid intima-media thickness progression in patients with type 2 diabetes mellitus. *Circulation* 2008; 117(16): 2123-30.

69. Gerstein HC, Yusuf S, Bosch J, Pogue J, Sheridan P, Dinccag N, *et al.* Effect of rosiglitazone on the frequency of diabetes in patients with impaired glucose tolerance or impaired fasting glucose: a randomised controlled trial. *Lancet* 2006; 368(9541): 1096-105.

70. Lonn EM, Gerstein HC, Sheridan P, Smith S, Diaz R, Mohan V, *et al.* Effect of ramipril and of rosiglitazone on carotid intima-media thickness in people with impaired glucose tolerance or impaired fasting glucose: STARR (STudy of Atherosclerosis with Ramipril and Rosiglitazone). *J Am Coll Cardiol* 2009; 53(22): 2028-35.

71. Kim SK, Hur KY, Kim HJ, Shim WS, Ahn CW, Park SW, *et al.* The increase in abdominal subcutaneous fat depot is an independent factor to determine the glycemic control after rosiglitazone treatment. *Eur J Endocrinol* 2007; 157(2): 167-74.

72. Nissen SE, Wolski K. Effect of rosiglitazone on the risk of myocardial infarction and death from cardiovascular causes. *N Engl J Med* 2007; 356(24): 2457-71.

73. Kahn SE, Haffner SM, Heise MA, Herman WH, Holman RR, Jones NP, *et al.* Glycemic durability of rosiglitazone, metformin, or glyburide monotherapy. *N Engl J Med* 2006; 355(23): 2427-43.

74. Home PD, Pocock SJ, Beck-Nielsen H, Curtis PS, Gomis R, Hanefeld M, *et al.* Rosiglitazone Evaluated for Cardiovascular Outcomes in Oral Agent Combination Therapy for Type 2 Diabetes (RECORD): a multicentre, randomised, open-label trial. *Lancet* 2009; 373(9681): 2125-35.

75. Vega GL. Management of atherogenic dyslipidemia of the metabolic syndrome: evolving rationale for combined drug therapy. *Endocrinol Metab Clin North Am* 2004; 33(3): 525-44, vi.

76. Knowler WC, Barrett-Connor E, Fowler SE, Hamman RF, Lachin JM, Walker EA, *et al.* Reduction in the incidence of type 2 diabetes with lifestyle intervention or metformin. *N Engl J Med* 2002; 346(6): 393-403.

77. Bray GA, Jablonski KA, Fujimoto WY, Barrett-Connor E, Haffner S, Hanson RL, *et al.* Relation of central adiposity and body mass index to the development of diabetes in the Diabetes Prevention Program. *Am J Clin Nutr* 2008; 87(5): 1212-8.

78. Orchard TJ, Temprosa M, Goldberg R, Haffner S, Ratner R, Marcovina S, *et al.* The effect of metformin and intensive lifestyle intervention on the metabolic syndrome: the Diabetes Prevention Program randomized trial. *Ann Intern Med* 2005; 142(8): 611-9.

79. Ross R, Dagnone D, Jones PJ, Smith H, Paddags A, Hudson R, *et al.* Reduction in obesity and related comorbid conditions after diet-induced weight loss or exercise-induced weight loss in men. A randomized, controlled trial. *Ann Intern Med* 2000; 133(2): 92-103.

80. Ohkawara K, Tanaka S, Miyachi M, Ishikawa-Takata K, Tabata I. A dose-response relation between aerobic exercise and visceral fat reduction: systematic review of clinical trials. *Int J Obes (Lond).* 2007; 31(12): 1786-97.

81. Rana JS, Arsenault BJ, Després JP, Côte M, Talmud PJ, Ninio E, *et al.* Inflammatory biomarkers, physical activity, waist circumference, and risk of future coronary heart disease in healthy men and women. *Eur Heart J* 2009; in press.

82. Mora S, Cook N, Buring JE, Ridker PM, Lee IM. Physical activity and reduced risk of cardiovascular events: potential mediating mechanisms. *Circulation* 2007; 116(19): 2110-8.

83. Arsenault BJ, Lachance D, Lemieux I, Alméras N, Tremblay A, Bouchard C, *et al.* Visceral adipose tissue accumulation, cardiorespiratory fitness, and features of the metabolic syndrome. *Arch Intern Med* 2007; 167(14): 1518-25.

84. Rhéaume C, Arsenault BJ, Bélanger S, Pérusse L, Tremblay A, Bouchard C, et al. Low cardiorespiratory fitness levels and elevated blood pressure. What Is the Contribution of Visceral Adiposity? *Hypertension* 2009; May 26: In press.

85. Myers J, Prakash M, Froelicher V, Do D, Partington S, Atwood JE. Exercise capacity and mortality among men referred for exercise testing. *N Engl J Med* 2002; 346(11): 793-801.

86. Blair SN, Kohl HW, 3rd, Paffenbarger RS, Jr., Clark DG, Cooper KH, Gibbons LW. Physical fitness and all-cause mortality. A prospective study of healthy men and women. *JAMA* 1989; 262(17): 2395-401.

87. Kodama S, Saito K, Tanaka S, Maki M, Yachi Y, Asumi M, et al. Cardiorespiratory fitness as a quantitative predictor of all-cause mortality and cardiovascular events in healthy men and women: a meta-analysis. *JAMA* 2009; 301(19): 2024-35.

88. Libby P. The forgotten majority: unfinished business in cardiovascular risk reduction. *J Am Coll Cardiol* 2005; 46(7): 1225-8.

89. Sjostrom L, Lindroos AK, Peltonen M, Torgerson J, Bouchard C, Carlsson B, et al. Lifestyle, diabetes, and cardiovascular risk factors 10 years after bariatric surgery. *N Engl J Med* 2004; 351(26): 2683-93.

90. Dixon JB, O'Brien PE, Playfair J, Chapman L, Schachter LM, Skinner S, et al. Adjustable gastric banding and conventional therapy for type 2 diabetes: a randomized controlled trial. *JAMA* 2008; 299(3): 316-23.

91. Cancello R, Henegar C, Viguerie N, Taleb S, Poitou C, Rouault C, et al. Reduction of macrophage infiltration and chemoattractant gene expression changes in white adipose tissue of morbidly obese subjects after surgery-induced weight loss. *Diabetes* 2005; 54(8): 2277-86.

92. Rubino F. Is type 2 diabetes an operable intestinal disease? A provocative yet reasonable hypothesis. *Diabetes Care* 2008; 31 Suppl 2: S290-6.

Chapter 11

What are the consequences of renal insufficiency or the nephrotic syndrome for lipid levels?

Christiane Drechsler [1] MD, Fellow, Nephrology and Clinical Research
Christoph Wanner [2] MD PhD, Professor of Nephrology
Ton Rabelink [1] MD PhD, Professor of Nephrology
1 Department of Nephrology, Leiden University Medical Center
Leiden, The Netherlands
2 Department of Medicine, Division of Nephrology
University Hospital Würzburg, Germany

Introduction

Chronic kidney disease is characterized by the failure of the kidneys to remove waste products and excess fluid from the body. It is defined by a sustained impairment of kidney function, as reflected by an abnormal excretion of urinary protein or a reduction of the glomerular filtration rate (GFR). When the glomerular filtration rate reaches levels below 15ml/min (corresponding to a reduction in kidney function by approximately 90%), patients require renal replacement therapy, which is provided in the form of dialysis or transplantation. The etiology of chronic kidney disease (CKD) is heterogeneous, involving both primary kidney diseases, and a variety of non-renal diseases, which affect the kidneys. The main causes among primary kidney diseases are glomerulonephritis and renal vascular diseases, while diabetes mellitus, hypertension, and atherosclerosis are the most frequent non-renal causes potentially leading to a loss of kidney function.

The National Kidney Foundation – Kidney Disease Outcomes Quality Initiative (NKF-K/DOQI) workgroup has defined CKD by a glomerular filtration rate <60ml/min/1.73m[2], or the presence of a marker of kidney damage [1, 2]. Based upon these definitions, a classification of CKD by stages has been recommended and internationally accepted (Table 1).

Chronic kidney disease represents a large public health problem. Its prevalence in the United States currently is about 13% [3, 4], with an increasing trend in the recent decade. Data from the United States Renal Data System (USRDS) furthermore show an increase in the incidence rate of end-stage renal disease, reaching 360 per million population in 2006. Accordingly, the number of patients entering the end-stage renal disease (ESRD) program

Table 1. Stages of chronic kidney disease.

Stage		GFR (ml/min/1.73m²)	Prevalence
1	Kidney damage with normal or increased GFR	≥90	3.3%
2	Kidney damage with mild decreased GFR	60 - 89	3.0%
3	Moderately decreased GFR	30 - 59	4.3%
4	Severely decreased GFR	15 - 29	0.2%
5	Kidney failure	<15 (or dialysis)	0.1%

GFR = glomerular filtration rate

rose from 106,912 in 2005 to 110,854 patients in 2006 [3, 5]. The costs of treatment, which in the form of dialysis represents one of the most expensive chronic therapies, put an enormous burden on health care resources. Prevention of disease progression and the associated complications therefore is highly important, requiring the knowledge of risk factors and appropriate treatment.

Dyslipidemia in the patient with kidney disease

Proteinuria-induced dyslipidemia

Abnormal lipid metabolism is common in patients with renal disease, and most prominent in the nephrotic syndrome. Studies have shown that about half of the patients with nephrotic syndrome (proteinuria >3g/day) had total cholesterol concentrations above 300mg/dL [6, 7], and 80% of the patients had LDL cholesterol levels above 130mg/dL [8].

The main abnormalities of lipid metabolism in the nephrotic syndrome include increases in total cholesterol, low-density lipoprotein (LDL) and very-low-density lipoprotein (VLDL) cholesterol, apolipoproteins B (ApoB), CIII and triglycerides, while ApoAI is reduced. Furthermore, the high-density lipoproteins are distributed abnormally (increased HDL3 fraction and decreased HDL2 fraction). Hyperlipidemia in the nephrotic syndrome results from increased hepatic synthesis and decreased catabolism of lipoproteins, whereby the contribution of each to establishing blood lipid levels has not been characterized in detail. Increased triglyceride-rich lipoprotein concentration, VLDL and intermediate-density lipoprotein (IDL) primarily results from decreased clearance [9], partly due to a reduced lipoprotein lipase (LPL) activity. Lipoprotein lipase is necessary for endothelial binding of VLDL and for normal lipolysis. The loss of the cofactor apoCII (a lipoprotein lipase activator), which is especially common in proteinuric renal disease, and a depletion of the endothelial bound lipoprotein lipase (LPL) pool [10] may contribute to the reduced LPL activity. In addition, both LDL and lipoprotein(a) [Lp(a)] synthesis are increased [9, 11], whereby evidence exists that LDL synthesis may be augmented through a mechanism bypassing its normal precursor VLDL. Finally, due to a decreased activity of lecithin:cholesterol acyltransferase (LCAT) in proteinuric renal disease [12], the number of mature spherical HDL particles is decreased. These particles are important carriers for several cofactors, amongst which apoCII, which affect LPL activity and VLDL level.

The impact of CKD on serum lipids and lipoproteins

Dyslipidemia in patients with CKD and no nephrotic syndrome can be characterized by high triglyceride levels and low HDL concentrations, while total and LDL cholesterol are normal or even low [13, 14]. Although the lipid abnormalities captured by routine laboratory measurements may not be impressive, more sophisticated analyses reveal profound disturbances in lipid metabolism. Mainly as a result of decreased catabolism, the concentration of triglyceride-rich lipoproteins (VLDL, IDL) is increased, in particular in the post-prandial phase. Lipolysis of the highly atherogenic VLDL and chylomicron (CM) remnants is impaired partly due to the decreased lipoprotein lipase (LPL) on the vascular endothelium, and partly due to increased levels of the major LPL inhibitory apolipoprotein, apoCIII. Furthermore, kidney failure is associated with a shift in the size distribution of LDL to increased content of small dense LDL. A reduction in LDL size, resulting in increased levels of small dense LDL, results from increased TG concentration, which via the action of cholesteryl ester transfer protein (CETP) and hepatic lipase (HL) [15] result in the formation of small dense LDL. Due to the increased oxidative stress in patients with CKD and the reduced clearance, the fraction of highly atherogenic oxidized LDL is increased.

Disorders in HDL maturation and catabolism add to the dyslipidemic profile in CKD patients. Processes favouring HDL maturation are associated with a greater abundance of large mature HDL and greater HDL levels. The adenosine triphosphate binding cassette 1 (ABCA1) is responsible for initial lipidation of apoAI and transfer of cholesterol to small (native) HDL particles. The formation of large, mature HDL particles is mediated by LCAT – resulting in the esterification of cholesterol – as well as by LPL. As previously mentioned, functional deficiencies in LCAT and LPL activity may therefore affect HDL maturation.

In addition, elevated levels of Lp(a) have been found in CKD [16-20], partly due to the diminished renal clearance [17]. Lp(a) is an LDL-like particle which has an additional protein, apolipoprotein(a), and constitutes an important risk factor for atherosclerosis. The mechanisms of lipid metabolism and alterations in renal failure are shown in Figure 1.

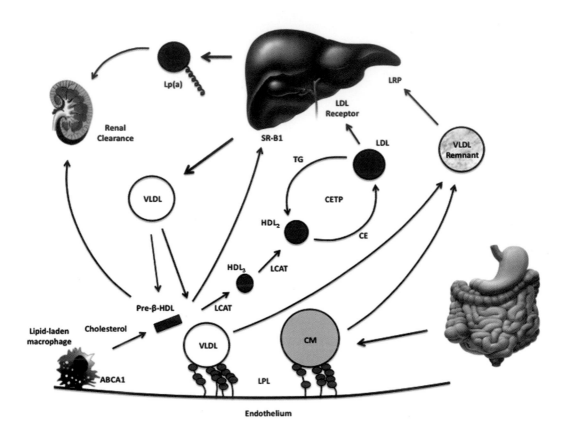

Figure 1. Triglyceride-rich lipoproteins are secreted by the gut (chylomicrons) or liver (VLDL) and then are processed on the vascular endothelium by lipoprotein lipase (LPL), yielding remnant particles. LPL is activated by apoCII and inhibited by apoCI and apoCIII. ApoCI and apoCIII are increased in chronic kidney disease (CKD). HDL formation is initiated by the combination of apoAI with cholesterol and phospholipids through interaction with the adenosine triphosphate binding cassette 1 (ABCA1). The nascent pre-β-HDL is then matured by cholesterol esterification through lecithin cholesterol ester transfer protein (LCAT), first to HDL3 and then to HDL2. HDL2 is taken up by the liver by the scavenger receptor B1 (SR-B1). Alternatively, it transfers its cholesterol ester-rich core to VLDL, creating LDL (via CETP activity). LCAT protein mass and activity are both reduced in CKD. This results in accumulation of pre-β or discoidal HDL and HDL3, which are subject to accelerated degradation in part by the kidney. While HDL3 is usually rich in the antioxidant enzyme paraoxonase 1 (PON1), this is not the case in HDL3 in patients having CKD. Lipoprotein(a) levels are increased in CKD as a result of decreased clearance. Abbreviations: TG = triglyceride; VLDL = very-low-density lipoprotein; LPL = lipoprotein lipase; CKD = chronic kidney disease; HDL = high-density lipoprotein; ABCA1 = adenosine triphosphate binding cassette 1; LCAT = lecithin cholesterol ester transfer protein; SR-B1 = scavenger receptor B1; CETP = cholesteryl ester transfer protein; Lp(a) = lipoprotein (a); LRP = lipoprotein-like receptor; CE = cholesteryl ester.

Lipid disorders in dialysis

The lipid abnormalities in CKD stages 2-4 as characterized by an increase in plasma triglycerides, VLDL and IDL, along with a reduction in HDL cholesterol, generally also apply for dialysis patients. Dyslipidemia becomes more pronounced as kidney failure advances to CKD stage 5 requiring dialysis.

Hemodialysis and peritoneal dialysis can both provide an adequate relief of uremic symptoms, but the two techniques appear to have different effects on uremic dyslipidemia [21, 22]. Patients on peritoneal dialysis (PD) show higher cholesterol, triglyceride, LDL and Lp(a) levels than patients on maintenance hemodialysis (HD). Possible reasons may be a considerable loss of protein (7-14g/day) into the peritoneal dialysate, and the absorption of glucose (150-200g/day) from the dialysis fluid. Plasma concentrations of apoB100 were shown to be increased in peritoneal dialysis patients, whereas normal concentrations of apoB100 were found in hemodialysis patients [21]. The increase in apoB100 thereby was most markedly in the VLDL fraction, and only to a minor extent in IDL and LDL. An overproduction of VLDL-1 and VLDL-2 apoB100 has been suggested secondary to reduced insulin sensitivity and increased free fatty acid availability in PD patients. This leads to an increase in the poolsize of triglycerides and apoB100 in the VLDL fraction of PD patients. Although lipid profiles differ between PD and HD patients, abnormalities in lipid metabolism qualitatively have similarities regarding the pathogenesis of atherosclerosis and endothelial dysfunction in these groups.

Lipid disorders after kidney transplantation

Lipid abnormalities in kidney transplant recipients are common, occurring in 60% to 70% of renal transplant recipients receiving immunosuppressive therapy [23, 24]. Major characteristics are the increases in levels of LDL, VLDL and triglycerides, while HDL is usually normal.

Risk factors contributing to the development of dyslipidemia after transplantation are age, male gender, proteinuria, obesity, pretransplant hyperlipidemia and diabetes mellitus. Furthermore, dyslipidemia following kidney transplantation is associated with the use and dose of immunosuppressive agents such as corticosteroids, calcineurin inhibitors, and inhibitors of the mammalian target of rapamycin (mTOR). The cumulative dose of corticosteroids thereby appears to be the most significant risk factor. Among calcineurin inhibitors, a higher incidence of hyperlipidemia was shown with the use of cyclosporine as compared to tacrolimus. Sirolimus and everolimus, however, both mTOR inhibitors, seem to even more impact on lipid metabolism with significant increases in triglyceride and cholesterol levels [25]. Mycophenolate mofetil is the only available immunosuppressive agent with no adverse effects on lipids.

Dyslipidemia and progression of kidney disease

Dyslipidemia, partly explained by its association with proteinuria, predicts progressive loss of kidney function [26]. This was seen particularly in early stages of diabetic nephropathy [27, 28]. Elevated levels of triglycerides seem to contribute to the progression of albuminuria [29], diabetic nephropathy [30], and retinopathy. They were furthermore associated with a higher risk of end-stage renal disease requiring renal replacement therapy [31]. In contrast, higher levels of HDL were found to be protective of albuminuria in type 1 diabetes [32].

Dyslipidemia, cardiovascular risk and mortality

Chronic kidney disease *per se* has been shown to be a strong risk factor for cardiovascular morbidity and mortality [33]. Patients with a moderately impaired kidney function already have a high risk to develop cardiovascular complications [34]. Cardiovascular risk further increases inversely proportionate to the decline in kidney function (Figure 2), and the majority of patients with chronic kidney disease die of cardiac and vascular events before reaching end-stage renal disease.

In patients on long-term dialysis, cardiac and vascular disease is the leading cause of death, accounting for 43% of all-cause mortality [3]. Compared to the general population, mortality from cardiovascular disease is excessively high: it ranges from a 500-fold increased risk in young patients aged 25-35 years to a 5-fold increased risk in individuals of a high age of 85 years or more [35]. Possible reasons may involve the increased prevalence of traditional risk factors as known from the general population, and further uremia-related risk factors. Lipid abnormalities, being common in patients with kidney disease, have been suggested to play a major role. Therefore, it is tempting to propose a general need for treatment of lipid disorders in this patient group.

However, while a loglinear relation between blood cholesterol levels and cardiovascular risk is well established in the general population, this is not the case in renal patients. Many studies in patients with CKD, mainly stage 5, have failed to show a similar, clear pattern of high plasma total cholesterol, LDL cholesterol and triglycerides being associated with increased cardiovascular mortality. In fact, a number of studies have even found that low (not high) serum total cholesterol was associated with increased mortality [36-39]. U-shaped curves, and recently, J-shaped curves, have been described for the relationship between serum cholesterol and mortality. This probably reflects the influence of malnutrition and chronic inflammation, resulting in the phenomenon known as reverse causation. Concomitant illnesses accompanied by inflammation are associated with an increased risk of death; when they furthermore induce a decrease in cholesterol synthesis, the result may be artifactually negative associations between cholesterol and mortality. Supporting this hypothesis, hypercholesterolemia was shown to be an independent risk factor for cardiovascular and all-cause mortality in dialysis patients without, but not in those with evidence of malnutrition or inflammation [40].

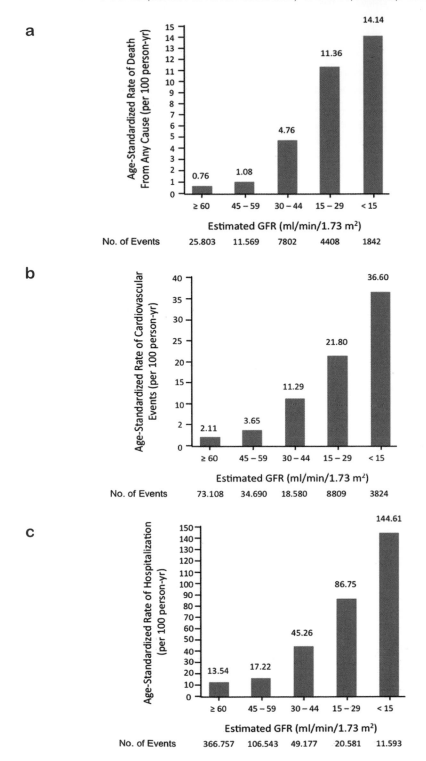

Figure 2. Age-standardized rates of death from any cause (a), cardiovascular events (b), and hospitalization (c), according to the estimated glomerular filtration rate (GFR). *Reproduced with permission from the Massachusetts Medical Society. Copyright © 2004. All rights reserved. From Go AS, et al [33].*

In general, caution is required on translating observational findings into possible therapeutic treatments. Furthermore, concern is also justified when applying recommendations for the treatment of lipid disorders from the general population – which are based upon many prospective randomized placebo-controlled trials – to patients with chronic kidney disease. Extrapolation of data from the general population may not meet the special disease pattern of kidney disease patients.

Despite cardiovascular deaths being a major cause of mortality in dialysis patients, the proportion of myocardial infarctions in cardiac deaths is much lower in patients with chronic kidney disease as compared to the general population. Only 25% of the cardiac deaths in hemodialysis patients can be attributed to myocardial infarctions, while the majority of events constitute sudden cardiac deaths [3]. Although sudden cardiac death may to some extent also result from infarctions and arrhythmias, other reasons such as structural heart diseases and/or electrolyte shifts presumably also play an important role. Whether these may be modifiable with cholesterol-lowering treatment, is unlikely.

Therefore, it is obvious that the classical guidelines, such as the National Cholesterol Education Program Adult Panel III cannot generally be applied to renal patients. In particular, treatment indications may differ according to the severity of chronic kidney disease. Further on in this chapter we present the available evidence for lipid-lowering therapy according to the stages of chronic kidney disease as defined by K/DOQI (Kidney Disease Outcomes Quality Initiative) (Table 1) [2, 41].

Lipid-lowering therapy in patients with the nephrotic syndrome

Studies have shown that patients with persistent nephrotic syndrome and hyperlipidemia are at increased risk for atherosclerotic disease, particularly if other risk factors are present [7, 42, 43]. Furthermore, it has been suggested from animal experiments and observations in humans that hyperlipidemia may also enhance the rate of progressive glomerular injury, possibly by promoting an intraglomerular equivalent of atherosclerosis. Thus, it appears reasonable that lowering lipid levels may both protect against systemic atherosclerosis and slow the progression of the underlying kidney disease. Studies have shown that statins can efficiently lower total and LDL cholesterol concentrations by 20% to 45%, and to a lesser extent triglyceride levels and Lp(a) levels [43-47]. Despite the lack of studies using 'hard' endpoints, statins are suggested as the treatment of choice for persistent hyperlipidemia in the nephrotic syndrome (IV/C). Due to side effects, other lipid-lowering medication such as nicotinic acid, fibric acid, probucol or bile acid sequestrants are not generally recommended. Instead, additional therapeutic options include dietary modification [48] and angiotensin inhibition (IV/C), the latter being associated with a 10% to 20% decline in the plasma levels of total and LDL-cholesterol and Lp(a) [49].

Statins in patients with chronic kidney disease

Early renal disease: CKD stage 1-3 (GFR ≥30ml/min/1.73m²)

The effects of a lipid-lowering therapy on cardiovascular, cerebrovascular and renal endpoints were investigated in a subgroup analysis of the Pravastatin Pooling Project, including 12,333 patients with mild CKD (stage 2) and 4491 patients with moderate CKD (stage 3). Pravastatin 40mg/day resulted in a significant 23% relative risk reduction in the combined endpoint of non-fatal myocardial infarction, cardiac death, percutaneous or surgical revascularizations in patients with moderate CKD. A similar effect was seen in patients with mild CKD, among whom even total mortality was reduced. The achieved relative risk reduction corresponds to the effect, which would have been expected in the general population without kidney disease. The corresponding absolute risk reduction was – due to the higher event rate – even more than twice as high compared to patients with normal kidney function (6.3 vs 2.9%) [50] **(IIb/B)**.

Furthermore, a prespecified subgroup analysis of 6517 patients with kidney dysfunction was performed among the Anglo-Scandinavian Cardiac Outcomes Trial (ASCOT), including 19,000 hypertensive patients with at least 3 other risk factors for coronary artery disease, and non-fasting cholesterol levels ≤6.5mmol/L. It showed that patients receiving 10mg atorvastatin per day had a significantly lower risk of reaching the composite primary endpoint, consisting of non-fatal myocardial infarction and cardiac death, compared to patients receiving placebo [51] **(IIb/B)**.

Similar results were obtained from analyses of 1329 patients with slightly elevated creatinine (110 to 200µmol/L) participating in the Heart Protection Study (HPS). A total of 268 of the patients receiving placebo experienced a vascular event vs. 182 of the simvastatin treated patients. This corresponds to a 25% relative risk reduction in the simvastatin group [52] **(IIb/B)**. Recent findings from the Treatment to New Targets (TNT) study confirmed that treatment of patients having less severe CKD does reduce the cardiovascular risk [53] **(IIb/B)**.

Finally, there are data suggesting that statins may also slow the rate of decline in kidney function and lower urinary protein excretion. One subanalysis within the GREACE study showed that in untreated patients with coronary heart disease, dyslipidemia and normal baseline creatinine, the glomerular filtration rate (GFR) decreased over a period of 3 years. Treatment with a statin could prevent this decline and lead to a significant improvement in kidney function [54]. In the TNT study, patients on 80mg atorvastatin per day had a significantly lower rate of decline of renal function than did patients receiving 10mg/day [55] **(IIb/B)**. Similarly, a post hoc subgroup analysis of the CARE study had shown a lower GFR decline in pravastatin as compared to placebo treated patients [56] **(IIb/B)**. The reduction of GFR decline as achieved by statins (reduction of 0.1ml/min/1.73m² per year in the latter study), however, is relatively small (in comparison: reductions of 3 to 4ml/min/1.73m² by the control of hypertension and ACE-inhibitor therapy in proteinuric patients [57, 58]).

Although some data also exist for fibrates suggesting beneficial effects on the rate of progression of renal disease and cardiovascular risk [59, 60] **(IIb/B)**, these drugs have been considered with caution in patients with CKD. This is mainly because most fibrates or their active metabolites accumulate in renal failure and occasionally cause rhabdomyolysis.

In conclusion, despite the absence of direct evidence from randomized controlled trials in patients with CKD, these data provide indirect evidence that patients with CKD stages 2 and 3 may benefit from a lipid-lowering intervention. Based on the above post hoc analyses of past statin trials on subcohorts of patients with early CKD, data are sufficiently suggestive to justify the administration of statins in these patients **(IIb/B)**.

Advanced renal disease: CKD stage 4-5 and dialysis patients

Unfortunately, patients with more advanced CKD (stage 4) were either absent in the above described subgroup analyses, or their numbers were too small to be analyzed. There is a complete lack of controlled studies addressing the effect of lipid-lowering medication on outcome in patients at CKD stage 4. These patients represent a population with advanced kidney failure, where all-cause mortality markedly increases and the pattern of cardiovascular disease may change, compared to CKD stages 2 and 3. One open study has been performed in a small group of patients (n=143) over 20 months, and showed that atorvastatin decreased the primary cardiac endpoint in patients with pre-end stage renal disease, while this was not the case in dialysis patients [61].

More definite evidence has been provided by the prospective, randomized controlled 4D study (The German Diabetes and Dialysis Study). This study evaluated the effect of 20mg atorvastatin / day vs placebo in 1255 hemodialysis patients with type 2 diabetes mellitus during 4 years of follow-up [62]. Although atorvastatin effectively lowered LDL cholesterol by 42%, the composite primary cardiovascular endpoint, consisting of death from cardiac causes, non-fatal myocardial infarction and stroke, was only reduced by 8%, which was not statistically significant (RR 0.92, 95% CI 0.77-1.10, p=0.37) **(Ib/A)**. Similarly, all-cause mortality was not significantly reduced (RR 0.93, 95% CI 0.79-1.08, p=0.33). There was a positive result, however, for the secondary endpoint of all cardiac events combined, which were lowered by 18% in the atorvastatin group as compared to the placebo group (RR 0.82, 95%CI 0.86-0.99, p=0.03). Further evidence was contributed by AURORA: A study to evaluate the Use of Rosuvastatin in subjects On Regular Dialysis: an Assessment of survival and cardiovascular events [63]. In this international prospective randomized controlled trial, 2776 hemodialysis patients were assigned to receive rosuvastatin 10mg daily or placebo, and followed for a median of 3.8 years. Despite the mean reduction in LDL cholesterol of 43% in the intervention group, the combined primary endpoint of death from cardiovascular causes, non-fatal myocardial infarction, or non-fatal stroke could not be reduced (HR 0.96, 95% CI 0.84-1.11, p=0.59) **(Ib/A)**. Rosuvastatin neither had an effect on individual components of the primary endpoint, nor on all-cause mortality (HR 0.96, 95% CI 0.86-1.07, p=0.51). It remains unclear whether these data can be generalized to peritoneal dialysis patients. This will be clarified by the ongoing Study of Heart and Renal Protection (SHARP), which is a large-scale randomized controlled trial comparing the use of simvastatin and ezetimibe vs. placebo in 9489 patients in CKD stage 4 and on dialysis – the results are awaited in 2011 [64].

In conclusion, the 4D and AURORA studies do not provide a rationale to start statin treatment in hemodialysis patients (Ib/A). Treatment aiming at primary prevention in the absence of signs and symptoms of coronary heart disease presumably comes too late once the patient has advanced to end-stage renal disease. It has been suggested, however, that patients who are already on statins when entering chronic dialysis should be left on the medication [14].

Patients after kidney transplantation

Recipients of kidney transplants had been investigated in the ALERT study, which was a randomized controlled trial comparing fluvastatin (40-80mg/day) vs. placebo in 2102 patients with long-term stable graft function. Despite a mean reduction in LDL cholesterol of 1mmol/L during 5.1 ± 1.1 years, there was no significant risk reduction for the combined primary endpoint, consisting of cardiac death, non-fatal myocardial infarction and coronary revascularization (RR 0.83 [95% CI 0.64-1.06], p=0.139) (Ib/A). Furthermore, total mortality and graft loss did not differ significantly between the groups (in the fluvastatin and placebo groups there were 143 deaths compared with 138, and 146 graft losses compared with 137, respectively). Rates in two of the three subcomponents of the primary endpoint – cardiac death and non-fatal myocardial infarction – were observed to be lower in the intervention group (RR 0.65 [0.48-0.88], p=0.005). The authors suggested that the trial may have been too small to detect a significant effect on the primary endpoint because the event rate was lower than expected [65].

A post hoc analysis of the ALERT trial showed that the success of a lipid-lowering therapy in kidney transplant recipients is dependent on when treatment is initiated. Indeed, a significant reduction in cardiac endpoints was observed in patients who started fluvastatin treatment within the first 4.5 years after renal transplantation (4.6% in fluvastatin group vs 9.2% in placebo group) [66] (IIb/B).

Despite the lack of direct evidence it can therefore be suggested that renal transplant recipients with hyperlipidemia should be treated with a statin so that target LDL cholesterol levels can be achieved (IIb/B). Importantly, for any statin therapy in renal transplant recipients, potential interactions with other medication and changes of immunosuppressive regimens should be taken into account. All statins, except pravastatin, primarily undergo metabolism by the CYP 450 isoenzymes in the liver. The CYP 2C9 isoenzyme is responsible for the metabolism of fluvastatin and rosuvastatin, whereas atorvastatin, lovastatin, and simvastatin are metabolized by the CYP 3A4 isoenzyme. Concomitant intake of further drugs being metabolized by the CYP 3A4 system – such as the immunosuppressant cyclosporine in renal transplant recipients, macrolide antibiotics or calcium channel blockers like verapamil – may dramatically increase the plasma concentration of the statin, placing patients at risk for adverse events like myopathy or rhabdomyolysis. Pravastatin and rosuvastatin are less likely to induce drug-drug interactions and are considered as more safe.

In summary, results from the 4D and ALERT trials do not necessarily doubt the validity of the subgroup analyses done for patients with CKD stages 2 and 3, in whom lipid-lowering therapy appears to be just as effective as in patients with normal kidney function. It remains less clear whether lipid-lowering therapy is still effective when started in patients with more advanced stages of chronic kidney disease.

Further therapeutic concepts for lipid-lowering in CKD

Nutritional interventions and physical activity

Nutritional interventions and physical activity play an important role as lipid-lowering treatments in the general population. They presumably have similar importance in patients with chronic kidney disease in early stages 1-3 **(IV/C)**.

In stage 4, reduction in nutrient intake without sufficient physical activity may lead to a catabolic state with reduction of muscle mass. Therefore, nutritional interventions should not generally be applied to patients in advanced stages of CKD, but carefully considered individually.

Antiproteinuric therapy

Any intervention leading to a reduction of urinary protein excretion also leads to a reduction in LDL-cholesterol and Lp(a). ACE inhibitors and AT1-receptor blockers have antiproteinuric properties, and thus result in a reduction of the microalbuminuria- or proteinuria-induced dyslipidemia.

Treatment guidelines

Guidelines including the European Best Practice Guidelines (EBPG) [67] and the US National Kidney Foundation's Kidney Disease Outcomes Quality Initiative (K/DOQI) [68, 69] have been difficult to define due to the lack of randomized controlled trials addressing dyslipidemia in chronic kidney disease. Kidney transplant recipients are represented by the Kidney Disease Improving Global Outcomes (KDIGO) [70] guideline, which for the treatment of dyslipidemia refers to K/DOQI. Table 2 summarizes guideline treatment recommendations, and – as the randomized controlled studies were still ongoing once the guidelines were developed – reflects that they are mainly based on opinion.

It is to be expected that further ongoing randomized controlled trials will add reliable evidence for the treatment of dyslipidemia especially in advanced chronic kidney disease (stages 4-5 and dialysis), so that new treatment guidelines with higher evidence levels may be established in the near future.

Table 2. Recommendations for the treatment of dyslipidemia according to the K/DOQI guidelines for patients with CKD and the KDIGO guidelines for kidney transplant recipients.

Treatment of patients with CKD stage 1-4

In general, the K/DOQI working group recommended that the NCEP/ATP III guidelines [71] were applicable to patients with CKD stages 1-4, with some specific aspects deserving further consideration:

- CKD should be classified as a CVD risk equivalent
- Complications of lipid-lowering therapies resulting from reduced kidney function should be anticipated
- It should be considered whether there may be indications for the treatment of dyslipidemia other than preventing CVD
- It should be determined whether the treatment of proteinuria may also be an effective treatment for dyslipidemias

Supporting the treatment of dyslipidemia, assessment and treatment of other modifiable traditional risk factors, such as hypertension, smoking, obesity and diabetes, should be performed

Treatment of patients with CKD stage 5

- For adults with stage 5 CKD and fasting triglycerides $\geq$500mg/dL ($\geq$5.65mmol/L) that cannot be corrected by removing an underlying cause, treatment with therapeutic lifestyle changes (TLC) and a triglyceride-lowering agent should be considered (C)
- For adults with stage 5 CKD and LDL $\geq$100mg/dL ($\geq$2.59mmol/L), treatment should be considered to reduce LDL to <100mg/dL (<2.59mmol/L) (B)
- For adults with stage 5 CKD and LDL <100mg/dL (<2.59mmol/L), fasting triglycerides $\geq$200mg/dL ($\geq$2.26mmol/L), and non-HDL cholesterol (total cholesterol minus HDL) $\geq$130mg/dL ($\geq$3.36mmol/L), treatment should be considered to reduce non-HDL cholesterol to <130mg/dL (<3.36mmol/L) (C)

Treatment of patients after kidney transplantation

- For patients with fasting triglycerides $\geq$500mg/dL ($\geq$5.65mmol/L) that cannot be corrected by removing an underlying cause, we suggest therapeutic lifestyle changes and a triglyceride-lowering agent [Based on KDOQI Recommendation 4.1 for patients with CKD stage 5, Evidence Level C]
- For patients with elevated low-density lipoprotein (LDL) cholesterol, we suggest: If LDL $\geq$100mg/dL ($\geq$2.59mmol/L), treat to reduce LDL to <100mg/dL (<2.59mmol/L) [Based on KDOQI Guideline 4.2 for patients with CKD stage 5, Evidence Level B]
- For patients with normal LDL cholesterol, elevated triglycerides and elevated non-HDL cholesterol, we suggest: If LDL <100mg/dL (<2.59mmol/L), fasting triglycerides $\geq$200mg/dL ($\geq$2.26mmol/L), and non-HDL $\geq$130mg/dL ($\geq$3.36mmol/L), treat to reduce non-HDL to <130mg/dL (<3.36mmol/L) [Based on KDOQI Guideline 4.3 for patients with CKD stage 5, Evidence Level C]

Conclusions

In conclusion, disturbances in lipid metabolism are common in patients with the nephrotic syndrome, patients with chronic kidney disease (CKD) and patients after kidney transplantation. The classical guidelines on lipid-lowering therapy – such as the National Cholesterol Education Program Adult Panel III – however, cannot generally be applied to renal patients, as extrapolation of data from the general population may not meet the special disease pattern of patients with CKD. Although post hoc analyses of statin trials support the administration of statins in patients with early stages of CKD (stages 1-3), patients with advanced chronic kidney disease do not benefit to the same extent from lipid-lowering therapy. In particular, there is no rationale to start statin treatment in patients, once they require maintenance hemodialysis.

Key points	Evidence level

Lipid abnormalities in the nephrotic syndrome and in renal insufficiency

- Abnormal lipid metabolism is common in patients with the nephrotic syndrome and in patients with chronic kidney disease (CKD) or after kidney transplantation.
- The main abnormalities of lipid metabolism in the nephrotic syndrome include increases in total cholesterol, low-density lipoprotein (LDL) and very-low-density lipoprotein (VLDL) cholesterol, apolipoproteins B, CIII and triglycerides, while apoAI is reduced.
- The profound disturbances in lipid metabolism in patients with chronic kidney disease include increased concentrations of triglyceride-rich lipoproteins, small dense and oxidized LDL, and impaired HDL maturation and catabolism. These alterations are not captured by routine laboratory measurements.
- Immunosuppressive therapy importantly contributes to the development of dyslipidemia after kidney transplantation.
- Chronic kidney disease *per se* is a strong risk factor for cardiovascular morbidity and mortality. Cardiovascular risk and mortality increase inversely proportionate to the decline in kidney function.

Continued overleaf

Key points *continued*	Evidence level

Treatment recommendations

- The classical guidelines on lipid-lowering therapy – such as the National Cholsterol Education Program Adult Panel III – cannot generally be applied to renal patients, as extrapolation of data from the general population may not meet the special disease pattern of patients with chronic kidney disease.

- Patients with the nephrotic syndrome should be treated with a statin. Additional therapeutic options include dietary modification and inhibition of the renin-angiotensin system (angiotensin-converting enzyme inhibitors). — IV/C

- Post hoc analyses of statin trials support the administration of statins in patients with early stages of chronic kidney disease (CKD stage 1-3). — IIb/B

- Patients with advanced chronic kidney disease do not benefit to the same extent from lipid-lowering therapy as do patients with early stages of CKD. In particular, there is no rationale to start statin treatment in patients, once they require maintenance hemodialysis. — Ib/A

- Despite the lack of direct evidence, it is suggested that renal transplant recipients with hyperlipidemia should be treated with a statin. Importantly, potential interactions with immunosuppressants and other medication should be taken into account. — IIb/B

- The present guidelines (EBPG and K/DOQI) on the treatment of lipid disorders in patients with chronic kidney disease do not reflect the current evidence.

References

1. National Kidney Foundation. K/DOQI clinical practice guidelines for chronic kidney disease: evaluation, classification and stratification. *Am J Kidney Dis* 2002; 39: S1.
2. Levey AS, Eckardt KU, Tsukamoto Y, *et al*. Definition and classification of chronic kidney disease: a position statement from Kidney Disease: Improving Global Outcomes (KDIGO). *Kidney Int* 2005 ;67: 2089-100.
3. U.S. Renal Data System, USRDS: 2006 Annual Report. National Institutes of Health, Bethesda, 2006.
4. Coresh J, Selvin E, Stevens LA, *et al*. Prevalence of chronic kidney disease in the United States. *JAMA* 2007; 298: 2038-47.
5. U.S. Renal Data System, USRDS: 2005 Annual Report. National Institutes of Health, Bethesda, 2005.
6. Kronenberg F, Lingenhel A, Lhotta K, *et al*. Lipoprotein(a) - and low-density lipoprotein-derived cholesterol in nephrotic syndrome: impact on lipid-lowering therapy? *Kidney Int* 2004; 66: 348-54.
7. Radhakrishnan J, Appel AS, Valeri A, Appel GB. The nephrotic syndrome, lipids, and risk factors for cardiovascular disease. *Am J Kidney Dis* 1993; 22: 135-42.
8. Weiner DE, Sarnak MJ. Managing dyslipidemia in chronic kidney disease. *J Gen Intern Med* 2004; 19: 1045-52.

9.   de Sain-van der Velden MG, Reijngoud DJ, Kaysen GA, *et al.* Evidence for increased synthesis of lipoprotein(a) in the nephrotic syndrome. *J Am Soc Nephrol* 1998; 9: 1474-81.

10. Attman PO, Samuelsson O, Alaupovic P. Lipid abnormalities in progressive renal insufficiency. *Contrib Nephrol* 1997; 120: 1-10.

11. de Sain-van der Velden MG, Kaysen GA, Barrett HA, *et al.* Increased VLDL in nephrotic patients results from a decreased catabolism while increased LDL results from increased synthesis. *Kidney Int* 1998; 53: 994-1001.

12. Kaysen GA, de Sain-van der Velden MG. New insights into lipid metabolism in the nephrotic syndrome. *Kidney Int* Suppl 1999; 71: S18-21.

13. Prinsen BH, de Sain-van der Velden MG, de Koning EJ, Koomans HA, Berger R, Rabelink TJ. Hypertriglyceridemia in patients with chronic renal failure: possible mechanisms. *Kidney Int Suppl* 2003; S121-4.

14. Ritz E, Wanner C. Lipid abnormalities and cardiovascular risk in renal disease. *J Am Soc Nephrol* 2008; 19: 1065-70.

15. Kaysen GA. New insights into lipid metabolism in chronic kidney disease: what are the practical implications? *Blood Purif* 2009; 27: 86-91.

16. Cressman MD, Heyka RJ, Paganini EP, O'Neil J, Skibinski CI, Hoff HF. Lipoprotein(a) is an independent risk factor for cardiovascular disease in hemodialysis patients. *Circulation* 1992; 86: 475-82.

17. Frischmann ME, Kronenberg F, Trenkwalder E, *et al. In vivo* turnover study demonstrates diminished clearance of lipoprotein(a) in hemodialysis patients. *Kidney Int* 2007; 71: 1036-43.

18. Kronenberg F, Konig P, Neyer U, *et al.* Multicenter study of lipoprotein(a) and apolipoprotein(a) phenotypes in patients with end-stage renal disease treated by hemodialysis or continuous ambulatory peritoneal dialysis. *J Am Soc Nephrol* 1995; 6: 110-20.

19. Levine DM, Gordon BR. Lipoprotein(a) levels in patients receiving renal replacement therapy: methodologic issues and clinical implications. *Am J Kidney Dis* 1995; 26: 162-9.

20. Longenecker JC, Klag MJ, Marcovina SM, *et al.* High lipoprotein(a) levels and small apolipoprotein(a) size prospectively predict cardiovascular events in dialysis patients. *J Am Soc Nephrol* 2005; 16: 1794-802.

21. Attman PO, Samuelsson OG, Moberly J, *et al.* Apolipoprotein B-containing lipoproteins in renal failure: the relation to mode of dialysis. *Kidney Int* 1999; 55: 1536-42.

22. Deighan CJ, Caslake MJ, McConnell M, Boulton-Jones JM, Packard CJ. Atherogenic lipoprotein phenotype in end-stage renal failure: origin and extent of small dense low-density lipoprotein formation. *Am J Kidney Dis* 2000; 35: 852-62.

23. Kobashigawa JA, Kasiske BL. Hyperlipidemia in solid organ transplantation. *Transplantation* 1997; 63: 331-8.

24. Ong CS, Pollock CA, Caterson RJ, Mahony JF, Waugh DA, Ibels LS. Hyperlipidemia in renal transplant recipients: natural history and response to treatment. *Medicine* (Baltimore) 1994; 73: 215-23.

25. Kasiske BL, de MA, Flechner SM, *et al.* Mammalian target of rapamycin inhibitor dyslipidemia in kidney transplant recipients. *Am J Transplant* 2008; 8: 1384-92.

26. Ozsoy RC, van der Steeg WA, Kastelein JJ, Arisz L, Koopman MG. Dyslipidaemia as predictor of progressive renal failure and the impact of treatment with atorvastatin. *Nephrol Dial Transplant* 2007; 22: 1578-86.

27. Earle KA, Harry D, Zitouni K. Circulating cholesterol as a modulator of risk for renal injury in patients with type 2 diabetes. *Diabetes Res Clin Pract* 2008; 79: 68-73.

28. Ficociello LH, Perkins BA, Silva KH, *et al.* Determinants of progression from microalbuminuria to proteinuria in patients who have type 1 diabetes and are treated with angiotensin-converting enzyme inhibitors. *Clin J Am Soc Nephrol* 2007; 2: 461-9.

29. Misra A, Kumar S, Kishore VN, Kumar A. The role of lipids in the development of diabetic microvascular complications: implications for therapy. *Am J Cardiovasc Drugs* 2003; 3: 325-38.

30. Hadjadj S, Duly-Bouhanick B, Bekherraz A, *et al.* Serum triglycerides are a predictive factor for the development and the progression of renal and retinal complications in patients with type 1 diabetes. *Diabetes Metab* 2004; 30: 43-51.

31. Cusick M, Chew EY, Hoogwerf B, *et al.* Risk factors for renal replacement therapy in the Early Treatment Diabetic Retinopathy Study (ETDRS), Early Treatment Diabetic Retinopathy Study Report No. 26. *Kidney Int* 2004; 66: 1173-9.

32. Molitch ME, Rupp D, Carnethon M. Higher levels of HDL cholesterol are associated with a decreased likelihood of albuminuria in patients with long-standing type 1 diabetes. *Diabetes Care* 2006; 29: 78-82.

33. Go AS, Chertow GM, Fan D, McCulloch CE, Hsu CY. Chronic kidney disease and the risks of death, cardiovascular events, and hospitalization. *N Engl J Med* 2004; 351: 1296-305.

34. Anavekar NS, McMurray JJ, Velazquez EJ, *et al.* Relation between renal dysfunction and cardiovascular outcomes after myocardial infarction. *N Engl J Med* 2004; 351: 1285-95.

35. Foley RN, Parfrey PS, Sarnak MJ. Clinical epidemiology of cardiovascular disease in chronic renal disease. *Am J Kidney Dis* 1998; 32: S112-9.

36. Habib AN, Baird BC, Leypoldt JK, Cheung AK, Goldfarb-Rumyantzev AS. The association of lipid levels with mortality in patients on chronic peritoneal dialysis. *Nephrol Dial Transplant* 2006; 21: 2881-92.

37. Iseki K, Yamazato M, Tozawa M, Takishita S. Hypocholesterolemia is a significant predictor of death in a cohort of chronic hemodialysis patients. *Kidney Int* 2002; 61: 1887-93.

38. Kilpatrick RD, McAllister CJ, Kovesdy CP, Derose SF, Kopple JD, Kalantar-Zadeh K. Association between serum lipids and survival in hemodialysis patients and impact of race. *J Am Soc Nephrol* 2007; 18: 293-303.

39. Kovesdy CP, Anderson JE, Kalantar-Zadeh K. Inverse association between lipid levels and mortality in men with chronic kidney disease who are not yet on dialysis: effects of case mix and the malnutrition-inflammation-cachexia syndrome. *J Am Soc Nephrol* 2007; 18: 304-11.

40. Liu Y, Coresh J, Eustace JA, *et al.* Association between cholesterol level and mortality in dialysis patients: role of inflammation and malnutrition. *JAMA* 2004; 291: 451-9.

41. Levey AS, Coresh J, Balk E, *et al.* National Kidney Foundation practice guidelines for chronic kidney disease: evaluation, classification, and stratification. *Ann Intern Med* 2003; 139: 137-47.

42. Ordonez JD, Hiatt RA, Killebrew EJ, Fireman BH. The increased risk of coronary heart disease associated with nephrotic syndrome. *Kidney Int* 1993; 44: 638-42.

43. Wheeler DC, Bernard DB. Lipid abnormalities in the nephrotic syndrome: causes, consequences, and treatment. *Am J Kidney Dis* 1994; 23: 331-46.

44. Brown CD, Azrolan N, Thomas L, *et al.* Reduction of lipoprotein(a) following treatment with lovastatin in patients with unremitting nephrotic syndrome. *Am J Kidney Dis* 1995; 26: 170-7.

45. Massy ZA, Ma JZ, Louis TA, Kasiske BL. Lipid lowering therapy in patients with renal disease. *Kidney Int* 1995; 48: 188-98.

46. Rabelink AJ, Hene RJ, Erkelens DW, Joles JA, Koomans HA. Effects of simvastatin and cholestyramine on lipoprotein profile in hyperlipidaemia of nephrotic syndrome. *Lancet* 1988; 2: 1335-8.

47. Thomas ME, Harris KP, Ramaswamy C, *et al.* Simvastatin therapy for hypercholesterolemic patients with nephrotic syndrome or significant proteinuria. *Kidney Int* 1993; 44: 1124-9.

48. Gentile MG, Fellin G, Cofano F, *et al.* Treatment of proteinuric patients with a vegetarian soy diet and fish oil. *Clin Nephrol* 1993; 40: 315-20.

49. Keilani T, Schlueter WA, Levin ML, Batlle DC. Improvement of lipid abnormalities associated with proteinuria using fosinopril, an angiotensin-converting enzyme inhibitor. *Ann Intern Med* 1993; 118: 246-54.

50. Tonelli M, Isles C, Curhan GC, *et al.* Effect of pravastatin on cardiovascular events in people with chronic kidney disease. *Circulation* 2004; 110: 1557-63.

51. Sever PS, Dahlof B, Poulter NR, *et al.* Prevention of coronary and stroke events with atorvastatin in hypertensive patients who have average or lower-than-average cholesterol concentrations, in the Anglo-Scandinavian Cardiac Outcomes Trial - Lipid Lowering Arm (ASCOT-LLA): a multicentre randomised controlled trial. *Lancet* 2003; 361: 1149-58.

52. MRC/BHF Heart Protection Study of cholesterol lowering with simvastatin in 20,536 high-risk individuals: a randomised placebo-controlled trial. *Lancet* 2002; 360: 7-22.

53. Shepherd J, Kastelein JJ, Bittner V, *et al.* Intensive lipid lowering with atorvastatin in patients with coronary heart disease and chronic kidney disease: the TNT (Treating to New Targets) study. *J Am Coll Cardiol* 2008; 51: 1448-54.

54. Athyros VG, Mikhailidis DP, Papageorgiou AA, *et al.* The effect of statins versus untreated dyslipidaemia on renal function in patients with coronary heart disease. A subgroup analysis of the Greek atorvastatin and coronary heart disease evaluation (GREACE) study. *J Clin Pathol* 2004; 57: 728-34.

55. Shepherd J, Kastelein JJ, Bittner V, *et al.* Effect of intensive lipid lowering with atorvastatin on renal function in patients with coronary heart disease: the Treating to New Targets (TNT) study. *Clin J Am Soc Nephrol* 2007; 2: 1131-9.

56. Tonelli M, Moye L, Sacks FM, Cole T, Curhan GC. Effect of pravastatin on loss of renal function in people with moderate chronic renal insufficiency and cardiovascular disease. *J Am Soc Nephrol* 2003; 14: 1605-13.

57. Randomised placebo-controlled trial of effect of ramipril on decline in glomerular filtration rate and risk of terminal renal failure in proteinuric, non-diabetic nephropathy. The GISEN Group (Gruppo Italiano di Studi Epidemiologici in Nefrologia). *Lancet* 1997; 349: 1857-63.

58. Klahr S, Levey AS, Beck GJ, *et al.* The effects of dietary protein restriction and blood-pressure control on the progression of chronic renal disease. Modification of Diet in Renal Disease Study Group. *N Engl J Med* 1994; 330: 877-84.

59. Nagai T, Tomizawa T, Nakajima K, Mori M. Effect of bezafibrate or pravastatin on serum lipid levels and albuminuria in NIDDM patients. *J Atheroscler Thromb* 2000; 7: 91-6.

60. Tonelli M, Collins D, Robins S, Bloomfield H, Curhan GC. Gemfibrozil for secondary prevention of cardiovascular events in mild to moderate chronic renal insufficiency. *Kidney Int* 2004; 66: 1123-30.

61. Stegmayr BG, Brannstrom M, Bucht S, *et al.* Low-dose atorvastatin in severe chronic kidney disease patients: a randomized, controlled endpoint study. *Scand J Urol Nephrol* 2005; 39: 489-97.

62. Wanner C, Krane V, Marz W, *et al.* Atorvastatin in patients with type 2 diabetes mellitus undergoing hemodialysis. *N Engl J Med* 2005; 353: 238-48.

63. Fellström BC, Jardine AG, Schmieder RE, *et al.* Rosuvastatin and cardiovascular events in patients undergoing hemodialysis. *N Engl J Med* 2009; 360: 1395-407.

64. Baigent C, Landry M. Study of Heart and Renal Protection (SHARP). *Kidney Int Suppl* 2003; S207-10.

65. Holdaas H, Fellstrom B, Jardine AG, *et al.* Effect of fluvastatin on cardiac outcomes in renal transplant recipients: a multicentre, randomised, placebo-controlled trial. *Lancet* 2003; 361: 2024-31.

66. Holdaas H, Fellstrom B, Jardine AG, *et al.* Beneficial effect of early initiation of lipid-lowering therapy following renal transplantation. *Nephrol Dial Transplant* 2005; 20: 974-80.

67. European Best Practice guidelines for hemodialysis (part 1). Section VII. Vascular disease and risk factors. *Nephrol Dial Transplant* 2002; 17(Suppl 7): 88-109.

68. National Kidney Foundation. K/DOQI Clinical Practice Guidelines for management of dyslipidemias in patients with kidney disease. *Am J Kidney Dis* 2003; 41 (4suppl 3): I-IV, S1-S91.

69. National Kidney Foundation. K/DOQI Clinical Practice Guidelines and Clinical Practice Recommendations for Diabetes and Chronic Kidney Disease. *Am J Kidney Dis* 2007; 49 (Suppl 2): S88-S95.

70. National Kidney Foundation. KDIGO Clinical Practice Guideline for the Care of Kidney Transplant Recipients, Public Review Draft, March 9, 2009; http://www.kdigo.org/clinical_practice_guidelines.

71. Executive summary of the Third Report of the National Cholesterol Education Program (NCEP) Expert Panel on Detection, Evaluation, and Treatment of High Blood Cholesterol in Adults (Adult Treatment Panel III). *JAMA* 2001; 285: 2486-97.

Chapter 12

The link between chronic inflammatory diseases and cardiovascular risk

Michael T. Nurmohamed MD PhD
Consultant Rheumatologist
Departments of Internal Medicine & Rheumatology
VU University Medical Centre;
Department of Rheumatology, Jan van Breemen Institute
Amsterdam, The Netherlands

Introduction

Over the last few decades it has become widely acknowledged that inflammation plays a pivotal role throughout all stages of atherogenesis, ranging from initial foam cell formation, lesion progression all the way through destabilization of the advanced lesions. Consequently, one could hypothesize that patients with chronic inflammatory disorders would be more susceptible to the development of atherosclerotic diseases in comparison to healthy persons. This would be particularly prominent in diseases with a high inflammatory burden, i.e. the chronic inflammatory rheumatic diseases, with rheumatoid arthritis (RA) as the most prevalent one. There is accumulating evidence to show that patients with RA have an increased cardiovascular risk. Therefore, in this chapter the link between inflammation and cardiovascular disease will be illustrated by reviewing the literature investigating cardiovascular disease, its underlying risk factors, and their relations to inflammation in RA. Moreover, the inflammatory aspects of atherosclerosis will be discussed.

Rheumatoid arthritis

Rheumatoid arthritis (RA) is a chronic inflammatory joint disease of unknown etiology, that affects around 1% of the population, which untreated may lead to severe disability and a shortened life expectancy. Hence, the treatment goal is to control the underlying inflammation in order to inhibit or even prevent joint destruction [1]. RA starts with thickening of the synovium and there are typical cellular infiltrates comprising macrophages and T-lymphocytes. Important cytokines involed in this inflammatory process are interleukin-1, tumor necrosis factor-α (TNF-α) and interleukin-6 (Figure 1).

Before the mid-eighties RA patients were first treated with a non-steroidal anti-inflammatory drug (NSAID) and later on disease-modifying antirheumatic drugs (DMARDs) were added (pyramid approach). More insight into the underlying pathophysiological mechanisms, showing destructive synovitis in the beginning of the disease, led to early and aggressive DMARD therapy. It was also shown that the combination of DMARDs, aiming at different levels of the underlying pathophysiological processes, provides additive efficacy without an increase of overall adverse effects.

In the last decade cytokine-specific biologic therapies have become widely available for clinical use. These agents aim to block essential cytokines such as tumor necrosis factor (TNF)-α, interleukin-1 or interleukin-6 and have shown to be the most effective antirheumatic drugs presently available.

Mortality

The overall standardized mortality ratio for RA is approximately two (ranging from 0.9 to 3.0) and numerous reports have demonstrated that excess mortality is mostly due to (atherosclerotic) cardiovascular disease [2, 3] (III/B).

Cardiovascular morbidity

In the last 20 years, several studies have witnessed an increased rate of cardiovascular diseases of atherosclerotic origin such as myocardial infarction, cerebrovascular disease and peripheral arterial disease, as well as heart failure, in RA patients in comparison to healthy controls. In a recent Dutch investigation, the size of this enhanced cardiovascular risk was studied by comparing prevalent cardiovascular disease in RA with that of type 2 diabetes [4]. Prevalences of atherosclerotic cardiovascular diseases were assessed in randomly selected RA patients (CARRÉ investigation), as well as in participants of a Dutch population-based cohort study on glucose metabolism and other cardiovascular risk factors (Hoorn investigation). RA patients without diabetes from the CARRÉ investigation (n=294) were compared to individuals without diabetes (n=258) and persons with diabetes (n=194) from the Hoorn investigation. The unadjusted prevalences of atherosclerotic cardiovascular diseases were 13% in non-diabetic RA patients, 5% in persons without diabetes, and 12% in individuals with diabetes, respectively. The age- and gender-adjusted odds ratios for cardiovascular disease were 3.1 in non-diabetic RA patients, and 2.3 in individuals with type 2 diabetes in comparison to persons without diabetes indicating that the prevalence of cardiovascular disease in RA is increased to a magnitude that is at least similar to that of type

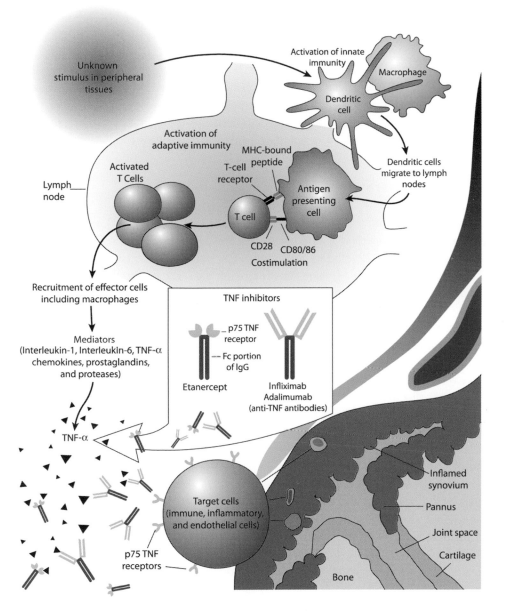

Figure 1. Pathophysiological role of cytokines and other mediators and their inhibitors in RA.

2 diabetes (**IIa/B**). Atherosclerotic cardiovascular events were encountered in 9% of the RA patients and in 4% of the controls from the general population, in the first 3 years of the prospective part of this study. This corresponds with an incidence rate of 3.3 per 100 patient-years for RA, and 1.5 per 100 person-years for the general population [5]. The age- and gender-adjusted hazard ratio was 1.9 (95% CI: 1.2-3.1).

Another prospective, 1-year follow-up investigation in 236 consecutive outpatients with RA revealed an incidence of 3.4 per 100 patient-years versus 0.6 per 100 person-years in the general population [6], corresponding to an adjusted hazard ratio of 3.2 (95% CI: 1.3-6.4).

Altogether, the presently available literature indicates an at least two-fold increased (atherosclerotic) cardiovascular risk in RA patients in comparison to general population subjects. As adjustment for cardiovascular risk factors only slightly attenuates the hazard ratios in RA in comparison to the general population, this indicates that RA itself should be considered an independent, important, cardiovascular risk factor **(IIa/B)**.

Preclinical atherosclerosis

It is well-known that carotid artery intima-media thickness (IMT) allows an adequate assessment of early, preclinical atherosclerosis and predicts for future CV disease. A recent review encompassing 22 studies with 1400 RA patients and 1200 controls revealed a 0.09mm (95% CI: 0.07-0.11) significantly greater IMT relative to controls [7]. Moreover, a significant relationship between IMT and disease activity was observed.

True longitudinal data about the IMT progression in RA are still lacking, but recently these were indirectly derived from cross-sectional data and it was observed that the IMT progression rate was related to disease duration and ranged from 0.15mm/10 years among patients with a disease duration less than 7 years to 0.30mm/10 years in patients with a more than 20 years disease duration [8]. Hence, RA patients with longstanding disease have more atherosclerosis than patients of the same age but with a shorter disease duration, which indicates that RA accelerates atherosclerosis.

The clinical implications of the above-mentioned preclinical atherosclerosis was recently assessed in a cohort of 47 RA patients who were at baseline when carotid IMT was assessed and free from CVD [9]. Cardiovascular events occurred in 17 patients during the 5-year follow-up period and when IMT was divided into quartiles, no cardiovascular events were observed in RA patients with an IMT less than 0.77mm, whereas a cardiovascular event was observed in 6 of the 10 RA patients with an IMT of more than 0.91mm. Obviously, further large-scale studies are mandatory for confirmation of these tempting findings.

Cardiovascular risk factors

This amplified cardiovascular burden in RA patients could be due to an increased prevalence of 'traditional' cardiovascular risk factors, such as smoking, hypercholesterolemia, diabetes mellitus, hypertension or impaired physical fitness [10-12]. Secondly, suboptimal or no treatment of (comorbid) cardiovascular risk factors may be important [13, 14]. Finally, RA itself, due to the chronic inflammation, may be an independent cardiovascular risk factor [15] **(III/B)**.

Dyslipidemia

Increased levels of total cholesterol (TC), low-density lipoprotein (LDL) cholesterol (LDL-C) and a decreased level of high-density lipoprotein (HDL) cholesterol (HDL-C) are related to an enhanced cardiovascular risk. The studies investigating lipids in RA patients are rather contradictory but nevertheless they point towards an inverse association between disease activity and lipid levels [16] **(III/B)**.

Active RA is characterized by loss of body cell mass due to decreasing skeletal muscle [17]. TNF and other proinflammatory cytokines are important mediators for this so-called rheumatoid cachexia and are also associated with depressed TC and HDL-C levels [18], resulting in an inverse relationship between disease activity and cholesterol levels, as a higher RA disease activity is associated with a lower TNF level.

Over the years apolipoprotein AI (apoAI) and apolipoprotein B (apoB) have emerged as important components of lipid metabolism. The protein apoAI is present on HDL-C, whereas the protein apoB is present on all atherogenic lipoporteins, including LDL-C, intermediate-density lipoprotein (IDL) and very-low-density lipoprotein (VLDL) particles. Therefore, these two apolipoproteins reflect the number of anti-atherogenic and atherogenic particles, respectively. There is some evidence that apoB might be a better predictor for cardiovascular events than LDL-C and that the apoB/apoAI ratio is an accurate prognostic indicator for cardiovascular disease [19]. In other words, apoAI might protect against cardiovascular disease, whereas apoB increases cardiovascular risk. Again, disease activity in RA patients had an adverse, inverse relationship with apoAI and HDL-C with disease activity [20] **(III/B)**.

Interestingly, beyond the tradional role of HDL as a key player in the reverse cholesterol transport (RCT), HDL has also been shown to exert a wide array of additional protective effects beyond the RCT pathway, comprising anti-inflammatory, anti-oxidative, anti-thrombotic and direct endothelial protective effects [21]. One of the anti-atherogenic functions of HDL-C is to protect LDL-C from oxidation by reactive oxygen species. This so called 'anti-inflammatory' HDL-C can be discerned from 'pro-inflammatory' HDL-C that lacks these properties and actually may enhance inflammation. Indeed, McMahon *et al* demonstrated that pro-inflammatory HDL-C was more frequently present in RA patients (n=48) than in controls (n=72), i.e. 20% versus 4%, respectively [22] **(III/B)**.

When does dyslipidemia start?

As dyslipidemia can already be detected in early active RA, the question arises as to when this phenomenon starts. Therefore, we studied the lipid profile and its relationship with inflammatory markers in persons who later developed RA [23].

Overall, these 'future' RA patients had 4% higher TC, 9% lower HDL-C, 17% higher triglyceride and 6% higher apoB concentrations in comparison to matched control subjects (p=0.05), 10 years or more before clinical disease onset. Although the differences in the various lipid concentrations appear small they do have clinical relevance, particularly in light of the results from other investigations with lipid-lowering drugs such as fibrates [24] **(IIb/B)**.

Antirheumatic treatment and lipid profile

A large number of studies in RA have investigated the relationship between the lipid profile and the use of antirheumatic drugs. It was demonstrated that treatment with DMARDs (including corticosteroids) has a favourable influence on the lipid profile in early RA patients with active disease activity, i.e. an increment of TC but a more pronounced increment of HDL-C. As a consequence, the atherogenic index (total/HDL cholesterol ratio), an important prognostic cardiovascular risk factor [25], improves (i.e. lower) **(IIb/B)**.

Studies with TNF-blockers show a transient increase of TC and HDL-C, mostly associated with a better atherogenic index, during the initial treatment months. Thereafter, the results differ between the investigations. This might be caused by differences in disease activity, (changing) comedication, particularly corticosteroids, diet and mobility. Conversely, it is in line with the expectation that HDL-C levels increase in cases of attenuating inflammatory activity, since HDL is an inverse acute phase reactant. Future studies should appropriately address these potential confounders to reach valid conclusions.

An intriguing question is whether or not the anti-atherogenic properties of HDL-C, that are lost in patients with active inflammation, are restored by antirheumatic drug treatment. This topic was investigated in ankylosing spondylitis (AS) [26], as patients with AS have an increased cardiovascular risk that approaches that of RA and that appears also to be inflammatory driven [27]. We investigated in 92 consecutive AS patients, in whom TNF-blocking therapy was initiated, lipid levels, inflammation markers (as C-reactive protein) and serum amyloid A (SAA) during the first 3 months of treatment. In a smaller subgroup, HDL-C composition was studied with surface-enhanced laser desorption/ionization time-of-flight (SELDI-TOF) analysis. During TNF-blocking therapy all inflammatory markers decreased, whereas TC, HDL-C and apoAI levels increased significantly with improved TC/HDL-C and apoB/apoA ratios. SELDI-TOF analysis revealed that initially SAA was present within HDL particles at high concentrations and declined during treatment with TNF-blocking therapy, concomitant with a decreased systemic inflammatory state. This is important as SAA replaces the anti-atherogenic apoAI in HDL particles, thereby jeopardizing the anti-atherogenic properties of HDL-C. Conversely, a declining SAA concentration within the HDL particle will restore the anti-atherogenic properties of HDL-C **(IIa/B)**.

Smoking, diabetes, metabolic syndrome, hypertension, body mass index and physical fitness

Smoking is one of the most important cardiovascular risk factors in the general population. It is possible that smoking plays a (cardiovascular) role in RA as it enhances the susceptibility for the development of RA as well its seriousness. A recent study showed more smoking in RA patients as well as a higher cardiovascular risk versus non-smoking RA patients **(II/B)**. However, it is important to recognize that the effect was significantly lower in comparison to the controls (hazard ratios for cardiovascular disease, 1.3 and 2.2, for smoking vs. non-smoking RA patients and smoking vs. non-smoking control subjects, respectively) [28].

Literature data about the prevalence of type 2 diabetes are not uniform but as there is mounting evidence for insulin resistance in RA, an increased prevalence of diabetes would be expected. In addition, several investigations show that the metabolic syndrome is more observed in RA patients versus control subjects, which appeared to have an inflammatory etiology [29-31]. In addition, the metabolic syndrome is amplified in hypothyroid RA patients, presumably due to an impaired microvascular function, also on an inflammatory basis [32] **(IIa/B)**.

Hypertension probably occurs more often in RA [33-35], but no conclusions can be reached with respect to the contribution of body mass index and physical fitness towards cardiovascular risk in RA **(III/B)**.

Atherosclerosis and inflammation

Formerly atherosclerosis has been considered as an accumulation of lipids within the arterial wall. However, nowadays atherosclerosis is considered a chronic inflammation of the artery (Figure 2). Endothelial dysfunction is the initiating step of atherogenesis and may be

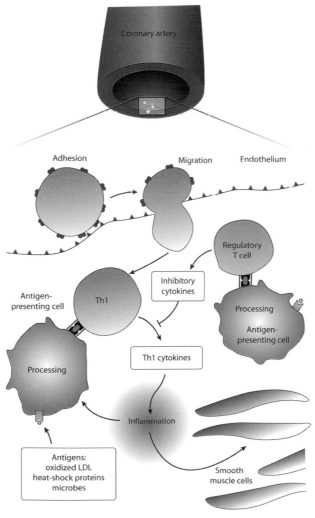

Figure 2. Effects of T-cell activation and plaque inflammation.

caused by several cardiovascular risk factors, e.g. oxidized LDL-C, smoking, diabetes or hypertension. The endothelium becomes more permeable, for example, lipoproteins, and becomes procoagulant instead of anticoagulant. The inflammation causes an influx of inflammatory and muscle cells, and subsequently inflammatory cytokines such as TNF and interleukin-1 cause an increased endothelial cell binding of (oxidized) LDL-C. This LDL cholesterol accumulates within macrophages and foam cells and fatty streaks are formed as a consequence. Thereafter, a fibrous cap is formed that separates the arterial lumen and the atherosclerotic plaque.

The lumen of this thickened arterial wall initially remains unaltered due to dilatation. Further activation and accumulation of macrophages and T-lymphocytes results in release of several mediators leading to further damage and narrowing of the artery lumen. Platelet activation by the impaired endothelium causes thromboxane formation leading to vasoconstriction and platelet aggregation. Finally, plaque rupture with thrombosis results in angina or myocardial infarction and this process is responsible for 70% of acute coronary syndromes. Endothelial erosion is the other main cause. The cellular interactions observed in the development of atherosclerosis resemble that of chronic inflammatory diseases such as RA [36], providing a plausible explanation for the amplified cardiovascular risk in RA patients and other inflammatory arthritis such as AS and psoriatic arthritis.

Endothelial progenitor cells (EPC) are essential for the repair of endothelial wall to retain vascular homeostasis and there is accumulated evidence to indicate that a lowered number of EPCs and/or hampered EPC function is associated with atherogenesis and new cardiovascular events. Furthermore, there is growing evidence for a lowered number of circulating EPCs in patients with (active) RA making them more susceptible to cardiovascular disease. It has been hypothesized that EPCs have been derived from the blood (thereby hampering endothelial restoration) and move to the inflamed synovium for neovascularisation.

Pathogenesis of the enhanced cardiovascular risk in RA

Altogether, traditional cardiovascular risk factors account partially for the observed excess cardiovascular risk in RA. As indicated above, the other key feature explaining the increased cardiovascular risk is thought to be inflammation, as it, on the one hand, plays an important role in different stages of atherogenesis, from early atheroma formation to plaque instability and thrombus development responsible for cardiovascular events, and, on the other hand, amplifies cardiovascular risk factors [37-40]. Moreover, there is strong evidence revealing that chronic inflammatory markers are independently associated with cardiovascular mortality and morbidity in RA patients [41-45]. Solomon and colleagues used a large registry cohort of almost 11,000 RA patients to investigate the contribution of RA-specific (i.e. inflammatory) factors and cardiovascular risk factors towards the occurrence of cardiovascular endpoints including myocardial infarction, stroke and transient ischemic attack. The median follow-up was 2 years, during which period there were 75 myocardial infarctions or strokes and it appeared that RA-specific factors had the same explanatory value as cardiovascular risk factors [46]. In other words, both inflammation and cardiovascular risk factors significantly contribute to the (increased) cardiovascular risk in RA (IIb/B).

Antirheumatic treatment and cardiovascular risk in RA

As indicated inflammation has a pivotal role in the development of excess cardiovascular risk in patients with RA. Likewise one would expect the suppression of the inflammatory process to lower the cardiovascular risk in RA. Commonly applied drugs in RA are discussed below.

Acetaminophen

Chan *et al* investigated the relationship of acetaminophen and major cardiovascular events in a prospective cohort of 70,971 women [47]. A total of 2041 major cardiovascular events were encountered in the 12-year follow-up period. It was demonstrated that frequent use of acetaminophen, i.e. 22 days/month or more, was associated with elevated risk of cardiovascular disease. The highest risk was observed with the use of 15 tablets per week or more (RR: 1.7 [95% CI, 1.1 to 2.6]) **(III/B)**. This association might be caused by inducing hypertension due to COX-2 inhibition [48].

Corticosteroids

The use of corticosteroids is a continuing matter of debate in view of their adverse cardiovascular risk profile that is particularly dose-related. For instance, hypertension was particularly observed in patients receiving 7.5mg or more prednisone daily for 6 months or longer [49]. In contrast, low-dose corticosteroids could have favourable effects on the lipid profile [50, 51].

Undoubtedly corticosteroids rapidly and effectively reduce the inflammatory process in RA and their use could be justified for a short period of time, e.g. for 'bridging' the time between the start and response to DMARDs [52], and obviously, the debate has yet to be settled.

NSAIDs and COXIBs

Over the last two decades there has been continuous discussion as to if and to what extent cyclo-oxygenase-2 inhibitors (COXIBs) are related to an amplified cardiovascular risk, in particular myocardial infarction, and large-scale placebo-controlled investigations have shown that COXIBs are indeed associated with a two-fold increased cardiovascular risk.

There are several observational registry investigations that suggest an indication of amplified cardiovascular risk (or not) with NSAIDs. Observational investigations are prone to methodological errors that can be only solved by large-scale randomized trials. However, such trials have not been performed with NSAIDs. At second best, one can use meta-analyses, with meta-regression techniques, of the comparative trials with NSAIDs and COXIBs to reach valid inferences regarding the cardiovascular risks of NSAIDs. It appears that non-naproxen NSAIDs have a comparable amplified cardiovascular risk compared with COXIBs [53] **(IIa/B)**.

DMARDs

There are some suggestions that effective suppression of the inflammatory process in RA decreases cardiovascular risk. Choi *et al* demonstrated in a cohort study in 1240 patients, where 190 patients died during 18 years of follow-up, that cardiovascular mortality was 70% lower in methotrexate treated patients in comparison to those who did not receive treatment [54]. Another study particularly showed that the methotrexate non-responders have a worse prognosis [55] **(III/B)**.

In two case control studies it appeared that not only cardiovascular mortality is reduced by methotrexate, but also cardiovascular morbidity [56, 57] **(III/B)**. Moreover, other traditional DMARDs, such as sulfasalazine and leflunomide, were associated with a lower cardiovascular risk in comparison to no treatment.

TNF-blocking agents

In view of the important role of TNF in both atherosclerosis and RA one would expect that TNF-blockers will also lower the cardiovascular risk in RA. However, the placebo-controlled registration trials with TNF-blocking have not considered cardiovascular endpoints and therefore we have to rely on database investigations.

Jacobsson *et al* coupled a Swedish database with 1430 RA patients, of which 921 patients were treated with TNF-blockade, with a national mortality register. There was a total of 188 deaths in the TNF-blockade group and the corrected hazard ratio for death was 0.65 when comparing TNF-blockade versus no TNF-blockade [58]. In another investigation, Jacobsson *et al* determined the incidence of first cardiovascular events coupling a database, with 983 RA patients, of which 531 received TNF-blockers, with registers of inpatient care and mortality [59]. Thirteen cardiovascular events were observed in patients treated with TNF-blockade, i.e. 14 cardiovascular events/1000 person-years, in comparison to 35 cardiovascular events/1000 person-years in RA patients not treated with TNF-blockade, resulting in an adjusted rate ratio of 0.46. In another, larger, cohort investigation it was demonstrated that the occurrence of myocardial infarction was by more than 60% when comparing responders to TNF-blockade with non-responders [60] **(III/B)**.

One could hypothesize that a potential favourable effect of TNF-blockers, as suggested above, on the cardiovascular risk might be mediated by attenuation of IMT progression (or even reduction of IMT) in view of the similarities of the underlying inflammatory processes of RA and atherosclerosis.

To date, a few studies have investigated the effect of TNF-blockade on IMT in RA patients [61-65]. Altogether, these studies point toward no progression or even regression of IMT. However, these investigations encompassed limited numbers of patients in addition to suboptimal methodological designs. Consequently, final conclusions are still not possible and this area certainly needs further exploration.

Cardiovascular risk management in RA

The cardiovascular risk in RA appears to be twice as high as in the general population and compares to type 2 diabetes, a well-known cardiovascular risk factor. The established cardiovascular risk factors only explain this excess cardiovascular risk to a limited extent. The other relevant factor appears to be the underlying inflammation in RA. Hence, RA should be considered as a new, independent, cardiovascular risk factor for which cardiovascular risk management is essential **(IIb/B)**. Generally, cardiovascular risk management starts with the determination of one's cardiovascular risk profile, i.e. assessment of smoking status, blood pressure, lipid profile, etc. With these risk factors, the 10 years absolute risk for a (fatal) cardiovascular event can then be determined with the aid of a cardiovascular risk formula, such as the Framingham risk calculator and the Systematic Coronary Risk Evaluation (SCORE). Treatment with statins and/or antihypertensives is then only started above a certain value, e.g. a 10-year cardiovascular mortality or morbidity risk of 10% or higher.

One could state that intervention studies in RA with statins and/or antihypertensives and cardiovascular endpoints are necessary before conclusions about their efficacy can be drawn. However, it is unlikely that the effect of these drugs would be lower in RA patients in comparison with the general population. Actually, the effects might be amplified as statins, and several antihypertensive agents also have anti-inflammatory properties. Recently, EULAR recommendations for cardiovascular risk management in rheumatoid and other inflammatory arthritis patients were published (Table 1) [66], that advocated yearly cardiovascular risk screening. Drug treatment with statins and/or antihypertensives is then dependent on the calculated 10-year cardiovascular risk. For RA it is recommended to adapt existing risk functions, such as SCORE, by a multiplier of 1.5 to achieve a more appropriate estimation of the 10-year cardiovascular risk. Finally, intensive suppression of the inflammatory process should be considered to further decrease the cardiovascular risk in patients with RA.

Conclusions

There is accumulating evidence that inflammation has an essential role in the development of atherosclerosis and this might explain the increased cardiovascular risk in the chronic inflammatory disease RA. Although increased prevalences of the 'traditional' cardiovascular risk factors also appear to be present, these cannot fully explain the increased propensity towards cardiovascular disease in RA patients.

Inflammation causes pro-atherogenic changes of the lipid profile that are counteracted by conventional DMARD treatment. TNF-blocking therapy induces beneficial effects on the lipid profile, but these might level off after the first few months of TNF-blocking therapy, probably due to changes in comedication, particularly corticosteroids.

Moreover, in inflammatory situations such as active RA or active AS, HDL-C loses its anti-atherogenic properties and becomes pro-atherogenic. Functionality of HDL-C might be restored by TNF-blocking therapy.

Table 1. EULAR recommendations for cardiovascular risk management in patients with rheumatoid arthritis.

- RA is a high-risk condition for cardiovascular disease, that is due to both an increased prevalence of traditional risk factors and the inflammatory burden

- Adequate control of disease activity is necessary to decrease the cardiovascular risk

- Annual cardiovascular risk assessment is recommended for all RA patients

- Risk score models should be adapted for RA patients by introducing a 1.5 multiplication

- TC/HDL cholesterol should be used when the SCORE model is used

- Intervention with lipid-lowering agents and antihypertensive drugs should be carried out according to national guidelines

- Statins, ACE inhibitors and/or AT-II blockers are preferred treatment options due to their potential pleiotropic effects

- The role of COXIBs and most NSAIDs regarding the cardiovascular risk is not well established and needs further investigation

- Corticosteroids: use the lowest dose possible

The increased cardiovascular risk in RA is linked to traditional cardiovascular risk factors as well as inflammation. Hence, cardiovascular risk management should be aimed at assessment (and treatment if indicated) of traditional cardiovascular risk factors as well as effective suppression of the inflammatory process.

Key points	Evidence level
◆ Cardiovascular mortality is doubled in patients with RA in comparison with the general population.	III/B
◆ Cardiovascular morbidity is also doubled and might be comparable to that of type 2 diabetes.	IIa/B
◆ RA itself is an independent (inflammatory) cardiovascular risk factor.	IIa/B
◆ An increased disease activity is associated with a more atherogenic lipid profile that improves during antirheumatic treatment.	IIb/B
◆ HDL-C becomes pro-atherogenic in inflammatory situations, and treatment with TNF-blocking agents might restore the atheroprotective properties of HDL-C.	IIb/B
◆ Hypertension, smoking and the metabolic syndrome probably occur more frequently in RA.	IIb/B
◆ Similarities on a cellular level of atherosclerosis and RA probably explain the increased cardiovascular risk in RA.	III/B
◆ DMARDs and TNF-blockers probably reduce the cardiovascular risk in RA.	III/B
◆ Cardiovascular risk management is mandatory for RA patients and this should focus on 'traditional' cardiovascular risk factors as well as suppression of the inflammatory process.	IIb/B

References

1. Alamanos Y, Voulgari PV, Drosos AA. Incidence and prevalence of rheumatoid arthritis, based on the 1987 American College of Rheumatology criteria: a systematic review. *Semin Arthritis Rheum* 2006; 36(3): 182-8.
2. van Doornum S, McColl G, Wicks IP. Accelerated atherosclerosis: an extraarticular feature of rheumatoid arthritis? *Arthritis Rheum* 2002; 46(4): 862-73.
3. Avina-Zubieta JA, Choi HK, Sadatsafavi M, Etminan M, Esdaile JM, Lacaille D. Risk of cardiovascular mortality in patients with rheumatoid arthritis: a meta-analysis of observational studies. *Arthritis Rheum* 2008; 59(12): 1690-7.
4. van Halm V, Peters MJ, Voskuyl AE, Boers M, Lems WF, Visser M, *et al*. Rheumatoid arthritis versus diabetes as a risk factor for cardiovascular disease: a cross-sectional study. The CARRÉ Investigation. *Ann Rheum Dis* 2009; 68(9): 1395-400.
5. Peters MJ, van Halm VP, Voskuyl AE, Boers M, Lems WF, Visser M, *et al*. Rheumatoid arthritis as important independent risk factor for incident cardiovascular disease. *Arthritis Rheum* 2009; 58(Suppl): 691.
6. del Rincon ID, Williams K, Stern MP, Freeman GL, Escalante A. High incidence of cardiovascular events in a rheumatoid arthritis cohort not explained by traditional cardiac risk factors. *Arthritis Rheum* 2001; 44(12): 2737-45.
7. van Sijl AM, Peters MJ, Knol DL, de Vet HC, Gonzalez-Gay MA, Smulders Y, *et al*. Carotid intima media thickness in rheumatoid arthritis as compared to control subjects - a meta-analysis. *Arthritis Rheum* 2009; 60 (Suppl 1): 600.

8. Del Rincon I, O'Leary DH, Freeman GL, Escalante A. Acceleration of atherosclerosis during the course of rheumatoid arthritis. *Atherosclerosis* 2007; 195: 354-60.

9. Gonzalez-Juanatey C, Llorca J, Martin J, Gonzalez-Gay MA. Carotid intima-media thickness predicts the development of cardiovascular events in patients with rheumatoid arthritis. *Semin Arthritis Rheum* 2009; 38(5): 366-71.

10. Goodson NJ, Solomon DH. The cardiovascular manifestations of rheumatic diseases. *Curr Opin Rheumatol* 2006; 18(2): 135-40.

11. Dessein PH, Joffe BI, Veller MG, Stevens BA, Tobias M, Reddi K, *et al.* Traditional and nontraditional cardiovascular risk factors are associated with atherosclerosis in rheumatoid arthritis. *J Rheumatol* 2005; 32(3): 435-42.

12. Pincus T, Callahan LF. Taking mortality in rheumatoid arthritis seriously - predictive markers, socioeconomic status and comorbidity. *J Rheumatol* 1986; 13(5): 841-5.

13. Boers M, Dijkmans B, Gabriel S, Maradit-Kremers H, O'Dell J, Pincus T. Making an impact on mortality in rheumatoid arthritis: targeting cardiovascular comorbidity. *Arthritis Rheum* 2004; 50(6): 1734-9.

14. Redelmeier DA, Tan SH, Booth GL. The treatment of unrelated disorders in patients with chronic medical diseases. *N Engl J Med* 1998; 338(21): 1516-20.

15. Maradit-Kremers H, Crowson CS, Nicola PJ, Ballman KV, Roger VL, Jacobsen SJ, *et al.* Increased unrecognized coronary heart disease and sudden deaths in rheumatoid arthritis: a population-based cohort study. *Arthritis Rheum* 2005; 52(2): 402-11.

16. White D, Fayez S, Doube A. Atherogenic lipid profiles in rheumatoid arthritis. *N Z Med J* 2006; 119(1240): U2125.

17. Walsmith J, Roubenoff R. Cachexia in rheumatoid arthritis. *Int J Cardiol* 2002; 85(1): 89-99.

18. Kotler DP. Cachexia. *Ann Intern Med* 2000; 133(8): 622-34.

19. Sniderman AD, Kiss RS. The strengths and limitations of the apoB/apoA-I ratio to predict the risk of vascular disease: a Hegelian analysis. *Curr Atheroscler Rep* 2007; 9(4): 261-5.

20. Park YB, Lee SK, Lee WK, Suh CH, Lee CW, Lee CH, *et al.* Lipid profiles in untreated patients with rheumatoid arthritis. *J Rheumatol* 1999; 26(8): 1701-4.

21. Barter PJ, Puranik R, Rye KA. New insights into the role of HDL as an anti-inflammatory agent in the prevention of cardiovascular disease. *Curr Cardiol Rep* 2007; 9(6): 493-8.

22. McMahon M, Grossman J, FitzGerald J, hlin-Lee E, Wallace DJ, Thong BY, *et al.* Proinflammatory high-density lipoprotein as a biomarker for atherosclerosis in patients with systemic lupus erythematosus and rheumatoid arthritis. *Arthritis Rheum* 2006; 54(8): 2541-9.

23. van Halm V, Nielen MM, Nurmohamed MT, van SD, Reesink HW, Voskuyl AE, *et al.* Lipids and inflammation: serial measurements of the lipid profile of blood donors who later developed rheumatoid arthritis. *Ann Rheum Dis* 2007; 66(2): 184-8.

24. Rubins HB, Robins SJ, Collins D, Fye CL, Anderson JW, Elam MB, Faas FH, Linares E, Schaefer EJ, Schectman G, Wilt TJ, Wittes J. Gemfibrozil for the secondary prevention of coronary heart disease in men with low levels of high-density lipoprotein cholesterol. Veterans Affairs High-Density Lipoprotein Cholesterol Intervention Trial Study Group. *N Engl J Med* 1999; 341(6): 410-8.

25. Nurmohamed MT. Atherogenic lipid profiles and its management in patients with rheumatoid arthritis. *Vasc Health Risk Manag* 2007; 3(6): 845-52.

26. van Eijk IC, de Vries MK, Levels JHM, Huizer EE, Dijkmans BAC, van der Horst-Bruinsma IE, *et al.* Improvement of lipid profile is accompanied by atheroprotective alterations in high density lipoprotein composition upon TNF blockade. *Arthritis Rheum* 2009; 60(5): 1324-30.

27. Peters MJ, van der Horst-Bruinsma I, Dijkmans BA, Nurmohamed MT. Cardiovascular risk profile of patients with spondylarthropathies, particularly ankylosing spondylitis and psoriatic arthritis. *Semin Arthritis Rheum* 2004; 34(3): 585-92.

28. Gonzalez A, Maradit Kremers H, Crowson CS, Ballman KV, Roger VL, Jacobsen SJ, *et al.* Do cardiovascular risk factors confer the same risk for cardiovascular outcomes in rheumatoid arthritis patients as in non-rheumatoid arthritis patients? *Ann Rheum Dis* 2008; 67(1): 64-9.

29. Karvounaris SA, Sidiropoulos PI, Papadakis JA, Spanakis EK, Bertsias GK, Kritikos HD, *et al.* Metabolic syndrome is common among middle-to-older aged Mediterranean patients with rheumatoid arthritis and correlates with disease activity: a retrospective, cross-sectional, controlled, study. *Ann Rheum Dis* 2007; 66(1): 28-33.

30. Dessein PH, Tobias M, Veller MG. Metabolic syndrome and subclinical atherosclerosis in rheumatoid arthritis. *J Rheumatol* 2006; 3(12): 2425-32.

31. Chung CP, Oeser A, Solus JF, Avalos I, Gebretsadik T, Shintani A, *et al.* Prevalence of the metabolic syndrome is increased in rheumatoid arthritis and is associated with coronary atherosclerosis. *Atherosclerosis* 2008; 196(2): 756-63.

32. Raterman HG, van Eijk IC, Voskuyl AE, Peters MJ, Dijkmans BA, van Halm V, *et al.* The metabolic syndrome is amplified in hypothyroid rheumatoid arthritis patients: a cross-sectional study. *Ann Rheum Dis* 2010; 69(1): 39-42.

33. Panoulas VF, Douglas KMJ, Milionis HJ, Stavropoulos-Kalinglou A, Nightingale P, Kita MD, *et al.* Prevalence and associations of hypertension and its control in patients with rheumatoid arthritis. *Rheumatology* (Oxford) 2007; 46(9): 1477-82.

34. Solomon DH, Curhan GC, Rimm EB, Cannuscio CC, Karlson EW. Cardiovascular risk factors in women with and without rheumatoid arthritis. *Arthritis Rheum* 2004; 50(11): 3444-9.

35. Goodson NJ, Silman AJ, Pattison DJ, Lunt M, Bunn D, Luben R, *et al.* Traditional cardiovascular risk factors measured prior to the onset of inflammatory polyarthritis. *Rheumatology* (Oxford) 2004; 43(6): 731-6.

36. Pasceri V, Yeh ET. A tale of two diseases: atherosclerosis and rheumatoid arthritis. *Circulation* 1999; 100(21): 2124-6.

37. Sattar N, McCarey DW, Capell H, McInnes IB. Explaining how 'high-grade' systemic inflammation accelerates vascular risk in rheumatoid arthritis. *Circulation* 2003; 108(24): 2957-63.

38. Ross R. Atherosclerosis - an inflammatory disease. *N Engl J Med* 1999; 340(2): 115-26.

39. Aubry MC, Maradit-Kremers H, Reinalda MS, Crowson CS, Edwards WD, Gabriel SE. Differences in atherosclerotic coronary heart disease between subjects with and without rheumatoid arthritis. *J Rheumatol* 2007; 34(5): 937-42.

40. Maradit-Kremers H, Nicola PJ, Crowson CS, Ballman KV, Gabriel SE. Cardiovascular death in rheumatoid arthritis: a population-based study. *Arthritis Rheum* 2005; 52(3): 722-32.

41. Gonzalez-Gay MA, Gonzalez-Juanatey C, Lopez-Diaz MJ, Pineiro A, Garcia Porrua C, Miranda-Filloy JA, *et al.* HLA-DRB1 and persistent chronic inflammation contribute to cardiovascular events and cardiovascular mortality in patients with rheumatoid arthritis. *Arthritis Rheum* 2007; 57(1): 125-32.

42. Goodson NJ, Symmons DP, Scott DG, Bunn D, Lunt M, Silman AJ. Baseline levels of C-reactive protein and prediction of death from cardiovascular disease in patients with inflammatory polyarthritis: a ten-year follow-up study of a primary care-based inception cohort. *Arthritis Rheum* 2005; 52(8): 2293-9.

43. Jacobsson LT, Turesson C, Hanson RL, Pillemer S, Sievers ML, Pettitt DJ, *et al.* Joint swelling as a predictor of death from cardiovascular disease in a population study of Pima Indians. *Arthritis Rheum* 2001; 44(5): 1170-6.

44. Maradit-Kremers H, Nicola PJ, Crowson CS, Ballman KV, Gabriel SE. Cardiovascular death in rheumatoid arthritis: a population-based study. *Arthritis Rheum* 2005; 52(3): 722-32.

45. Wallberg-Jonsson S, Johansson H, Ohman ML, Rantapaa-Dahlqvist S. Extent of inflammation predicts cardiovascular disease and overall mortality in seropositive rheumatoid arthritis. A retrospective cohort study from disease onset. *J Rheumatol* 1999; 26(12): 2562-71.

46. Solomon D, Greenberg J, Reed G, Setoguchi S, Tsao P, Kremer J. Cardiovascular risk among patients with RA in Corrona: comparing the explanatory value of traditional cardiovascular risk factors with RA factors. *Ann Rheum Dis* 2008; 67(Suppl II): 482.

47. Chan AT, Manson JE, Albert CM, Chae CU, Rexrode KM, Curhan GC, *et al.* Nonsteroidal antiinflammatory drugs, acetaminophen, and the risk of cardiovascular events. *Circulation* 2006; 113(12): 1578-87.

48. Hinz B, Cheremina O, Brune K. Acetaminophen (paracetamol) is a selective cyclooxygenase-2 inhibitor in man. *FASEB J* 2008; 22(2): 383-90.

49. Panoulas VF, Douglas KMJ, Stavropoulos-Kalinoglou A, Metsios GS, Nightingale P, Kita MD, *et al.* Long-term exposure to medium-dose glucocorticoid therapy associates with hypertension in patients with rheumatoid arthritis. *Rheumatology* (Oxford) 2008; 47(1): 72-5.

50. Boers M, Nurmohamed MT, Doelman CJA, Lard LR, Verhoeven AC, Voskuyl AE, *et al.* Influence of glucocorticoids and disease activity on total and high density lipoprotein cholesterol in patients with rheumatoid arthritis. *Ann Rheum Dis* 2003; 62(9): 842-5.

51. Vis M, Nurmohamed MT, Wolbink G, Voskuyl AE, de Koning M, van de Stadt R, *et al.* Short term effects of infliximab on the lipid profile in patients with rheumatoid arthritis. *J Rheumatol* 2005; 32(2): 252-5.

52. Kirwan JR. Systemic low-dose glucocorticoid treatment in rheumatoid arthritis. *Rheum Dis Clin North Am* 2001; 27(2): 389-x.

53. Kearney PM, Baigent C, Godwin J, Halls H, Emberson JR, Patrono C. Do selective cyclo-oxygenase-2 inhibitors and traditional non-steroidal anti-inflammatory drugs increase the risk of atherothrombosis? Meta-analysis of randomised trials. *BMJ* 2006; 332(7553): 1302-8.

54. Choi HK, Hernan MA, Seeger JD, Robins JM, Wolfe F. Methotrexate and mortality in patients with rheumatoid arthritis: a prospective study. *Lancet* 2002; 359(9313): 1173-7.

55. Krause D, Schleusser B, Herborn G, Rau R. Response to methotrexate treatment is associated with reduced mortality in patients with severe rheumatoid arthritis. *Arthritis Rheum* 2000; 43(1): 14-21.

56. van Halm VP, Nurmohamed MT, Twisk JWR, Dijkmans BAC, Voskuyl AE. Disease-modifying antirheumatic drugs are associated with a reduced risk for cardiovascular disease in patients with rheumatoid arthritis: a case control study. *Arthritis Res Ther* 2006; 8(5): R151.

57. Suissa S, Bernatsky S, Hudson M. Antirheumatic drug use and the risk of acute myocardial infarction. *Arthritis Rheum* 2006; 55(4): 531-6.

58. Jacobsson LTH, Turesson C, Nilsson JA, Petersson IF, Lindqvist E, Saxne T, *et al.* Treatment with TNF blockers and mortality risk in patients with rheumatoid arthritis. *Ann Rheum Dis* 2007; 66(5): 670-5.

59. Jacobsson LTH, Turesson C, Gulfe A, Kapetanovic MC, Petersson IF, Saxne T, *et al.* Treatment with tumor necrosis factor blockers is associated with a lower incidence of first cardiovascular events in patients with rheumatoid arthritis. *J Rheumatol* 2005; 32(7): 1213-8.

60. Dixon WG, Watson KD, Lunt M, Hyrich KL, Silman AJ, Symmons DPM. Reduction in the incidence of myocardial infarction in patients with rheumatoid arthritis who respond to anti-tumor necrosis factor alpha therapy: results from the British Society for Rheumatology Biologics Register. *Arthritis Rheum* 2007; 56(9): 2905-12.

61. Del Porto F, Lagana B, Lai S, Nofroni I, Tinti F, Vitale M, *et al.* Response to anti-tumour necrosis factor alpha blockade is associated with reduction of carotid intima-media thickness in patients with active rheumatoid arthritis. *Rheumatology* (Oxford) 2007; 46: 1111-5.

62. Gonzalez-Juanatey C, Llorca J, Garcia-Porrua C, Martin J, Gonzalez-Gay MA. Effect of anti-tumor necrosis factor alpha therapy on the progression of subclinical atherosclerosis in severe rheumatoid arthritis. *Arthritis Rheum* 2006; 55: 150-3.

63. Wong M, Oakley SP, Young L, Jiang B, Wierzbicki AS, Panayi G, *et al.* Infliximab improves vascular stiffness in patients with rheumatoid arthritis 6. *Ann Rheum Dis* 2009; 68(8): 1277-84.

64. Sidiropoulos PI, Siakka P, Pagonidis K, Raptopoulou A, Kritikos H, Tsetis D, *et al.* Sustained improvement of vascular endothelial function during anti-TNFalpha treatment in rheumatoid arthritis patients 3. *Scand J Rheumatol* 2009; 38(1): 6-10.

65. Ferrante A, Giardina AR, Ciccia F, Parrinello G, Licata G, Avellone G, *et al.* Long-term anti-tumour necrosis factor therapy reverses the progression of carotid intima-media thickness in female patients with active rheumatoid arthritis. *Rheumatol Int* 2009; Apr 23 [Epub ahead of print].

66. Peters MJ, Symmons DPM, McCarey DW, Nurmohamed MT. Cardiovascular risk management in patients with rheumatoid arthritis and other types of inflammatory arthritis - A EULAR task force. *Ann Rheum Dis* 2010; 69(2): 325-31.

Chapter 13

What is the evidence for a physiological and pathogenic role of lipoprotein (a)?

Sotirios Tsimikas MD FACC FAHA FSCAI, Professor of Medicine
Division of Cardiology, Vascular Medicine Program
University of California San Diego, La Jolla, California

"It is a riddle, wrapped in a mystery, inside an enigma;
but perhaps there is a key......."

Winston Churchill, 1939

Introduction

Lipoprotein (a) [Lp(a)] is a unique lipoprotein which has no known physiological function, despite nearing 50 years since its discovery. Plasma Lp(a) concentrations are primarily mediated by the *LPA* gene locus and are not generally affected by environmental influences. Elevated levels of Lp(a), which occur in up to 30% of whites and 70% of blacks, have been associated with cardiac death, myocardial infarction, stroke and peripheral arterial disease, particularly in subjects with small apolipoprotein (a) isoforms. Lp(a) is a modest risk factor when elevated in isolation, but its cardiovascular risk is strongly accentuated by additional cardiac risk factors. Its high homology to plasminogen makes it a potential mediator of atherothrombosis, yet *in vivo* clinical data for this property is lacking. Compared to other lipoproteins, Lp(a) has been unexpectedly found to be a preferential carrier of oxidized phospholipids in plasma. Currently, no specific therapy exists to lower Lp(a) levels, but there is growing interest in this area, particularly as antisense oligonucleotides and cholesterol ester transport protein inhibitors have been recently shown to lower Lp(a) levels in humans. This chapter will review the genetics of apolipoprotein (a), the metabolism of Lp(a), the clinical data linking it to atherothrombosis and analyze future directions in this enigmatic lipoprotein.

Genetics of the *LPA* locus and lipoprotein (a) protein architecture

Lp(a) was first described in 1962 by Kare Berg (Dr Berg passed away in 2009) as an antigenic determinant in humans when he immunized rabbits with human low-density lipoprotein (LDL) derived from a single human donor [1]. He noted that approximately one third of human plasma samples reacted to the anti-serum from the immunized rabbits, including the plasma from the donor of the LDL. Subsequently, Lp(a) has been discovered to consist of apolipoprotein (a) which is covalently bound to apolipoprotein B-100 (apoB) by a single disulfide bond formed by cysteine 4057 of apo(a) and cysteine 4326 of apoB [2, 3].

The *LPA* gene codes for unique apo(a) structures called kringles (K) that contain three disulfide bonds and resemble a Danish pastry. Kringles are common motifs in the protein structure of coagulation and growth factors and are present in plasminogen, urokinase, tissue plasminogen activator, prothrombin, angiostatin, hepatocyte growth Factor, Factor XII and macrophage stimulating Factor, among others. *LPA* codes for KIV, KV and a protease-like domain which is inactive [4]. Apo(a) KIV is composed of 10 subtypes, of which KIV-2 is present in multiple copies (from 3 to >40) (Figure 1). The *apo(a)* gene sits opposite the plasminogen gene (*PMG*) on chromosome 6 and has high homology to it (75-94%). *PMG* differs from

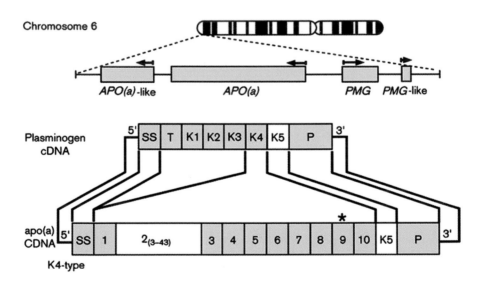

Figure 1. Genetic architecture and biological characteristics of *apo(a)*. The apolipoprotein (a) locus is present on chromosome 6. The *apo(a)* gene is approximately 50kb from the plasminogen gene and is flanked by two pseudogenes. The apo(a) and plasminogen cDNA structures are compared. The known functional roles of the K4 repeats are indicated (see text). * = free cysteine; K = kringle; Lp(a) = lipoprotein(a); P = protease domain; PMG = plasminogen; SS = signal sequence; T = tail. *Reproduced with permission from Hobbs HH, et al [2].*

apo(a) by containing coding sequences for five kringles (KI-V) which lack the repeats present in apo(a) and also does not bind to apoB. The PMG gene also has an active protease domain that is cleaved by tissue plasminogen activator to form plasmin. PMG is 92Kda in size, whereas apo(a) has marked size heterogeneity (167 to >650Kda) among individuals due largely to the variable number of KIV-2 repeats and additional polymorphisms in other areas of the LPA gene locus. Multiple apo(a) KIV isoforms exist ranging from 12 to >50 copies (one KIV-1, one each of KIV-3-10, 3-40 KIV-2 repeats and KV). Furthermore, most subjects (~80%) have two distinct apo(a) alleles that may also vary significantly in size. These issues have led to significant challenges in developing in vitro assays to quantitate plasma Lp(a) levels as variability in Lp(a) size exists not only among different individuals but also within the same individual [5].

The LPA gene and thus the apo(a) protein is only present in humans, non-human primates and Old World monkeys. An unrelated apo(a) gene is also present in European hedgehogs which is composed of 37 copies of K3, that is postulated to have occurred through divergent evolution [6]. Apo(a) is unlike other apolipoproteins in that it is hydrophilic and carbohydrate-rich and projects into the aqueous phase when bound to apoB. Lp(a) levels are largely determined genetically and are not affected by LDL receptor activity [7, 8]. Additional genetic polymorphisms in the apo(a) gene may also account for some of this variability [9-14]. Plasma Lp(a) levels may vary by 1000-fold (from <0.1 to >250mg/dL) between individuals and are generally inversely associated with the size of the smaller apo(a) allele **(IIa/B)**. Subjects of African and South Asian descent have 2-3-fold higher levels of Lp(a) than Caucasians, but the underlying reasons are not fully understood [15]. There is no standardized method yet accepted to measure Lp(a). Plasma Lp(a) levels are generally measured as the mass of the entire Lp(a) particle, with a variety of methods using specific antibodies and presented in mg/dL with the levels being derived from a standard curve of human plasma. More recently, with the recognition of the multiple KIV repeats interfering with the assay, it has been appropriately recommended that data be presented in mmol/L using molar standards of known apo(a) size [16]. Some groups have also reported assays measuring or estimating Lp(a) cholesterol content, similar to LDL-C, but these assays are not yet fully validated. It is to be emphasized that all clinically available LDL-C assays contain the cholesterol content of Lp(a) within the LDL-C value.

Lp(a) metabolism

The mechanisms mediating apo(a) synthesis are well known, but the mechanisms underlying Lp(a) clearance are less well understood. Figure 2 summarizes some of the characteristics of Lp(a) [17]. Apo(a) is synthesized in hepatocytes and the rate of synthesis is primarily related to apo(a) gene transcription [2]. Post-translational regulation, such as formation of the three disulfide bonds for each kringle subtype and N-linked glycation, is important for proper apo(a) folding and transport out of the endothelial reticulum (ER), which may take up to 120 minutes and is dependent of apo(a) size. Once apo(a) exits the ER, it is transported to the Golgi apparatus for further post-translational modification, and finally to the hepatocyte cell surface. Lp(a) is then assembled from newly synthesized apoB (LDL), first by low affinity, non-covalent interactions between KIV-5-8, and then through a disulfide bond

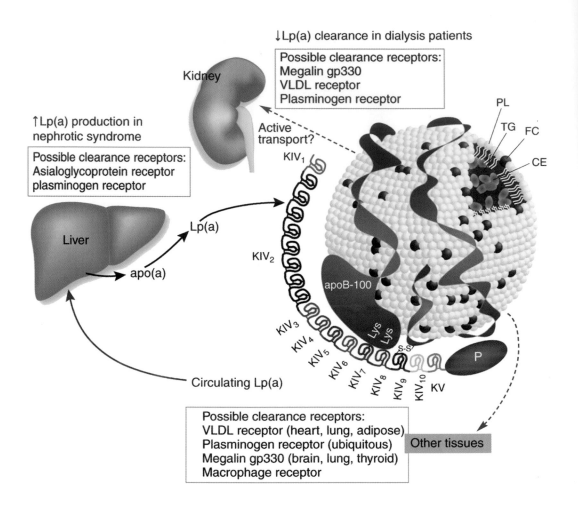

Figure 2. Schematic representation of proposed pathways for lipoprotein(a) catabolism. Circulating lipoprotein(a) [Lp(a)] is derived from apolipoprotein (a) that is synthesized and secreted by the liver (black arrows); proposed routes of Lp(a) removal from the circulation are shown by red arrows. Although the pathways of Lp(a) catabolism *in vivo* are unclear, the liver seems to play a major role in this process (solid red arrow). Additionally, the kidney (dashed red arrow) appears to contribute to Lp(a) clearance, as is evidenced, for example, by the decreased fractional catabolic rate observed in hemodialysis patients with compromised renal function. Peripheral tissues (dashed red arrow) also may contribute to Lp(a) removal from the circulation. For all routes of catabolism, possible clearance receptors are listed, although their respective contributions to Lp(a) clearance *in vivo* remain to be determined. apoB-100 = apolipoprotein B-100; PL = phospholipids; TG = triglycerides; FC = free cholesterol; CE = cholesterol ester. *Reproduced with permission from Albers JJ, et al* [17]. *Nature Publishing Group ©* *2007.*

between unpaired cysteine residues on KIV-9 on apo(a) and cysteine 4326 on the C-terminal region of apoB. Because small isoform apo(a) particles are more easily synthesized and secreted, and because different sized isoforms are cleared at similar rates, it is believed that subjects with small apo(a) isoforms have higher Lp(a) levels.

Mechanisms of Lp(a) atherogenicity

Lp(a) is thought to act as a cardiovascular disease risk factor at three major etiological levels: pro-atherogenic, pro-thrombotic and pro-inflammatory (Figure 3). The pro-atherogenic properties are mediated by several pathways, including the delivery of

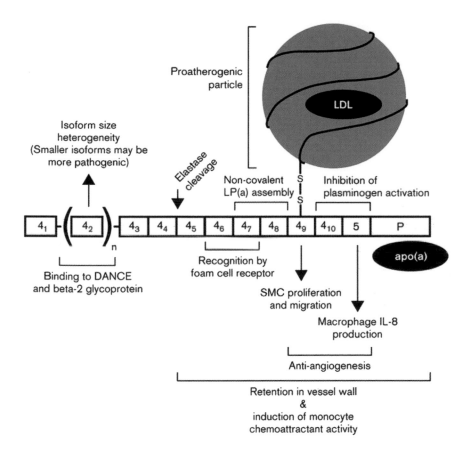

Figure 3. Specific functions have been mapped to discrete structural units in lipoprotein(a). Using a combination of the expression of recombinant forms of apolipoprotein(a) [apo(a)] and elastase cleavage of apolipoprotein(a)/lipoprotein(a) [Lp(a)], functional domains in apolipoprotein (a) have been identified. These domains are potentially involved in the promotion of atherosclerosis and inflammation, the inhibition of angiogenesis and fibrinolysis, and lipoprotein(a) assembly. The LDL-like moiety promotes foam cell formation by virtue of the interaction of apolipoprotein (a) kringle 4 types 6 and 7, with a specific receptor expressed on foam cells. *Reproduced with permission from Koschinsky ML, et al [70].*

cholesterol esters to the vessel wall by Lp(a) and the high affinity of apo(a) to proteins and proteoglycans on the endothelial surface and in the arterial wall, which is mediated by lysine binding sites on apo(a) [18, 19]. In fact, Lp(a) is quite difficult to dissociate from atherosclerotic lesions once it is bound to proteins. The biological significance of this property is illustrated by showing that mice overexpressing mutant apo(a) lacking a competent lysine binding site on KIV-10 develop significantly less atherosclerosis compared to mice with wild-type apo(a) [20]. Lp(a) has also been postulated to inhibit spontaneous fibrinolysis by virtue of its high homology to plasminogen. *In vitro* studies have demonstrated that Lp(a) affects several pathways of fibrinolysis, including direct effects on plasminogen activity [21, 22] and activation of tissue factor activity [23]. It also mediates activation of platelets through the thrombin receptor [24]. However, conclusive evidence of its pro-thrombotic effects in humans is lacking and has been mainly noted in non-randomized, retrospective studies that are limited by significant selection bias. In addition, the plasma levels of plasminogen are significantly higher than Lp(a) levels in most patients, thus the clinical relevance of these studies remains to be determined. Finally, *in vitro* studies have shown that apo(a) alone is pro-inflammatory and its exposure to macrophages results in increased IL-8 levels, a pro-inflammatory cytokine [25, 26].

A novel hypothesis on the atherogenicity of Lp(a) as a carrier of pro-inflammatory oxidized phospholipids

Our research has shown that Lp(a), compared to other lipoproteins, preferentially binds oxidized phospholipids (OxPL) measured in human plasma with antibody E06 [27-31]. We have recently proposed the alternative hypothesis that a unique physiological role of Lp(a) may be to bind pro-inflammatory OxPL, which may also explain its pathophysiological role as a risk factor for CVD. When present at high plasma concentrations, Lp(a) would be more atherogenic than native LDL, as it binds with increased affinity to arterial intimal proteoglycans resulting in increased intimal concentration of LDL with associated proinflammatory OxPL.

OxLDL and OxPL are highly immunogenic, present in atherosclerotic lesions of humans and animals, and intimately involved in plaque vulnerability and plaque destabilization, being present in much higher quantities (70-fold) in plaque than plasma [31]. OxPL, key components of minimally oxidized LDL, fully oxidized LDL, apoptotic cells and atherosclerotic lesions, are important contributors to early events in atherogenesis by activating pro-inflammatory genes, leading to inflammatory cascades in the vessel wall [32-34]. We have developed a chemiluminescent ELISA to detect OxPL on human apolipoprotein B-100 particles (OxPL/apoB) in plasma using antibody E06. Following a series of large clinical studies we have determined that OxPL/apoB levels correlate with Lp(a) levels [27, 35-40]. However, this relationship is strongly dependent on the underlying size of the apo(a) isoforms, where small isoforms are strongly associated with high OxPL/apoB levels, but large isoforms are weakly associated [39, 41].

Work from our laboratory has also shown that elevated plasma levels of OxPL/apoB are associated with anatomical CVD and worse CVD outcomes (reviewed by Fraley *et al* [42]). For example, OxPL/apoB levels are elevated in patients with coronary, carotid and femoral artery disease [38, 39], acute coronary syndromes [35], and following percutaneous coronary intervention [36]. Increased levels of OxPL/apoB are also associated with the progression of carotid and femoral atherosclerosis [39] and predict new cardiovascular events [43, 44]. For example, in the Bruneck study (Figure 4) [43], a prospective population-based survey of 40-79-year-old men and women, baseline levels of OxPL/apoB were evaluated for CVD events in a multivariable analysis, which included traditional risk factors, hsCRP and Lp-PLA2 activity. Cumulative hazard plots demonstrate that OxPL/apoB strongly predicted new CVD events, defined as cardiovascular death, myocardial infarction, stroke and transient ischemic attack. Interestingly, OxPL/apoB levels were independent of all known risk factors, except for Lp(a). Moreover, OxPL/apoB levels predicted future CVD events beyond the information provided by the Framingham Risk Score (Figure 5). We have further confirmed this finding in the prospective EPIC-Norfolk cohort of apparently healthy men and women aged 45-79 years followed for 6 years [44].

Another interesting aspect related to the potential pathophysiological role of Lp(a) is that of its relationship to events. If Lp(a) indeed has any beneficial function in its risk to cardiovascular disease, it would be expected to show a non-linear relationship. In fact, we

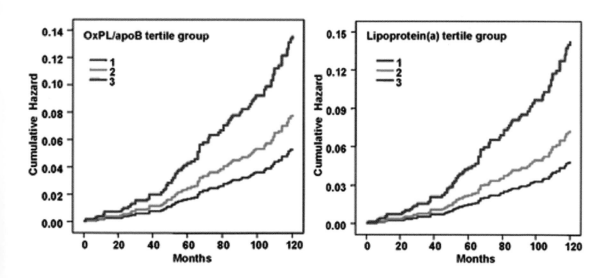

Figure 4. Cumulative rate of death, myocardial infarction and stroke based on tertiles of baseline values of OxPL/apoB (left panel) and Lp(a) (right panel) in the prospective 10-year follow-up of the Bruneck Study. *Reproduced with permission from Kiechl S, et al* [43].

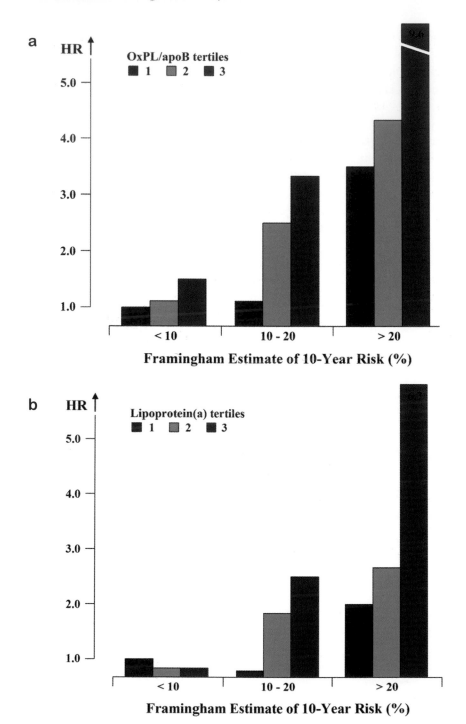

Figure 5. Relationship between tertile groups of OxPL/apoB (<0.0379, 0.0379-0.0878, >0.0878) (a) and Lp(a) (<6.9, 6.9-23.8, >23.8)(b) and CVD risk within each Framingham Risk Score Group. Framingham Risk Score was calculated as low risk (<10% risk of events over 10 years), moderate risk (10%-20%) and high risk (>20%). *Reproduced with permission from Kiechl S, et al* [43].

recently showed in the Bruneck study that a J-shaped curve was present in the relationship to future (10 years) risk of death, myocardial infarction and stroke **(IIa/B)** (Figure 6). A close look at this relationship demonstrates that the lowest sextile (levels <2.7mg/dL) was actually associated with a higher hazard ratio of new CVD events than the second lowest sextile (2.7-6.8mg/dL). In fact, the risk did not rise until Lp(a) levels were greater than >24mg/dL. Remarkably, this is the level at which cardiovascular risk rises based on epidemiological studies. In support of this notion, Berg *et al* [45] showed that the optimal benefit from simvastatin in the 4S study was not in the lowest Lp(a) quartile, but the second lowest. These intriguing findings suggest the hypothesis that Lp(a) may indeed have a vestigial or primordial physiological function at very low levels in binding and transporting OxPL. However, when Lp(a) levels are elevated and these OxPL cannot be removed, then it is atherogenic, particularly with its strong predilection for the vessel wall, where it may deliver pro-inflammatory OxPL, among the other pro-atherogenic properties mentioned above.

Another interesting insight into this potential aspect of Lp(a) was recently demonstrated by noting a synergistic effect between Lp(a), and OxPL/apoB, and lipoprotein-associated

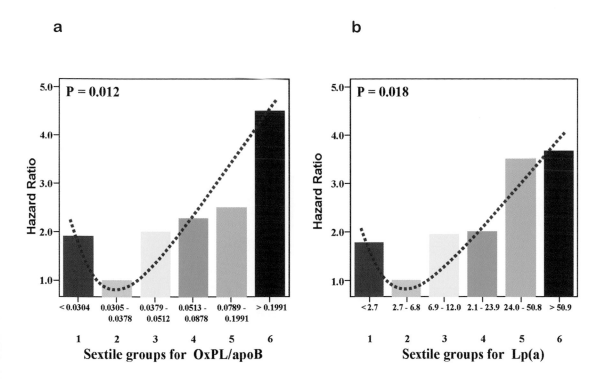

Figure 6. Plots of hazard ratios for incident CVD according to OxPL/apoB (a) and Lp(a) (b) sextile groups. *Reproduced with permission from Kiechl S, et al* [43].

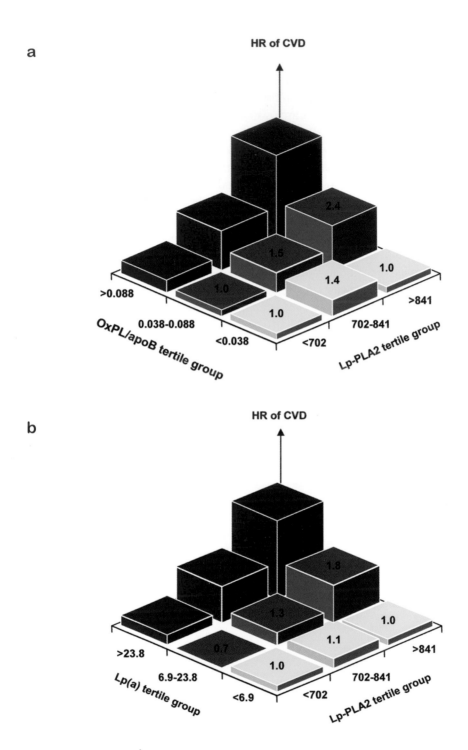

Figure 7. Relationship between OxPL/apoB (a) and Lp(a) (b) tertile groups and CVD risk according to tertiles of Lp-PLA2 activity (p=0.018 and p=0.008 for interaction of OxPL/apoB and Lp(a), respectively). *Reproduced with permission from Kiechl S, et al* [43].

phospholipase A2 (Lp-PLA2) activity (Figure 7). For example, when either OxPL/apoB (or Lp(a)) and Lp-PLA2 levels were low, there was essentially no association of either with CVD. However, at the highest tertiles of Lp-PLA2 and either Lp(a) or OxPL/apoB the hazard ratio was approximately doubled. This finding implies that these measures may be related pathophysiologically and provide complementary information in predicting new CVD events. These findings suggest that OxPL are preferentially transferred to and sequestered by Lp(a) and thus may be subjected to degradation by the Lp(a)-associated Lp-PLA2 [46]. This concept implies that under normal conditions, some minimal level of Lp(a) in the circulation may be beneficial as it may function as a transporter and scavenger of OxPL. Under these conditions, the pro-inflammatory lyso-PC, which derives from the degradation of OxPL catalyzed by Lp-PLA2, could then be transferred from Lp(a) to albumin, which represents the major carrier of lyso-PC in plasma. However, under conditions of acute inflammation and oxidative stress, the Lp(a)-associated Lp-PLA2 activity may become insufficient to respond to the increased sequestration of OxPL on Lp(a). In cases of increased Lp(a) plasma levels, this lipoprotein may become pro-atherogenic, particularly due to its enhanced binding to the vessel wall matrix [46, 47].

Clinical studies on Lp(a) as a cardiovascular risk factor

Multiple cross-sectional and prospective studies have demonstrated that Lp(a) is an independent risk factor for CVD death, myocardial infarction, stroke and peripheral arterial disease **(Ia/A)** [48, 49]. As with most genetic risk factors that initiate risk at birth, it is a stronger CVD risk factor in young patients, in those with highly elevated levels and in those with additional atherogenic risk factors, particularly elevated LDL-cholesterol [38, 43, 50]. Interestingly, apo(a) isoforms may provide enhanced predictive value beyond knowledge of Lp(a) levels, even in black subjects, where Lp(a) alone is not a strong a risk factor [15, 51-57]. The literature on the cardiovascular risk of Lp(a) was nicely summarized in a recent meta-analysis by Bennet et al [58] (Figure 8). Analyzing data from 9870 incident cases of CVD showed an odds ratio of 1.45 (95% CI 1.32-1.58) for individuals in the top tertile compared to the bottom tertile.

More recently, two additional large studies [59, 60] have provided convincing evidence of Lp(a) as an independent risk factor for myocardial infarction and cardiovascular disease. Kamstrup et al [60] evaluated 9330 men and women from the general population in the Copenhagen City Heart Study over 10 years of follow-up where 498 participants developed MI. Following adjustment for multiple other risk factors, they demonstrated a progressive increase in risk of MI according to the level of Lp(a) in both men and women. In women, hazard ratios for MI for elevated lipoprotein(a) levels were 1.1 for 5 to 29mg/dL (22nd to 66th percentile), 1.7 for 30 to 84mg/dL (67th to 89th percentile), 2.6 for 85 to 119mg/dL (90th to 95th percentile), and 3.6 for > or =120mg/dL (>95th percentile) versus levels <5mg/dL (<22nd percentile). In men, hazard ratios were 1.5, 1.6 , 2.6 , and 3.7, respectively. Absolute 10-year risks of MI were 10% and 20% in smoking, hypertensive women aged >60 years with lipoprotein(a) levels of <5 and > or =120mg/dL, respectively. Equivalent values in men were 19% and 35%.

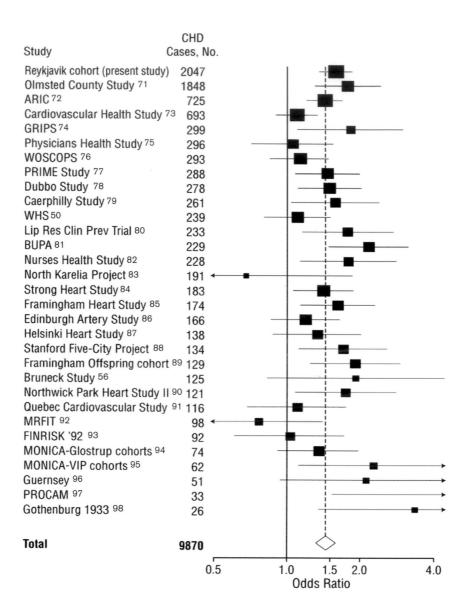

Study	CHD Cases, No.
Reykjavik cohort (present study)	2047
Olmsted County Study [71]	1848
ARIC [72]	725
Cardiovascular Health Study [73]	693
GRIPS [74]	299
Physicians Health Study [75]	296
WOSCOPS [76]	293
PRIME Study [77]	288
Dubbo Study [78]	278
Caerphilly Study [79]	261
WHS [50]	239
Lip Res Clin Prev Trial [80]	233
BUPA [81]	229
Nurses Health Study [82]	228
North Karelia Project [83]	191
Strong Heart Study [84]	183
Framingham Heart Study [85]	174
Edinburgh Artery Study [86]	166
Helsinki Heart Study [87]	138
Stanford Five-City Project [88]	134
Framingham Offspring cohort [89]	129
Bruneck Study [56]	125
Northwick Park Heart Study II [90]	121
Quebec Cardiovascular Study [91]	116
MRFIT [92]	98
FINRISK '92 [93]	92
MONICA-Glostrup cohorts [94]	74
MONICA-VIP cohorts [95]	62
Guernsey [96]	51
PROCAM [97]	33
Gothenburg 1933 [98]	26
Total	**9870**

0.5   1.0   1.5   2.0   4.0

Odds Ratio

Figure 8. Odds ratios for coronary heart disease (CHD) (top third vs. bottom third) in each of 31 published prospective studies of Lp(a) in essentially general populations. Heterogeneity: χ^2 30 = 52.6; p=0.007: I^2 = 43% (95% confidence interval [CI], 12%-63%). ARIC = Atherosclerosis Risk in Communities; BUPA = British United Provident Association; GRIPS = Göttingen Risk, Incidence and Prevalence Study; Lip Res Clin Prev Trial = Lipid Research Clinics Coronary Primary Prevention Trial; MONICA = Monitoring Trends and Determinants in Cardiovascular Disease; MRFIT = Multiple Risk Factor Intervention Trial; PRIME = Prospective Epidemiological Study of Myocardial Infarction; PROCAM = Prospective Cardiovascular Münster Study; VIP = Västerbotten Intervention Project; WHS = Women's Health Study; and WOSCOPS = West of Scotland Coronary Prevention Study. Error bars represent 95% CIs. *Reproduced with permission from Bennet A, et al* [58]. *Copyright © 2008 American Medical Association. All rights reserved.*

In another study from the Emerging Risk Factor Collaboration group [59], individual records from 126,634 participants without a history of CHD in 36 prospective studies were evaluated including 1.3 million person-years of follow-up, 22,076 first-ever fatal or non-fatal vascular disease outcomes or non-vascular deaths, including 9336 CHD outcomes, 1903 ischemic strokes, 338 hemorrhagic strokes, 751 unclassified strokes, 1091 other vascular deaths, 8114 non-vascular deaths, and 242 deaths of unknown cause. The risk ratio for CHD, adjusted for age and sex, lipids and other conventional risk factors was approximately 1.3 or 1.13 per 3.5-fold higher usual Lp(a) concentration (i.e. per 1SD). The corresponding adjusted risk ratios for ischemic stroke were similar and there was no increased risk for non-vascular mortality or cancer deaths **(IIa/B)**.

Drug therapy and Lp(a)

Because no pharmacological agents are currently available to specifically lower Lp(a) levels without affecting other lipoproteins, no human studies exist to assess whether lowering Lp(a) levels also lowers atherosclerosis or CVD risk. In subjects at high risk or with prior CVD events, LDL apheresis is quite useful in not only reducing LDL-C, but also Lp(a). LDL apheresis also reduces other pro-atherogenic and pro-thrombotic constituents. However, studies evaluating CVD events following prolonged apheresis treatment have not been reported. Niacin reduces Lp(a) levels up to 30%, particularly in individuals with highly elevated Lp(a) levels **(IIa/B)** [61-63]. Steroid hormones tend to lower Lp(a), and in fact post-menopausal women generally have an increase in Lp(a) levels. Statins have been recommended to lower risk of CVD in patients at risk for new or recurrent events based on post hoc analyses showing that the risk of high Lp(a) is ameliorated when a statin is used to treat high LDL-C. Interestingly, several studies have shown that statins tend to increase Lp(a) modestly (5-50%), often in a dose response manner [37, 40, 64, 65]. We have previously noted that this effect of statins, and also of low-fat diets [40, 66], is always associated with an increase in OxPL/apoB, suggesting that this may reflect a beneficial function of Lp(a). In animal models (without Lp(a)) a similar increase in OxPL/apoB is associated with loss of OxPL from the vessel wall and concomitant evidence of plaque stabilization [67]. Whether this will be a useful marker of clinical benefit awaits to be determined in large-scale prospective studies.

Finally, recent animal studies suggest that more direct approaches to lower Lp(a) are on the horizon. For example, we recently demonstrated that the antisense oligonucleotide (ASO), mipomersen, directed to human apoB-100, significantly reduced human apoB-100 levels in Lp(a)-transgenic mice (expressing human apoB-100 and apo(a) to make authentic Lp(a) particles), as expected [68]. However, over the 11-week treatment period, compared to baseline, it also reduced Lp(a) levels by ~75% in a time-dependent fashion. This was primarily due to limiting the availability of apoB-100 to bind to apo(a). Furthermore, it significantly reduced plasma levels of OxPL on apoB and apo(a) particles. If ultimately approved for human use, mipomersen may represent a novel therapeutic approach in not only reducing apoB-100 and LDL-C, but also in reducing Lp(a) and their associated OxPL. Another study has also recently showed that the cholesterol ester transfer protein inhibitor, anacetrapib, significantly lowered Lp(a) levels in a dose response manner [69]. Although the underlying mechanism of this finding is not understood at this point, it does suggest additional avenues of treatment if these agents are ultimately approved for clinical use.

Recommendations on measuring Lp(a) in clinical practice

Because pharmacological agents specifically targeting Lp(a) do not yet exist and clinical trials to test the hypothesis that lowering Lp(a) alone have not been performed, Lp(a) continues to remain an emerging risk factor rather than an established one. However, substantial evidence exists that should make clinicians feel comfortable that it is a strong and independent cardiovascular risk factor. In addition, because it a genetic risk factor, it theoretically only has to be measured once, with the only caveat that it can act as an acute phase reactant. For example, Lp(a) levels can remain elevated up to 6 months following acute coronary syndromes [35].

Despite the fact that Lp(a) is an independent risk factor, widespread screening for elevated Lp(a) levels in the general population is not currently recommended by consensus panels. However, many physicians measure Lp(a) routinely in patients they are considering treating with lipid-lowering therapy. It is to be emphasized that a substantial segment of the population has elevated Lp(a) levels (30% of Caucasians and 70% of blacks have levels >30mg/dL or 75nmol/L) and this recommendation may change in the future as more therapeutic studies are reported (IIa/B). Measurement of Lp(a) is suggested in selected patients at risk, such as those with high LDL-C or apoB levels where the cardiovascular risk is already increased, in subjects with a strong family history and particularly those in whom CVD was present in younger family members, in subjects with premature CVD with relatively normal lipid profiles and in subjects that do not respond well to statins (IIa/B). When elevated Lp(a) levels are noted, they may allow further refinement of CVD risk, as noted above in the case of the Framingham Risk Score estimates [43].

Several key points related to the pathophysiology, clinical use of Lp(a) and level of evidence regarding each parameter are described in the following table.

Conclusions

It can be strongly argued that elevated Lp(a) levels can now be regarded as an established, rather than an emerging, risk factor for cardiovascular disease, particularly with the accumulation of data presented in large meta-analyses and recent genetic studies using Mendelian randomization approaches. Although the underlying mechanisms through which elevated Lp(a) levels mediate atherothrombosis are not fully established, Lp(a) likely plays a role in lipid, oxidative, inflammatory and pro-thrombotic pathways. With the development of specific therapies targeting Lp(a) lowering, it may be feasible in the near future to test the hypothesis that lowering elevated Lp(a) levels will result in reduced cardiovascular risk.

Key points	Evidence level
◆ An inverse association exists between Lp(a) levels and apo(a) isoforms and subjects with both high Lp(a) and small apo(a) isoforms are at particularly high risk, independent of race.	IIa/B
◆ Elevated Lp(a) levels are considered to be >30mg/dL or >75nmol/L and are present in 30-70% of individuals.	IIa/B
◆ Lp(a) levels are not generally affected by traditional risk factors or environmental influences.	IIa/B
◆ A J-shaped curve is present in some studies on the relationship between Lp(a) levels and CVD risk.	IIa/B
◆ Lp(a) is an independent risk factor for CVD events in well subjects as well as those with prior CVD.	Ia/A
◆ Selected screening for high Lp(a) in high-risk individuals is recommended.	IIa/B
◆ Niacin in combination with a statin is the optimal treatment for subjects at high risk or with established CVD and elevated Lp(a) levels.	IIa/B

References

1. Berg K. A new serum type system in man - the LP system. *Acta Pathol Microbiol Scand* 1963; 59: 369-82.
2. Hobbs HH, White AL. Lipoprotein(a): intrigues and insights. *Curr Opin Lipidol* 1999; 10: 225-36.
3. Anuurad E, Boffa MB, Koschinsky ML, *et al*. Lipoprotein(a): a unique risk factor for cardiovascular disease. *Clin Lab Med* 2006; 26: 751-72.
4. McLean JW, Tomlinson JE, Kuang WJ, *et al*. cDNA sequence of human apolipoprotein(a) is homologous to plasminogen. *Nature* 1987; 330: 132-7.
5. Marcovina SM, Albers JJ, Scanu AM, *et al*. Use of a reference material proposed by the International Federation of Clinical Chemistry and Laboratory Medicine to evaluate analytical methods for the determination of plasma lipoprotein(a). *Clin Chem* 2000; 46: 1956-67.
6. Lawn RM, Boonmark NW, Schwartz K, *et al*. The recurring evolution of lipoprotein(a). *J Biol Chem* 1995; 270: 24004-9.
7. Boerwinkle E, Leffert CC, Lin J, *et al*. Apolipoprotein(a) gene accounts for greater than 90% of the variation in plasma lipoprotein(a) concentrations. *J Clin Invest* 1992; 90: 52-60.
8. Utermann G. Genetic architecture and evolution of the lipoprotein(a) trait. *Curr Opin Lipidol* 1999; 10: 133-41.
9. Luke MM, Kane JP, Liu DM, *et al*. A polymorphism in the protease-like domain of apolipoprotein(a) is associated with severe coronary artery disease. *Arterioscler Thromb Vasc Biol* 2007; 27: 2030-6.
10. Ober C, Nord AS, Thompson EE, *et al*. Genome-wide association study of plasma lipoprotein(a) levels identifies multiple genes on chromosome 6q. *J Lipid Res* 2009; 50: 798-806.
11. Tregouet DA, Konig IR, Erdmann J, *et al*. Genome-wide haplotype association study identifies the SLC22A3-LPAL2-LPA gene cluster as a risk locus for coronary artery disease. *Nat Genet* 2009; 41: 283-5.
12. Ogorelkova M, Kraft HG, Ehnholm C *et al*. Single nucleotide polymorphisms in exons of the apo(a) kringles IV types 6 to 10 domain affect Lp(a) plasma concentrations and have different patterns in Africans and Caucasians. *Hum Mol Genet* 2001; 10: 815-24.

13. Valenti K, Aveynier E, Leaute S, *et al.* Contribution of apolipoprotein(a) size, pentanucleotide TTTTA repeat and C/T(+93) polymorphisms of the apo(a) gene to regulation of lipoprotein(a) plasma levels in a population of young European Caucasians. *Atherosclerosis* 1999; 147: 17-24.

14. Kraft HG, Windegger M, Menzel HJ, *et al.* Significant impact of the +93 C/T polymorphism in the apolipoprotein(a) gene on Lp(a) concentrations in Africans but not in Caucasians: confounding effect of linkage disequilibrium. *Hum Mol Genet* 1998; 7: 257-64.

15. Paultre F, Pearson TA, Weil HF, *et al.* High levels of Lp(a) with a small apo(a) isoform are associated with coronary artery disease in African American and white men. *Arterioscler Thromb Vasc Biol* 2000; 20: 2619-24.

16. Marcovina SM, Koschinsky ML, Albers JJ, *et al.* Report of the National Heart, Lung, and Blood Institute Workshop on Lipoprotein(a) and Cardiovascular Disease: recent advances and future directions. *Clin Chem* 2003; 49: 1785-96.

17. Albers JJ, Koschinsky ML, Marcovina SM. Evidence mounts for a role of the kidney in lipoprotein(a) catabolism. *Kidney Int* 2007; 71: 961-2.

18. Cushing GL, Gaubatz JW, Nava ML, *et al.* Quantitation and localization of apolipoproteins [a] and B in coronary artery bypass vein grafts resected at re-operation. *Arteriosclerosis* 1989; 9: 593-603.

19. Dangas G, Mehran R, Harpel PC, *et al.* Lipoprotein(a) and inflammation in human coronary atheroma: association with the severity of clinical presentation. *J Am Coll Cardiol* 1998; 32: 2035-42.

20. Boonmark NW, Lou XJ, Yang ZJ, *et al.* Modification of apolipoprotein(a) lysine binding site reduces atherosclerosis in transgenic mice. *J Clin Invest* 1997; 100: 558-64.

21. Sangrar W, Bajzar L, Nesheim ME, *et al.* Antifibrinolytic effect of recombinant apolipoprotein(a) in vitro is primarily due to attenuation of tPA-mediated Glu-plasminogen activation. *Biochemistry* 1995; 34: 5151-7.

22. Feric NT, Boffa MB, Johnston SM, *et al.* Apolipoprotein(a) inhibits the conversion of glu-plasminogen to lys-plasminogen: a novel mechanism for lipoprotein(a)-mediated inhibition of plasminogen activation. *J Thromb Haemost* 2008; 6: 2113-20.

23. Caplice NM, Panetta C, Peterson TE, *et al.* Lipoprotein (a) binds and inactivates tissue factor pathway inhibitor: a novel link between lipoproteins and thrombosis. *Blood* 2001; 98: 2980.

24. Rand ML, Sangrar W, Hancock MA, *et al.* Apolipoprotein(a) enhances platelet responses to the thrombin receptor-activating peptide SFLLRN. *Arterioscler Thromb Vasc Biol* 1998; 18: 1393-9.

25. Edelstein C, Pfaffinger D, Hinman J, *et al.* Lysine-phosphatidylcholine adducts in kringle V impart unique immunological and potential pro-inflammatory properties to human apolipoprotein(a). *J Biol Chem* 2003; 278: 52841-7.

26. Klezovitch O, Edelstein C, Scanu AM. Stimulation of interleukin-8 production in human THP-1 macrophages by apolipoprotein(a). Evidence for a critical involvement of elements in its C-terminal domain. *J Biol Chem* 2001; 276: 46864-9.

27. Bergmark C, Dewan A, Orsoni A, *et al.* A novel function of lipoprotein [a] as a preferential carrier of oxidized phospholipids in human plasma. *J Lipid Res* 2008;4 9: 2230-9.

28. Friedman P, Hörkkö S, Steinberg D, *et al.* Correlation of antiphospholipid antibody recognition with the structure of synthetic oxidized phospholipids: Importance of Schiff base formation and Aldol condensation. *J Biol Chem* 2001; 277: 7010-20.

29. Hörkkö S, Bird DA, Miller E, *et al.* Monoclonal autoantibodies specific for oxidized phospholipids or oxidized phospholipid-protein adducts inhibit macrophage uptake of oxidized low-density lipoproteins. *J Clin Invest* 1999; 103: 117-28.

30. Palinski W, Hörkkö S, Miller E, *et al.* Cloning of monoclonal autoantibodies to epitopes of oxidized lipoproteins from apolipoprotein E-deficient mice. Demonstration of epitopes of oxidized low density lipoprotein in human plasma. *J Clin Invest* 1996; 98: 800-14.

31. Tsimikas S, Witztum JL. The role of oxidized phospholipids in mediating lipoprotein(a) atherogenicity. *Curr Opin Lipidol* 2008; 19: 369-77.

32. Gargalovic PS, Imura M, Zhang B, *et al.* Identification of inflammatory gene modules based on variations of human endothelial cell responses to oxidized lipids. *Proc Natl Acad Sci USA* 2006; 103: 12741-6.

33. Leitinger N. Oxidized phospholipids as modulators of inflammation in atherosclerosis. *Curr Opin Lipidol* 2003; 14: 421-30.

34. Navab M, Ananthramaiah GM, Reddy ST, *et al*. Thematic review series: the pathogenesis of atherosclerosis: The oxidation hypothesis of atherogenesis: the role of oxidized phospholipids and HDL. *J Lipid Res* 2004; 45: 993-1007.

35. Tsimikas S, Bergmark C, Beyer RW, *et al*. Temporal increases in plasma markers of oxidized low-density lipoprotein strongly reflect the presence of acute coronary syndromes. *J Am Coll Cardiol* 2003; 41: 360-70.

36. Tsimikas S, Lau HK, Han KR, *et al*. Percutaneous coronary intervention results in acute increases in oxidized phospholipids and lipoprotein(a): short-term and long-term immunologic responses to oxidized low-density lipoprotein. *Circulation* 2004; 109: 3164-70.

37. Tsimikas S, Witztum JL, Miller ER, *et al*. High-dose atorvastatin reduces total plasma levels of oxidized phospholipids and immune complexes present on apolipoprotein B-100 in patients with acute coronary syndromes in the MIRACL trial. *Circulation* 2004; 110: 1406-12.

38. Tsimikas S, Brilakis ES, Miller ER, *et al*. Oxidized phospholipids, Lp(a) lipoprotein, and coronary artery disease. *N Engl J Med* 2005; 353: 46-57.

39. Tsimikas S, Kiechl S, Willeit J, *et al*. Oxidized phospholipids predict the presence and progression of carotid and femoral atherosclerosis and symptomatic cardiovascular disease: five-year prospective results from the Bruneck study. *J Am Coll Cardiol* 2006; 47: 2219-28.

40. Rodenburg J, Vissers MN, Wiegman A, *et al*. Oxidized low-density lipoprotein in children with familial hypercholesterolemia and unaffected siblings: effect of pravastatin. *J Am Coll Cardiol* 2006; 47: 1803-10.

41. Tsimikas S, Clopton P, Brilakis ES, *et al*. Relationship of oxidized phospholipids on apolipoprotein B-100 particles to race/ethnicity, apolipoprotein(a) isoform size, and cardiovascular risk factors: results from the Dallas Heart Study. *Circulation* 2009; 119: 1711-9.

42. Fraley AE, Tsimikas S. Clinical applications of circulating oxidized low-density lipoprotein biomarkers in cardiovascular disease. *Curr Opin Lipidol* 2006; 17: 502-9.

43. Kiechl S, Willeit J, Mayr M, *et al*. Oxidized phospholipids, lipoprotein(a), lipoprotein-associated phospholipase A2 activity, and 10-year cardiovascular outcomes: prospective results from the Bruneck Study. *Arterioscler Thromb Vasc Biol* 2007; 27: 1788-95.

44. Tsimikas S, Mallat Z, Talmud PJ, *et al*. Elevated oxidized phospholipids on apolipoprotein B-100 particles are associated with future cardiovascular events in the EPIC-Norfolk Study: potentiation of risk with lipoprotein-associated (Lp-PLA2) and secretory phospholipase A2 (sPLA2) activity. *Circulation* 2008; AHA abstract Nov 2008.

45. Berg K, Dahlen G, Christophersen B, *et al*. Lp(a) lipoprotein level predicts survival and major coronary events in the Scandinavian Simvastatin Survival Study. *Clin Genet* 1997; 52: 254-61.

46. Tsimikas S, Tsironis LD, Tselepis AD. New insights into the role of lipoprotein(a)-associated lipoprotein-associated phospholipase A2 in atherosclerosis and cardiovascular disease. *Arterioscler Thromb Vasc Biol* 2007; 27: 2094-9.

47. Karabina SA, Elisaf MC, Goudevenos J, *et al*. PAF-acetylhydrolase activity of Lp(a) before and during Cu(2+)-induced oxidative modification *in vitro*. *Atherosclerosis* 1996; 125: 121-34.

48. Danesh J, Collins R, Peto R. Lipoprotein(a) and coronary artery disease. Meta-analysis of prospective studies. *Circulation* 2000; 102: 1082-5.

49. Maher VM, Brown BG, Marcovina SM, *et al*. Effects of lowering elevated LDL cholesterol on the cardiovascular risk of lipoprotein(a). *JAMA* 1995; 274: 1771-4.

50. Suk DJ, Rifai N, Buring JE, *et al*. Lipoprotein(a), measured with an assay independent of apolipoprotein(a) isoform size, and risk of future cardiovascular events among initially healthy women. *JAMA* 2006; 296: 1363-70.

51. Marcovina SM, Koschinsky ML. Lipoprotein(a) as a risk factor for coronary artery disease. *Am J Cardiol* 1998; 82: 57U-66U.

52. Kraft HG, Lingenhel A, Kochl S, *et al*. Apolipoprotein(a) kringle IV repeat number predicts risk for coronary heart disease. *Arterioscler Thromb Vasc Biol* 1996; 16: 713-9.

53. Parlavecchia M, Pancaldi A, Taramelli R, *et al*. Evidence that apolipoprotein(a) phenotype is a risk factor for coronary artery disease in men <55 years of age. *Am J Cardiol* 1994; 74: 346-51.

54. Sandholzer C, Saha N, Kark JD, *et al*. Apo(a) isoforms predict risk for coronary heart disease. A study in six populations. *Arterioscler Thromb* 1992; 12: 1214-26.

55. Seed M, Hoppichler F, Reaveley D, *et al.* Relation of serum lipoprotein(a) concentration and apolipoprotein(a) phenotype to coronary heart disease in patients with familial hypercholesterolemia. *N Engl J Med* 1990; 322: 1494-9.

56. Kronenberg F, Kronenberg MF, Kiechl S, *et al.* Role of lipoprotein(a) and apolipoprotein(a) phenotype in atherogenesis: prospective results from the Bruneck study. *Circulation* 1999; 100: 1154-60.

57. Moliterno DJ, Jokinen EV, Miserez AR, *et al.* No association between plasma lipoprotein(a) concentrations and the presence or absence of coronary atherosclerosis in African-Americans. *Arterioscler Thromb Vasc Biol* 1995; 15: 850-5.

58. Bennet A, Di Angelantonio E, Erqou S, *et al.* Lipoprotein(a) levels and risk of future coronary heart disease: large-scale prospective data. *Arch Intern Med* 2008; 168: 598-608.

59. The Emerging Risk Factors Collaboration. Lipoprotein(a) concentration and the risk of coronary heart disease, stroke, and nonvascular mortality. *JAMA* 2009; 302: 412-23.

60. Kamstrup PR, Benn M, Tybjaerg-Hansen A, *et al.* Extreme lipoprotein(a) levels and risk of myocardial infarction in the general population: the Copenhagen City Heart Study. *Circulation* 2008; 117: 176-84.

61. Scanu AM, Bamba R. Niacin and lipoprotein(a): facts, uncertainties, and clinical considerations. *Am J Cardiol* 2008; 101: S44-7.

62. Guyton JR, Brown BG, Fazio S, *et al.* Lipid-altering efficacy and safety of ezetimibe/simvastatin coadministered with extended-release niacin in patients with type IIa or type IIb hyperlipidemia. *J Am Coll Cardiol* 2008; 51: 1564-72.

63. Guyton JR. Niacin in cardiovascular prevention: mechanisms, efficacy, and safety. *Curr Opin Lipidol* 2007; 18: 415-20.

64. Kostner GM, Gavish D, Leopold B, *et al.* HMG CoA reductase inhibitors lower LDL cholesterol without reducing Lp(a) levels. *Circulation* 1989; 80: 1313-9.

65. Choi SH, Chae A, Miller E, *et al.* Relationship between biomarkers of oxidized low-density lipoprotein, statin therapy, quantitative coronary angiography, and atheroma: volume observations from the REVERSAL (Reversal of Atherosclerosis with Aggressive Lipid Lowering) study. *J Am Coll Cardiol* 2008; 52: 24-32.

66. Silaste ML, Rantala M, Alfthan G, *et al.* Changes in dietary fat intake alter plasma levels of oxidized low-density lipoprotein and lipoprotein(a). *Arterioscler Thromb Vasc Biol* 2004; 24: 498-503.

67. Tsimikas S, Aikawa M, Miller FJ, Jr., *et al.* Increased plasma oxidized phospholipid: apolipoprotein B-100 ratio with concomitant depletion of oxidized phospholipids from atherosclerotic lesions after dietary lipid-lowering: a potential biomarker of early atherosclerosis regression. *Arterioscler Thromb Vasc Biol* 2007; 27: 175-81.

68. Merki E, Graham MJ, Mullick AE, *et al.* Antisense oligonucleotide directed to human apolipoprotein B-100 reduces lipoprotein(a) levels and oxidized phospholipids on human apolipoprotein B-100 particles in lipoprotein(a) transgenic mice. *Circulation* 2008; 118: 743-53.

69. Bloomfield D, Carlson GL, Sapre A, *et al.* Efficacy and safety of the cholesteryl ester transfer protein inhibitor anacetrapib as monotherapy and coadministered with atorvastatin in dyslipidemic patients. *Am Heart J* 2009; 157: 352-60.

70. Koschinsky ML, Marcovina SM. Structure-function relationships in apolipoprotein(a): insights into lipoprotein(a) assembly and pathogenicity. *Curr Opin Lipidol* 2004; 15: 167-74.

71. Nguyen TT, Ellefson RD, Hodge DO, Bailey KR, Kottke TE, Abu-Lebdeh HS. Predictive value of electrophoretically detected lipoprotein(a) for coronary heart disease and cerebrovascular disease in a community-based cohort of 9936 men and women. *Circulation* 1997; 96(5): 1390-7.

72. Sharrett AR, Ballantyne CM, Coady SA, *et al.* Coronary heart disease prediction from lipoprotein cholesterol levels, triglycerides, lipoprotein(a), apolipoproteins A-I and B, and HDL density subfractions: the Atherosclerosis Risk in Communities (ARIC) Study. *Circulation* 2001; 104(10): 1108-13.

73. Ariyo AA, Thach C, Tracy R. Lp(a) lipoprotein, vascular disease, and mortality in the elderly. *N Engl J Med* 2003; 349(22): 2108-15.

74. Cremer P, Nagel D, Mann H, *et al.* Ten-year follow-up results from the Goettingen Risk, Incidence and Prevalence Study (GRIPS), I: risk factors for myocardial infarction in a cohort of 5790 men. *Atherosclerosis* 1997; 129(2): 221-30.

75. Ridker PM, Hennekens CH, Stampfer MJ. A prospective study of lipoprotein(a) and the risk of myocardial infarction. *JAMA* 1993; 270(18): 2195-9.

76. Gaw A, Brown EA, Docherty G, Ford I. Is lipoprotein(a)-cholesterol a better predictor of vascular disease events than total lipoprotein(a) mass? a nested case control study from the West of Scotland Coronary Prevention Study. *Atherosclerosis* 2000; 148(1): 95-100.

77. Luc G, Bard JM, Arveiler D, *et al.* Lipoprotein (a) as a predictor of coronary heart disease: the PRIME Study. *Atherosclerosis* 2002; 163(2): 377-84.

78. Simons LA, Simons J, Friedlander Y, McCallum J. Risk factors for acute myocardial infarction in the elderly (the Dubbo study). *Am J Cardiol* 2002; 89(1): 69-72.

79. Sweetnam PM, Bolton CH, Downs LG, *et al.* Apolipoproteins A-I, A-II and B, lipoprotein(a) and the risk of ischaemic heart disease: the Caerphilly study. *Eur J Clin Invest* 2000; 30(11): 947-56.

80. Schaefer EJ, Lamon-Fava S, Jenner JL, *et al.* Lipoprotein(a) levels and risk of coronary heart disease in men: the Lipid Research Clinics Coronary Primary Prevention Trial. *JAMA* 1994; 271(13): 999-1003.

81. Wald NJ, Law M, Watt HC, *et al.* Apolipoproteins and ischaemic heart disease: implications for screening. *Lancet* 1994; 343(8889): 75-9.

82. Shai I, Rimm EB, Hankinson SE, *et al.* Lipoprotein(a) and coronary heart disease among women: beyond a cholesterol carrier? *Eur Heart J* 2005; 26(16): 1633-9.

83. Alfthan G, Pekkanen J, Jauhiainen M, *et al.* Relation of serum homocysteine and lipoprotein(a) concentrations to atherosclerotic disease in a prospective Finnish population based study. *Atherosclerosis* 1994; 106(1): 9-19.

84. Wang W, Hu D, Lee ET; *et al.* Lipoprotein(a) in American Indians is low and not independently associated with cardiovascular disease: the Strong Heart Study. *Ann Epidemiol* 2002; 12(2): 107-14.

85. Bostom AG, Gagnon DR, Cupples LA, *et al.* A prospective investigation of elevated lipoprotein(a) detected by electrophoresis and cardiovascular disease in women: the Framingham Heart Study. *Circulation* 1994; 90(4): 1688-95.

86. Price JF, Lee AJ, Rumley A, Lowe GD, Fowkes FG. Lipoprotein(a) and development of intermittent claudication and major cardiovascular events in men and women: the Edinburgh Artery Study. *Atherosclerosis* 2001; 157(1): 241-9.

87. Jauhiainen M, Koskinen P, Ehnholm C, *et al.* Lipoprotein (a) and coronary heart disease risk: a nested case-control study of the Helsinki Heart Study participants. *Atherosclerosis* 1991; 89(1): 59-67.

88. Wild SH, Fortmann SP, Marcovina SM. A prospective case control study of lipoprotein(a) levels and apo(a) size and risk of coronary heart disease in Stanford Five-City Project participants. *Arterioscler Thromb Vasc Biol* 1997; 17(2): 239-45.

89. Bostom AG, Cupples LA, Jenner JL, *et al.* Elevated plasma lipoprotein(a) and coronary heart disease in men aged 55 years and younger: a prospective study. *JAMA* 1996; 276(7): 544-8.

90. Seed M, Ayres KL, Humphries SE, Miller GJ. Lipoprotein(a) as a predictor of myocardial infarction in middle-aged men. *Am J Med* 2001; 110(1): 22-7.

91. Cantin B, Despres JP, Lamarche B, *et al.* Association of fibrinogen and lipoprotein(a) as a coronary heart disease risk factor in men (The Quebec Cardiovascular Study). *Am J Cardiol* 2002; 89(6): 662-6.

92. Evans RW, Shpilberg O, Shaten BJ, Ali S, Kamboh MI, Kuller LH. Prospective association of lipoprotein(a) concentrations and apo(a) size with coronary heart disease among men in the Multiple Risk Factor Intervention Trial. *J Clin Epidemiol* 2001; 54(1): 51-7.

93. Rajecki M, Pajunen P, Jousilahti P, Rasi V, Vahtera E, Salomaa V. Hemostatic factors as predictors of stroke and cardiovascular diseases: the FINRISK '92 Hemostasis Study. *Blood Coagul Fibrinolysis* 2005; 16(2): 119-24.

94. Klausen IC, Sjol A, Hansen PS, *et al.* Apolipoprotein(a) isoforms and coronary heart disease in men: a nested case-control study. *Atherosclerosis* 1997; 132(1): 77-84.

95. Thøgersen AM, Soderberg S, Jansson JH, *et al.* Interactions between fibrinolysis, lipoproteins and leptin related to a first myocardial infarction. *Eur J Cardiovasc Prev Rehabil* 2004; 11(1): 33-40.

96. Coleman MP, Key TJ, Wang DY, *et al.* A prospective study of obesity, lipids, apolipoproteins and ischaemic heart disease in women. *Atherosclerosis* 1992; 92(2-3): 177-85.

97. Assmann G, Schulte H, von Eckardstein A. Hypertriglyceridemia and elevated lipoprotein(a) are risk factors for major coronary events in middle-aged men. *Am J Cardiol* 1996; 77(14): 1179-84.

98. Rosengren A, Wilhelmsen L, Eriksson E, Risberg B, Wedel H. Lipoprotein(a) and coronary heart disease: a prospective case-control study in a general population sample of middle aged men. *BMJ* 1990; 301(6763): 1248-51.

Chapter 14

Sitosterolemia; xenophobia for the body

Shailendra B. Patel BM ChB DPhil FRCP, Professor of Medicine
Medical College of Wisconsin, and the Clement J. Zablocki
Veterans Affairs Medical Center, Milwaukee, Wisconsin, USA

Gerald Salen MD, Professor of Medicine
University of Medicine and Dentistry of New Jersey
New Jersey Medical School, Newark, New Jersey, USA

Introduction

In 1973, Bhattacharyya and Connor reported two sisters who presented with tendon xanthomas, who did not have elevated plasma cholesterol (as would be expected for a diagnosis of familial hypercholesterolemia [FH]), but who had increased levels of plant sterols (sitosterol, campesterol and stigmasterol) in plasma [1]. Sitosterol was the most abundant plant sterol identified in these patients and, consequently, they named the disease β-sitosterolemia. Since all natural sitosterol exists only as the 3β isomer, the addition of 'β' is not needed. Plant sterols (xenosterols) are unique to plants, are not synthesized in mammalian species and are usually not found in our bodies in any appreciable amounts. A typical western diet contains 250-500mg of cholesterol, of which an average of 50% is absorbed in the intestine [2], and 300mg of plant sterols [3], of which in fact <1% of the plant sterols are taken up [4]. Thus, although our diets are equally rich in cholesterol and plant sterols, only cholesterol is allowed entry and retention, whereas plant sterols are excluded [5]. Further characterization of these sisters suggested that the disease was genetic, likely autosomal recessive, and hinted at a sophisticated mechanism important in dietary sterol trafficking [1]. Since this early description, more than 100 cases have been reported world-wide. Plant sterols differ from cholesterol by having the same cyclopentane phenanthrene ring, 3β-hydroxy group, and an 8-carbon side chain, but in addition, contain an extra methyl constituent on carbon 24 to form campesterol, or an extra ethyl group on carbon 24 to form sitosterol, or an extra ethyl group on carbon 24 along with a double bond between carbons 22 and 23 to form stigmasterol (Figure 1). Although this disease is commonly called sitosterolemia or phytosterolemia, it is scientifically more accurate to call it 'xenosterolemia', though this term is unlikely to gain popularity. We emphasize the word 'xenosterol', since there are not only more than 20 different species of

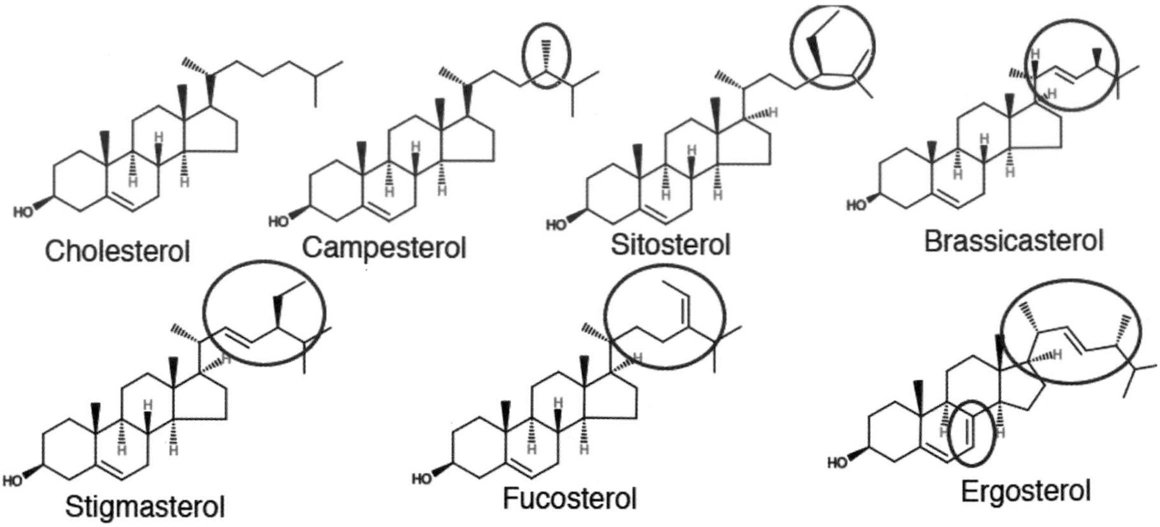

Figure 1. Sterol structures. The red circles highlight the difference between cholesterol, and the remaining xenosterols (plant sterols). Note that campesterol is the least different, with a methyl addition in the 'R' tail compared to cholesterol, whereas more rare sterols, such as stigmasterol or fucosterol show differences in the R tail moieties as well as the saturation level in the phenanthrene rings. Ergosterol is the major sterol species in yeast, not plants and is shown to highlight the spectrum of xenosterols present in our diets.

plant sterols known, but also sterols found in shell-fish are excluded by our bodies, but can be retained by subjects with sitosterolemia [6]. Thus, we seem to have a mechanism to allow us to exclude xenosterols in general. Sitosterolemia is caused by mutations in one of two genes, *ABCG5* or *ABCG8* that comprise the sitosterolemia locus, *STSL*, on human chromosome 2p21 [7-9]. Uncovering the genetic basis for this disease not only revolutionized our understanding of how dietary cholesterol is absorbed, how xenosterols are kept out of the body, but led also to important knowledge as to how the intestine and the liver excrete cholesterol. We now know that ABCG5 and ABCG8 function together to pump all sterols out of the body, with a presumed predilection for xenosterols. Up until this point, how the liver (and intestine) excreted cholesterol was not known [10].

Clinical features

Although there are a number of clinical features that may alert the astute physician to this diagnosis (Table 1), an affected person may have none or only one of any of these features.

Table 1. Clinical features of sitosterolemia.	
Signs and symptoms	**Relative frequency***
Arthralgia	Common
Tendon or tuberous xanthomas	Common
Mildly elevated total cholesterol	Common
Mild anemia	Common
Thrombocytopenia	Common
Elevated liver enzymes (<3 ULN)	Common
Valvular thickening	Infrequent
Carotid bruits	Infrequent
Premature coronary artery disease	Infrequent
Severe hypercholesterolemia	In childhood only
Sudden death <40y age	Rare
Endocrine insufficiency	Very rare
Progressive liver disease	Very rare

* Based upon clinical observations reported only, no formal study available. Based upon the ezetimibe studies, we define common as ~30%, infrequent as <10%, rare as ~1% and very rare as <1%.

A number of these symptoms and signs merit discussion. Young children (ages 3-8 years old) with sitosterolemia may present with very high plasma cholesterol levels; we showed that some children previously diagnosed as having pseudo-homozygous familial hypercholesterolemia (because no defect in the LDL-receptors could be identified) had sitosterolemia [7, 11, 12] **(IIb/B)**. Hemolysis is a frequent problem in affected individuals, especially in adolescents and young adults, and is likely related to the plasma levels of phytosterols. Subjects may have periods of increased hemolysis, separated by periods with relatively normal hematocrits. However, some individuals may only present with hematological features such as stomatocytosis and macrothrombocytopenia [13]. An important clinical feature in sitosterolemic subjects is the development of serious symptomatic coronary and aortic atherosclerosis at a very young age, often ending in lethal myocardial infarction **(III/B)**. One of the authors (GS) was caring for a family of four sitosterolemic siblings, when the 17-year-old affected brother died suddenly of an acute myocardial infarction [14, 15]. At post mortem, the coronary arteries were extensively atherosclerotic and subsequent tissue analyses showed very elevated levels of sitosterol. An Amish boy of 13 years old was also reported to have died from coronary atherosclerosis [16] and subsequently many other cases with premature coronary artery disease have been reported [17-20]. In this regard, it is important to note that not only male but also female subjects with sitosterolemia are susceptible to premature obstructing atherosclerosis of the coronary vessels, carotids and aorta [18, 19, 21]. Involvement of the aortic valve, with concomitant clinical signs [21], is not infrequent. Thus, premature atherosclerosis can be a presenting feature. However, considering that coronary artery disease is one of the commonest of human disorders, diagnosing a rare disease, especially one that requires a specialized biochemical test (gas chromatography [GC] or high performance liquid chromatography [HPLC] analyses), will remain a clinical challenge. The presence of tendon or tuberous xanthomas in a patient <u>without</u> elevated LDL-cholesterol levels >200mg/dL (>5mmol/L) should increase suspicion for sitosterolemia (III/B). As is common with rare diseases, the full spectrum of signs and symptoms may not be fully known; case reports indicate that endocrine dysfunction [22] or idiopathic cirrhosis of the liver may also occur [23], but it is not clear if these are coincidental or truly associated features.

Genetics and pathophysiology

Sitosterolemia is an autosomal recessive disease [24]; parents of affected children do not seem to have any specific health concerns or have increased risk for coronary artery disease. Parents of affected children have normal levels of plasma plant sterols, but may have transiently increased levels when fed pharmacological amounts (>1g) of plant sterols [25, 26]. Historically, pharmacological amounts of plant sterols were used to treat hypercholesterolemia [27-30], as it was known that these sterols are not absorbed [5] and retained in men but also prevent intestinal absorption of cholesterol. This therapy fell out of favour after the invention of statins, though it has been revived recently by the addition of plant sterols and stanols in functional foods [31]. Although the disease was mapped to a single locus, STSL, on human chromosome 2p21 [11, 32], the surprise was that two highly homologous genes, ABCG5 and ABCG8, arranged in a head-to-head organization, comprise this locus [7]. These proteins belong to the ATP-binding cassette family G. All affected individuals have two defective copies of ABCG5 or two defective copies of ABCG8, but to date no individual has been described that has a defective copy of each gene [7]. Genetic evidence exists that ABCG5 and ABCG8 act as obligate heterodimers, and this has now been confirmed biochemically [33]. An illustration depicting the mutations, as well as common polymorphisms identified in normal subjects, is shown in Figure 2. Many of the reported mutations suggest there is a founder effect in most communities, indicating that these mutations have been present for a long time [34]. We have estimated that some of these mutations may be as old as 2,500 years and some of the natural variations observed as old as 40,000 years [35]. There is some dichotomy with respect to the ethnic distributions of mutations; almost all Caucasian sitosterolemia subjects have mutations affecting ABCG8, whereas all Asian subjects have mutations affecting ABCG5 [7, 10]. It is unclear if this is a result of a founder effect, or whether there is some biological significance exerting selection pressure. In the normal population, there is genetic variation in these two genes and these may play a biological role from susceptibility to gall stones [36], to contributing to plasma lipid levels as shown by genome wide scans [37, 38]. The latter is known to be a risk factor for atherosclerotic cardiovascular disease, although how these genes may play a role in doing so remains to be determined. Additionally, while levels of plasma plant sterols are very low (<0.5mg/dL) in normal individuals (and these are under genetic influence [39, 40]), it is controversial as to whether only small increases in plant sterol levels confer a risk of cardiovascular disease. Some observational studies have indicated they do [41-45] whereas others have suggested they do not [46-49]. On balance, plant

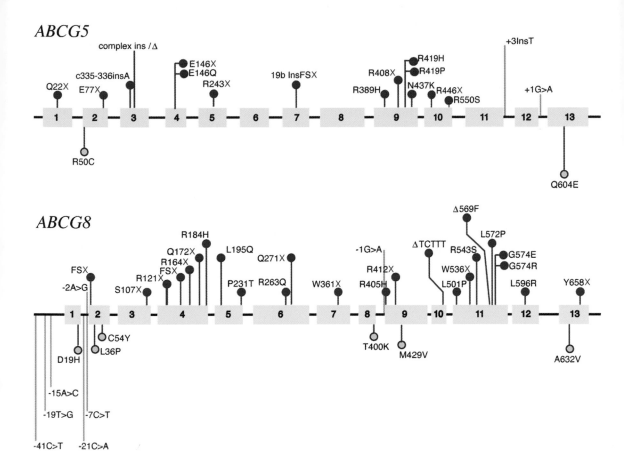

Figure 2. Mutations and polymorphisms at the *STSL* locus, encoding *ABCG5* and *ABCG8*. The two genes, *ABCG5* and *ABCG8*, have 13 exons each and are arranged in a head-to-head organization, and transcribed in opposite direction. For clarity, the genes are shown separately. Mutations are annotated above the gene structure, whereas the common polymorphic variants identified are shown below the gene structure. Rare variants are not shown.

sterols found in normal subjects are likely to play no significant role in the pathophysiology of cardiovascular disease. However, it is unclear if raising such levels, as can occur with pharmacological intervention by using functional foods, will prove to be beneficial or harmful, as there are no endpoint studies.

The new biology of dietary sterol trafficking

ABCG5 and ABCG8 are obligate heterodimers and are transmembrane proteins expressed in the apical membranes of the small intestine (especially in the duodenum and jejunum) and in the hepatocytes [50, 51]. These proteins constitute the long sought sterol export pump in the liver, pumping cholesterol into bile, but seem to have a preference for non-cholesterol sterols when these are present. Thus, in the intestine, they act to pump sterols back out into the lumen of the intestine, and in the liver they efflux sterols into the biliary tree, in synchrony with bile salt and phospholipid secretion. The current model of how they may regulate dietary sterol trafficking now involves the protein Niemann-Pick C1-like 1 (NPC1L1), which plays a role in the uptake of sterols (cholesterol and plant sterols) into the enterocytes (Figure 3). In an uncharacterized mechanism, cholesterol is allowed to proceed into a metabolic channel that eventually allows cholesterol (and its ester) to get incorporated into chylomicrons and secreted into lymph. Xenosterols, such as plant sterols, are prevented from entering the chylomicron pathway (though a small quantity seems to make it in), and are excreted back into the intestinal lumen via ABCG5/ABCG8. The small amount of xenosterols that are contained in the chylomicrons and enter the blood stream will be taken up as remnant particles by the liver, which efficiently excretes these plant sterols back into bile via ABCG5/ABCG8, and thus back into the intestinal lumen for eventual excretion. The preference for human liver to excrete sitosterol compared to cholesterol was demonstrated in the rapid clearance of injected labelled sitosterol compared to labelled cholesterol [52]. The liver takes up cholesterol from the blood via receptor-mediated lipoprotein uptake, and excess cholesterol is excreted via ABCG5/ABCG8 into bile. Loss of ABCG5/ABCG8 results in a defect in both the intestine and the liver; plant sterols enter at the intestinal level with no excretion back into the lumen, and the liver is unable to excrete the absorbed xenosterols or cholesterol into bile, thus allowing accumulation of these sterols [52]. Interestingly, plasma cholesterol levels are not elevated in adult subjects with sitosterolemia [12]. One explanation for this is that whole body cholesterol synthesis is reduced [53], in part by a direct suppression of HMG CoA reductase activity by plant sterols [54-57], but also because the expression of LDL-receptors in the liver was upregulated, not suppressed [58]. Thus, the liver can continue to clear cholesterol which is presumed to be lost via conversion to bile acids and excreted in bile. Why this does not occur in some affected children, who can have very elevated levels of plasma cholesterol, is not clear.

Animal models to mimic sitosterolemia have now been reported [50, 59, 60]. These have been shown to recapitulate almost all of the clinical features of sitosterolemia; these animals show hyperabsorption of all sterols [61], show a failure to excrete sterols into bile [50, 60] and exhibit hemolysis and macrothrombocytopenia [62]. However, increased atherosclerosis has not been reported to occur in these animals [63].

Biochemical abnormalities and diagnosis

Plant sterols or xenosterols are barely detectable in normal human plasma. In sitosterolemia, plant sterols accumulate at levels comparable to cholesterol [12] **(Ib/A)**. To detect these sterols, techniques to separate the various sterols need to be employed [15]. The

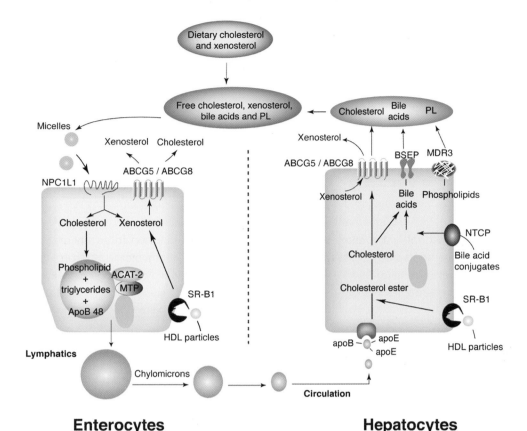

Enterocytes   Hepatocytes

Figure 3. Model for absorption and secretion of cholesterol and xenosterols (plant sterols). The process of digestion of sterols begins in the duodenum, with the mixing of digested dietary sterol, and bile containing free sterols, phospholipids and bile acids to form micelles. This physical mixing is absolutely for absorption of sterols. Once micelles are formed, they interact (a process not elucidated) with the enterocyte, where sterols are allowed to enter the cell in a step that is dependent upon NPC1L1 function. Once the sterols are in the cell, cholesterol is allowed to enter the metabolic pathway, where it is esterified (by acyl cholesterol; acyl transferase, ACAT-2) and then re-packaged into chylomicrons with triglyceride and phospholipids, a process catalyzed by microsomal triglyceride transfer protein (MTP). A very small amount of xenosterols (unesterified) escapes this quality control and is also packaged into chylomicrons. The vast majority of xenosterols, primarily plant sterols from our diets, are directed towards ABCG5/ABCG8 and pumped back out into the lumen of the intestine, destined to be lost in the faeces. Chylomicrons are secreted into lymph, which eventually enters the circulation and the triglycerides are progressively depleted by lipases, generating a cholesterol-enriched remnant particle that is recognized by the liver and rapidly cleared. The dietary sterols (primarily cholesterol) in the liver can be re-packaged and secreted into VLDL (not shown) or can be broken down to bile acids and pumped into bile via the bile salt export pump (BSEP). Cholesterol, as well as any xenosterols, can also be exported as free sterols into bile by the action of ABCG5/ABCG8. It should be pointed out that HDL also delivers sterols to the liver and intestine (and thus delivers such sterols from the periphery to the liver) for disposal. Phospholipids found in the bile are exported by the action of the multiple drug resistance protein 3 (MDR3). Additionally, bile salts re-enter the liver (as part of the enterohepatic circulation) via sodium/taurocholate co-transporter (NTCP) and join the pool of bile acids re-excreted by BSEP. Note that the net effect of these pathways is to keep xenosterols at a very low level, while ensuring cholesterol balance. *Adapted from Lu K, et al* [74].

standard clinical 'cholesterol' test uses a bacterial enzyme, cholesterol oxidase, which does not distinguish between plant sterols and cholesterol. Since normal human blood contains >99% cholesterol, this assay is valid and reliable under normal circumstances. However, when the plasma contains significant amounts of non-cholesterol sterols, such tests will report all of these as 'cholesterol'. Thus, a subject with sitosterolemia may be reported to have a plasma total cholesterol of 200mg/dL (5.13mmol/L), whereas by GC analyses, these results would be a total cholesterol of 150mg/dL (3.85mmol/L), and a sitosterol value of 50mg/dL (1.28mmol/L). This may explain why many diagnoses are made late in the course of the disease and may still be a reason for a missed diagnosis. One can envisage a clinical scenario where a 45-year-old man presents with a fatal myocardial infarct, and if a total cholesterol value is measured at post mortem of 6mmol/L, most clinicians have seen such cases before, will assume that this was probably a tragic, but not unexpected event and the mildly elevated cholesterol was only a single risk factor. Thus, no further investigations are likely to be carried out in the relatives of this individual. Clearly, when tendon or tuberous xanthomas are detected and the level of plasma cholesterol is not in the expected range of familial hypercholesterolemia, the diagnosis of sitosterolemia will be considered. Thus, increased awareness may lead to an increased diagnosis of this seemingly rare disease.

GC or HPLC techniques separate the various different sterol species and the diagnosis of sitosterolemia is relatively simple as all of the affected individuals have dramatically elevated plant sterol levels (>10mg/dL), whereas normal subjects have levels that are <0.5mg/dL. To date, no other disease is known that leads to an elevation of plasma plant sterol levels. The only clinical scenario in which elevated plant sterols can be detected is during total parenteral nutrition [64], as some of these preparations contain plant-derived lipid emulsions.

The GC (or HPLC) profiles will typically show a cholesterol peak, as well as peaks for the various plant sterols (Figure 4). In addition, although most of the plant sterols are not metabolized to any extent in our bodies, they can be modified by 5α-reductase, generating the stanol derivatives such as campestanol and sitostanol, etc [15]. In fact, about 15% of these plant sterols are present as stanols (Figure 4).

Tissues taken at post mortem from sitosterolemic subjects show that plant sterols accumulate in almost all tissues, except the brain, as it is relatively protected by the blood-brain barrier [14, 15]. The concept that our metabolism effectively excretes xenosterols in general is highlighted by studies that show that when sitosterolemia subjects are fed a diet rich in shellfish sterols, these too accumulate and can be detected in the circulation as well [6].

Treatment

Previous treatments generally consisted of reducing intake of foods rich in plant sterols and the administration of bile-acid resins, such as cholestyramine [65, 66], to promote sterol excretion which is effective, but not well tolerated [67, 68] **(IIa/B)**. Statin drugs have been used to treat sitosterolemia patients and although these are effective at lowering cholesterol levels, these drugs have limited effects on lowering plasma plant sterol levels [67, 68] **(IIb/B)**. Diet

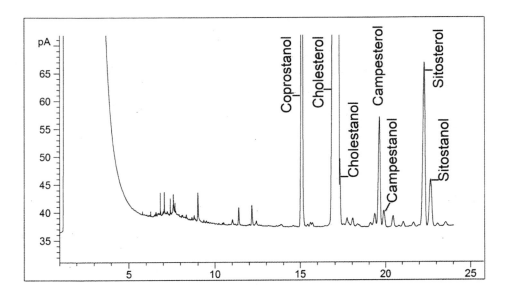

Figure 4. Chromatogram of a plasma sample from a subject with sitosterolemia. Sterols from an affected subject were extracted and analyzed by GC. An internal standard (coprostanol) is added prior to extraction to allow for quantitation of the separated sterol species. The y-axis shows the detector response and the x-axis shows the retention time in the capillary. The identities of the various sterols are as indicated. For comparison, in an unaffected subject, the peaks of cholestanol, sitosterol and campesterol would be in the range that is shown for the campestanol peak in this profile, and no plant stanols would be detectable. Thus, the elevations of these xenosterols is readily appreciable.

therapies aimed at eliminating all plant foods from the diet can lower the plasma plant sterol levels and have been reported to show improvement in some cases [66, 69] (III/B). Such therapies are difficult to maintain, given the severity of dietary restrictions needed; all of these are based upon case studies and none of these document the exact diet used. The breakthrough in therapy came as a result of a development of a drug, ezetimibe [70], that blocked dietary cholesterol absorption, but whose mechanism of action, at that time, was unknown. Coincidental with the discovery of ABCG5/ABCG8, these were hypothesized as being a potential target and as a result, to test this hypothesis, subjects with sitosterolemia were enrolled to test if this drug was effective or not in them [71]. Ezetimibe was not only effective in these subjects at reducing plasma cholesterol levels, it dramatically lowered plant sterol levels in a randomized double-blind, placebo-controlled study over 8 weeks [71] (Ib/A). The lowering of plasma plant sterol levels was irrespective of gender, baseline sitosterol concentrations, or concomitant therapy with bile acid-binding resins, or statins. A 2-year extension of this study showed that plant sterols were reduced progressively for up to 24 weeks and then remained stable, although sitosterol levels were not reduced to normal **(IIb/B)**. Ezetimibe remains the most effective therapy, as judged by plasma plant sterol levels. Clearly, this is a surrogate endpoint and it is not clear if the use of this drug will lead to a prolongation of life-expectancy and a reduction in cardiovascular events. However, anecdotal reports suggest that by lowering these plant sterols with ezetimibe, xanthomas regress, cardiac murmurs are improved, hemolysis and anemia resolve and cardiac dysfunction is improved [21] **(III/B)**. In the 2-year open-label extension study, ezetimibe did not show a significant effect on tendon xanthoma **(IIb/B)**. Ezetimibe is now known to inhibit NPC1L1, and the discovery of this protein has allowed for the development of the current model shown in Figure 3.

Conclusions

Sitosterolemia is a rare, autosomal recessive sterol storage disorder caused by mutations in one of two genes, *ABCG5* or *ABCG8*. The disease can present with relatively common clinical manifestations, such as atherosclerosis, hemolysis, as well as with rare signs such as tendon and tuberous xanthomas or severe hypercholesterolemia in childhood. The disease results in progressive accumulation of xenosterols, primarily sitosterol, as this is the most abundant xenosterol in our diets, in all tissues of the body, except in the central nervous system. Additionally, body pools of cholesterol are also expanded as ABCG5 and ABCG8 are responsible for exporting cholesterol out into the biliary tree. The loss of these proteins allows the accumulation of all of the dietary sterols and thus the diet dictates the type of sterol that is accumulated. Early diagnosis is important, as there is now an effective drug, ezetimibe, which can block dietary sterol entry in the intestine and leads to dramatic lowering of plant sterols. Therapy with ezetimibe has been validated in a randomized, placebo-controlled double-blind study, with long-term follow-up, with improvement in biochemical as well as hematological parameters [71-73] **(Ib/A)**. Long-term effects on morbidity and mortality are not available. Although the diagnostic test is highly specific and very sensitive, it requires specialized testing, such as sterol analyses by GC or HPLC. Identification of the genetic defect in sitosterolemia has also led us to uncover physiological pathways not known before and allowed us to understand better how cholesterol traffics in our bodies. Since many of the clinical features are frequently found in common disorders, the increased awareness of this disease is of importance.

Key points	Evidence level

◆ Rare, autosomal recessive genetic disorder. **Ib/A**

Presenting features

◆ Hypercholesterolemia during childhood. **IIb/B**
◆ Tendon or tuberous xanthomas in the absence of elevated LDL-C. **IIb/B**
◆ Normal or mildly elevated cholesterol levels. **Ib/A**
◆ Anemia, hemolytic episodes and macrothrombocytopenia. **Ib/A**
◆ Premature atherosclerosis, coronary artery disease and/or valvular involvement. **III/B**
◆ Abnormal liver function tests. **IIb/B**

Diagnosis

◆ Have to consider as differential diagnosis. **IV/C**
◆ Need GC or HPLC for sterol analyses. **Ib/A**
◆ Diagnostically elevated plant sterols. **Ib/A**

Therapy

◆ Ezetimibe, FDA approved, is effective. **Ib/A**
◆ Statin use. **IIb/B**
◆ Bile acid sequestrants. **IIb/B**
◆ Ileal bypass. **IIb/B**
◆ LDL apheresis. **IV/C**

References

1. Bhattacharyya AK, Connor WE. Beta-sitosterolemia and xanthomatosis. A newly described lipid storage disease in two sisters. *J Clin Invest* 1974; 53(4): 1033-43.
2. Bosner MS, Lange LG, Stenson WF, Ostlund RE, Jr. Percent cholesterol absorption in normal women and men quantified with dual stable isotopic tracers and negative ion mass spectrometry. *J Lipid Res* 1999; 40(2): 302-8.
3. Andersson SW, Skinner J, Ellegard L, Welch AA, Bingham S, Mulligan A, *et al*. Intake of dietary plant sterols is inversely related to serum cholesterol concentration in men and women in the EPIC Norfolk population: a cross-sectional study. *Eur J Clin Nutr* 2004; 58(10): 1378-85.
4. Gould RG, Jones RJ, LeRoy GV, Wissler RW, Taylor CB. Absorbability of beta-sitosterol in humans. *Metab* 1969; 18(8): 652-62.
5. Schoenheimer R. Uber die Bedeutung der Pflanzensterine fur den tierischen Organismus. *Hoppe-Seyler's Z für physiol Chem* 1929; 180: 1-5.
6. Gregg RE, Connor WE, Lin DS, Brewer H, Jr. Abnormal metabolism of shellfish sterols in a patient with sitosterolemia and xanthomatosis. *J Clin Invest* 1986; 77(6): 1864-72.

7. Lu K, Lee M-H, Hazard S, Brooks-Wilson A, Hidaka H, Kojima H, *et al*. Two genes that map to the *STSL* locus cause sitosterolemia: genomic structure and spectrum of mutations involving sterolin-1 and sterolin-2, encoded by *ABCG5* and *ABCG8* respectively. *Am J Hum Genet* 2001; 69: 278-90.

8. Lee M-H, Lu K, Hazard S, Yu H, Shulenin S, Hidaka H, *et al*. Identification of a gene, *ABCG5*, important in the regulation of dietary cholesterol absorption. *Nat Genet* 2001; 27: 79-83.

9. Berge KE, Tian H, Graf GA, Yu L, Grishin NV, Schultz J, *et al*. Accumulation of dietary cholesterol in sitosterolemia caused by mutations in adjacent ABC transporters. *Science* 2000; 290(5497): 1771-5.

10. Kidambi S, Patel SB. Cholesterol and non-cholesterol sterol transporters: ABCG5, ABCG8 and NPC1L1: a review. *Xenobiotica* 2008; 38(7-8): 1119-39.

11. Patel SB, Salen G, Hidaka H, Kwiterovich PO, Stalenhoef AF, Miettinen TA, *et al*. Mapping a gene involved in regulating dietary cholesterol absorption. The sitosterolemia locus is found at chromosome 2p21. *J Clin Invest* 1998; 102(5): 1041-4.

12. Lee MH, Lu K, Patel SB. Genetic basis of sitosterolemia. *Curr Opin Lipidol* 2001; 12(2): 141-9.

13. Rees DC, Iolascon A, Carella M, O'Marcaigh AS, Kendra JR, Jowitt SN, *et al*. Stomatocytic haemolysis and macrothrombocytopenia (Mediterranean stomatocytosis/macrothrombocytopenia) is the haematological presentation of phytosterolaemia. *Br J Haematol* 2005; 130(2): 297-309.

14. Salen G, Horak I, Rothkopf M, Cohen JL, Speck J, Tint GS, *et al*. Lethal atherosclerosis associated with abnormal plasma and tissue sterol composition in sitosterolemia with xanthomatosis. *J Lipid Res* 1985; 26(9): 1126-33.

15. Salen G, Shefer S, Nguyen L, Ness GC, Tint GS, Shore V. Sitosterolemia. *J Lipid Res* 1992; 33(7): 945-55.

16. Kwiterovich P, Jr., Bachorik PS, Smith HH, McKusick VA, Connor WE, Teng B, *et al*. Hyperapobetalipoproteinaemia in two families with xanthomas and phytosterolaemia. *Lancet* 1981; 1(8218): 466-9.

17. Wang J, Joy T, Mymin D, Frohlich J, Hegele RA. Phenotypic heterogeneity of sitosterolemia. *J Lipid Res* 2004; 45(12): 2361-7.

18. Mymin D, Wang J, Frohlich J, Hegele RA. Image in cardiovascular medicine. Aortic xanthomatosis with coronary ostial occlusion in a child homozygous for a nonsense mutation in ABCG8. *Circulation* 2003; 107(5): 791.

19. Kolovou G, Voudris V, Drogari E, Palatianos G, Cokkinos DV. Coronary bypass grafts in a young girl with sitosterolemia. *Eur Heart J* 1996; 17(6): 965-6.

20. Berger GM, Deppe WM, Marais AD, Biggs M. Phytosterolaemia in three unrelated South African families. *Postgrad Med J* 1994; 70(827): 631-7.

21. Solca C, Stanga Z, Pandit B, Diem P, Greeve J, Patel SB. Sitosterolaemia in Switzerland: molecular genetics links the US Amish-Mennonites to their European roots. *Clin Genet* 2005; 68(2): 174-8.

22. Mushtaq T, Wales JK, Wright NP. Adrenal insufficiency in phytosterolaemia. *Eur J Endocrinol* 2007; 157 Suppl 1: S61-5.

23. Miettinen TA, Klett EL, Gylling H, Isoniemi H, Patel SB. Liver transplantation in a patient with sitosterolemia and cirrhosis. *Gastroenterology* 2006; 130(2): 542-7.

24. Beaty TH, Kwiterovich P, Jr., Khoury MJ, White S, Bachorik PS, Smith HH, *et al*. Genetic analysis of plasma sitosterol, apoprotein B, and lipoproteins in a large Amish pedigree with sitosterolemia. *Am J Hum Genet* 1986; 38(4): 492-504.

25. Kwiterovich PO, Jr., Chen SC, Virgil DG, Schweitzer A, Arnold DR, Kratz LE. Response of obligate heterozygotes for phytosterolemia to a low-fat diet and to a plant sterol ester dietary challenge. *J Lipid Res* 2003; 44(6): 1143-55.

26. Hidaka H, Nakamura T, Aoki T, Kojima H, Nakajima Y, Kosugi K, *et al*. Increased plasma plant sterol levels in heterozygotes with sitosterolemia and xanthomatosis. *J Lipid Res* 1990; 31(5): 881-8.

27. Farquhar JW, Smith RE, Dempsey ME. The effect of beta-sitosterol on serum lipids of young men with arteriosclerotic heart disease. *Circulation* 1956; 14: 77-82.

28. Best MM, Duncan CH, VanLoon EJ, Wathen JD. The effects of sitosterol in lipids. *Am J Med* 1955; 19: 61-70.

29. Best MM, Duncan CH, VanLoon EJ, Wathen JD. Lowering of serum cholesterol by the administration of a plant sterol. *Circulation* 1954; 10(8): 201-6.

30. Pollack OJ. Reduction of blood cholesterol in man. *Circulation* 1953; 7: 703-6.

31. Katan MB, Grundy SM, Jones P, Law M, Miettinen T, Paoletti R. Efficacy and safety of plant stanols and sterols in the management of blood cholesterol levels. *Mayo Clin Proc* 2003; 78(8): 965-78.

32. Lu K, Lee M-H, Carpten JD, Sekhon M, Patel SB. High-resolution physical and transcript map of human chromosome 2p21 containing the sitosterolemia locus. *Eur J Hum Genet* 2001; 9: 364-74.

33. Graf GA, Yu L, Li WP, Gerard R, Tuma PL, Cohen JC, *et al.* ABCG5 and ABCG8 are obligate heterodimers for protein trafficking and biliary cholesterol excretion. *J Biol Chem* 2003; 278(48): 48275-82.

34. Lee M-H, Gordon D, Ott J, Lu K, Ose L, Miettinen T, *et al.* Fine mapping of a gene responsible for regulating dietary cholesterol absorption; founder effects underlie cases of phytosterolemia in multiple communities. *Eur J Hum Genet* 2001; 9: 375-84.

35. Pandit B, Ahn GS, Hazard SE, Gordon D, Patel SB. A detailed hapmap of the sitosterolemia locus spanning 69 kb; differences between Caucasians and African-Americans. *BMC Med Genet* 2006; 7: 13.

36. Buch S, Schafmayer C, Volzke H, Becker C, Franke A, von Eller-Eberstein H, *et al.* A genome-wide association scan identifies the hepatic cholesterol transporter ABCG8 as a susceptibility factor for human gallstone disease. *Nat Genet* 2007; 39(8): 995-9.

37. Kathiresan S, Melander O, Guiducci C, Surti A, Burtt NP, Rieder MJ, *et al.* Six new loci associated with blood low-density lipoprotein cholesterol, high-density lipoprotein cholesterol or triglycerides in humans. *Nat Genet* 2008; 40(2): 189-97.

38. Willer CJ, Sanna S, Jackson AU, Scuteri A, Bonnycastle LL, Clarke R, *et al.* Newly identified loci that influence lipid concentrations and risk of coronary artery disease. *Nat Genet* 2008; 40(2): 161-9.

39. Boomsma DI, Princen HM, Frants RR, Gevers Leuven JA, Kempen HJ. Genetic analysis of indicators of cholesterol synthesis and absorption: lathosterol and phytosterols in Dutch twins and their parents. *Twin Res* 2003; 6(4): 307-14.

40. Berge KE, von Bergmann K, Lutjohann D, Guerra R, Grundy SM, Hobbs HH, *et al.* Heritability of plasma noncholesterol sterols and relationship to DNA sequence polymorphism in *ABCG5* and *ABCG8*. *J Lipid Res* 2002; 43(3): 486-94.

41. Glueck CJ, Speirs J, Tracy T, Streicher P, Illig E, Vandegrift J. Relationships of serum plant sterols (phytosterols) and cholesterol in 595 hypercholesterolemic subjects, and familial aggregation of phytosterols, cholesterol, and premature coronary heart disease in hyperphytosterolemic probands and their first-degree relatives. *Metab* 1991; 40(8): 842-8.

42. Rajaratnam RA, Gylling H, Miettinen TA. Independent association of serum squalene and noncholesterol sterols with coronary artery disease in postmenopausal women. *J Am Coll Cardiol* 2000; 35(5): 1185-91.

43. Sudhop T, Gottwald BM, von Bergmann K. Serum plant sterols as a potential risk factor for coronary heart disease. *Metab* 2002; 51(12): 1519-21.

44. Assmann G, Cullen P, Erbey J, Ramey DR, Kannenberg F, Schulte H. Plasma sitosterol elevations are associated with an increased incidence of coronary events in men: results of a nested case-control analysis of the Prospective Cardiovascular Munster (PROCAM) study. *Nutr Metab Cardiovasc Dis* 2006; 16(1): 13-21.

45. Matthan NR, Pencina M, Larocque JM, Jacques PF, D'Agostino RB, Schaefer EJ, *et al.* Alterations in cholesterol absorption / synthesis characterize Framingham offspring study participants with CHD. *J Lipid Res* 2009; 50 (9): 1927-35.

46. Wilund KR, Yu L, Xu F, Vega GL, Grundy SM, Cohen JC, *et al.* No association between plasma levels of plant sterols and atherosclerosis in mice and men. *Arterioscler Thromb Vasc Biol* 2004; 24(12): 2326-32.

47. Pinedo S, Vissers MN, Bergmann K, Elharchaoui K, Lutjohann D, Luben R, *et al.* Plasma levels of plant sterols and the risk of coronary artery disease: the prospective EPIC-Norfolk Population Study. *J Lipid Res* 2007; 48(1): 139-44.

48. Fassbender K, Lutjohann D, Dik MG, Bremmer M, Konig J, Walter S, *et al.* Moderately elevated plant sterol levels are associated with reduced cardiovascular risk - the LASA study. *Atherosclerosis* 2008; 196(1): 283-8.

49. Windler E, Zyriax BC, Kuipers F, Linseisen J, Boeing H. Association of plasma phytosterol concentrations with incident coronary heart disease data from the CORA study, a case-control study of coronary artery disease in women. *Atherosclerosis* 2009; 203 (1): 284-90.

50. Klett EL, Lu K, Kosters A, Vink E, Lee MH, Altenburg M, *et al.* A mouse model of sitosterolemia: absence of ABCG8/sterolin-2 results in failure to secrete biliary cholesterol. *BMC* Med 2004; 2(1): 5.

51. Klett EL, Lee MH, Adams DB, Chavin KD, Patel SB. Localization of ABCG5 and ABCG8 proteins in human liver, gall bladder and intestine. *BMC Gastroenterol* 2004; 4(1): 21.

52. Salen G, Shore V, Tint GS, Forte T, Shefer S, Horak I, *et al.* Increased sitosterol absorption, decreased removal, and expanded body pools compensate for reduced cholesterol synthesis in sitosterolemia with xanthomatosis. *J Lipid Res* 1989; 30(9): 1319-30.

53. Miettinen TA. Phytosterolaemia, xanthomatosis and premature atherosclerotic arterial disease: a case with high plant sterol absorption, impaired sterol elimination and low cholesterol synthesis. *Eur J Clin Invest* 1980; 10(1): 27-35.

54. Shefer S, Salen G, Bullock J, Nguyen LB, Ness GC, Vhao Z, *et al*. The effect of increased hepatic sitosterol on the regulation of 3-hydroxy-3-methylglutaryl-coenzyme A reductase and cholesterol 7 alpha-hydroxylase in the rat and sitosterolemic homozygotes. *Hepatology* 1994; 20(1 Pt 1): 213-9.

55. Nguyen LB, Salen G, Shefer S, Bullock J, Chen T, Tint GS, *et al*. Deficient ileal 3-hydroxy-3-methylglutaryl coenzyme A reductase activity in sitosterolemia: sitosterol is not a feedback inhibitor of intestinal cholesterol biosynthesis. *Metab Clin & Exp* 1994; 43(7): 855-9.

56. Nguyen LB, Salen G, Shefer S, Tint GS, Shore V, Ness GC. Decreased cholesterol biosynthesis in sitosterolemia with xanthomatosis: diminished mononuclear leukocyte 3-hydroxy-3-methylglutaryl coenzyme A reductase activity and enzyme protein associated with increased low-density lipoprotein receptor function. *Metab Clin & Exp* 1990; 39(4): 436-43.

57. Honda A, Salen G, Nguyen LB, Tint GS, Batta AK, Shefer S. Down-regulation of cholesterol biosynthesis in sitosterolemia: diminished activities of acetoacetyl-CoA thiolase, 3-hydroxy-3-methylglutaryl-CoA synthase, reducatse, squalene synthase and 7-dehydrocholesterol delta-7 reductase in liver and mononuclear leucocytes. *J Lipid Res* 1998; 39: 44-50.

58. Nguyen LB, Shefer S, Salen G, Ness GC, Tint GS, Zaki FG, *et al*. A molecular defect in hepatic cholesterol biosynthesis in sitosterolemia with xanthomatosis. *J Clin Invest* 1990; 86(3): 923-31.

59. Yu L, Hammer RE, Li-Hawkins J, Von Bergmann K, Lutjohann D, Cohen JC, *et al*. Disruption of ABCG5 and ABCG8 in mice reveals their crucial role in biliary cholesterol secretion. *Proc Natl Acad Sci USA* 2002; 99(25): 16237-42.

60. Plosch T, Bloks VW, Terasawa Y, Berdy S, Siegler K, Van Der Sluijs F, *et al*. Sitosterolemia in ABC-Transporter G5-deficient mice is aggravated on activation of the liver-X receptor. *Gastroenterology* 2004; 126(1): 290-300.

61. Wang HH, Patel SB, Carey MC, Wang DQ. Quantifying anomalous intestinal sterol uptake, lymphatic transport, and biliary secretion in Abcg8(-/-) mice. *Hepatology* 2007; 45(4): 998-1006.

62. Kruit JK, Drayer AL, Bloks VW, Blom N, Olthof SG, Sauer PJ, *et al*. Plant sterols cause macrothrombocytopenia in a mouse model of sitosterolemia. *J Biol Chem* 2008; 283(10): 6281-7.

63. Wilund KR, Yu L, Xu F, Vega G, Grundy S, Cohen JC, *et al*. No association between plasma levels of plant sterols and atherosclerosis in mice and men. *Arterioscler Thromb Vasc Biol* 2004; 24 (12): 2326-32.

64. Clayton PT, Bowron A, Mills KA, Massoud A, Casteels M, Milla PJ. Phytosterolemia in children with parenteral nutrition-associated cholestatic liver disease. *Gastroenterology* 1993; 105(6): 1806-13.

65. Parsons HG, Jamal R, Baylis B, Dias VC, Roncari D. A marked and sustained reduction in LDL sterols by diet and cholestyramine in beta-sitosterolemia. *Clin & Invest Med; Med Cliniq et Exp* 1995; 18(5): 389-400.

66. Belamarich PF, Deckelbaum RJ, Starc TJ, Dobrin BE, Tint GS, Salen G. Response to diet and cholestyramine in a patient with sitosterolemia. *Pediatrics* 1990; 86(6): 977-81.

67. Cobb MM, Salen G, Tint GS, Greenspan J, Nguyen LB. Sitosterolemia: opposing effects of cholestyramine and lovastatin on plasma sterol levels in a homozygous girl and her heterozygous father. *Metab Clin & Exp* 1996; 45(6): 673-9.

68. Nguyen LB, Cobb M, Shefer S, Salen G, Ness GC, Tint GS. Regulation of cholesterol biosynthesis in sitosterolemia: effects of lovastatin, cholestyramine, and dietary sterol restriction. *J Lipid Res* 1991; 32(12): 1941-8.

69. Mannucci L, Guardamagna O, Bertucci P, Pisciotta L, Liberatoscioli L, Bertolini S, *et al*. Beta-sitosterolaemia: a new nonsense mutation in the *ABCG5* gene. *Eur J Clin Invest* 2007; 37(12): 997-1000.

70. Patel SB. Ezetimibe: a novel cholesterol-lowering agent that highlights novel physiologic pathways. *Curr Cardiol Rep* 2004; 6(6): 439-42.

71. Salen G, von Bergman K, Lutjohann D, Kwiterovich P, Kane J, Patel SB, *et al*. Ezetimibe effectively reduces plasma plant sterols in patients with sitosterolemia. *Circulation* 2004; 109(8): 966-71.

72. Lutjohann D, von Bergmann K, Sirah W, Macdonell G, Johnson-Levonas AO, Shah A, *et al*. Long-term efficacy and safety of ezetimibe 10mg in patients with homozygous sitosterolemia: a 2-year, open-label extension study. *Int J Clin Pract* 2008; 62(10): 1499-510.

73. Musliner T, Cselovszky D, Sirah W, McCrary Sisk C, Sapre A, Salen G, *et al*. Efficacy and safety of ezetimibe 40mg vs. ezetimibe 10mg in the treatment of patients with homozygous sitosterolaemia. *Int J Clin Pract* 2008; 62(7): 995-1000.

74. Lu K, Lee M, Patel SB. Dietary cholesterol absorption; more than just bile. *Trends Endo Metab* 2001; 12(7): 314-20.

Chapter 15

How can we deal with inborn errors in cholesterol and bile acid biosynthesis?

Hester van Meer MD, Paediatrician, Fellow Paediatric Gastroenterology
Vincent W. Bloks, Research Officer
Folkert Kuipers PhD, Professor, Dean of Faculty of Medical Sciences
Henkjan J. Verkade MD, Professor, Paediatric Gastroenterologist and
Chair, Department of Paediatrics
Center for Liver, Digestive and Metabolic Diseases, Beatrix Children's Hospital -
University Medical Center Groningen, University of Groningen, The Netherlands

Introduction

There is a multitude of cholesterol and bile acid synthesis defects. Their frequency is relatively rare, and individual diseases frequently require different approaches. This chapter provides an overview of the most relevant defects in cholesterol and bile acid biosynthesis and their presentation, and diagnostic and therapeutic approaches.

Cholesterol metabolism

Cholesterol is essential for eukaryotic cells as a structural component of plasma and organelle membranes. Cholesterol is also the precursor for biologically important compounds such as steroid hormones and bile acids. Additionally, cholesterol activates Sonic Hedgehog [1], a signalling protein essential for normal embryonic development. Cholesterol is derived from the diet, but can also be synthesized *de novo*. Particularly during rapid fetal growth, significant amounts of cholesterol are required, which can be derived from the mother via placental supply, or via fetal or placental synthesis. Cholesterol is synthesized by all nucleated mammalian cells. Biosynthesis occurs from acetyl-CoA via the mevalonate pathway in which several enzymatic steps are involved (Figure 1 shows a simplified scheme of the pathway). The first step is the formation of 3-hydroxy-3-methylglutaryl-CoA (HMG-CoA) from acetyl-CoA and acetoacetyl-CoA, catalyzed by the enzyme HMG-CoA synthase. HMG-CoA is then converted to mevalonate by HMG-CoA-reductase, which represents the rate-controlling step. Mevalonate is converted to isopentenyl-5-pyrophosphate, condensated to squalene and further metabolized to lanosterol. Conversion of lanosterol into cholesterol takes another 19 enzymatic reactions. The importance of the cholesterol synthesis pathway is evident from the profound effects of several inborn errors in cholesterol synthesis. As most inborn errors in cholesterol synthesis are very rare, evidence for the treatment of these inborn errors is limited.

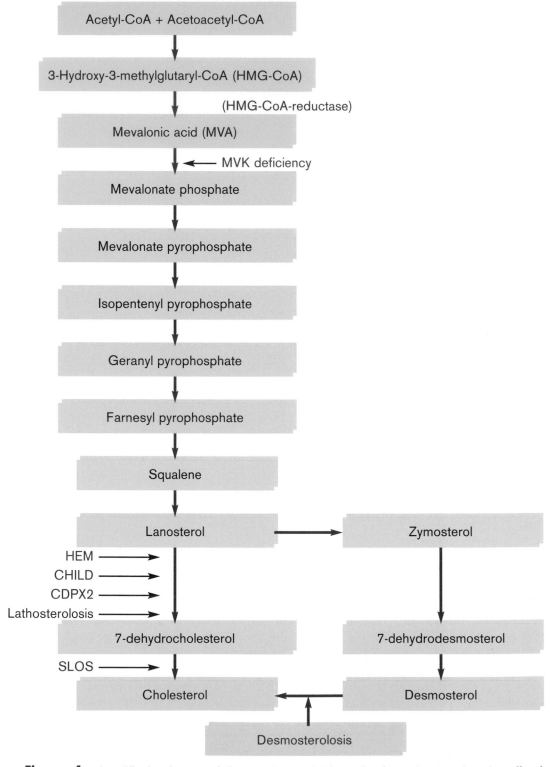

Figure 1. Simplified scheme of the cholesterol biosynthesis pathway. The described inborn errors in cholesterol biosynthesis are depicted in blue. *Adapted from Herman GE. Human Molecular Genetics 2003; 12: R75-88.*

Bile acid metabolism

Bile acids are synthesized from cholesterol in the liver exclusively. The enzymatic conversion of cholesterol can occur via two pathways (Figure 2). In the neutral or classical

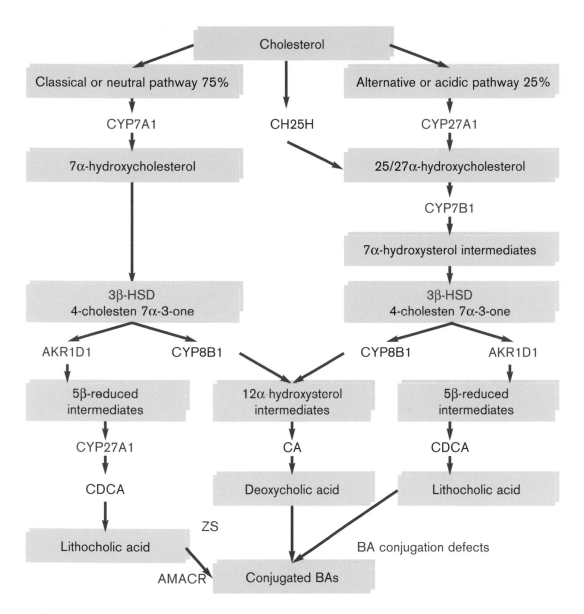

Figure 2. Pathway for the biosynthesis of the primary bile acids. Inborn errors of bile acid synthesis are depicted in blue. CYP7A1 = cholesterol 7α-hydroxylase; CYP27A1 = sterol 27-hydroxylase; CYP7B1 = oxysterol 7α-hydroxylase; 3β-HSD = 3β-hydroxy-Δ^5-C27-steroid dehydrogenase; CYP8B1 = sterol 12-α-hydroxylase; AKR1D1 = 5βRD: 3-oxo-Δ^4-steroid 5β-reductase; CH25H = cholesterol 25-hydroxylase. *Adapted from Lefebvre P, et al. Role of bile acids and bile acid receptors in metabolic regulation. Physiol Rev 2009; 89(1): 147-91; Thomas C, et al. Targeting bile-acid signalling for metabolic diseases. Nat Rev Drug Discov 2008; 7(8): 678-93; Liver Disease in Children, 3rd edition. Suchy FJ, Sokol RJ, Balistreri WF, Eds. Chapter 31, Setchell KDR.*

pathway, the steroid nucleus is modified by hydroxylation reactions prior to the side-chain shortening. Cholesterol 7α-hydroxylase (CYP7A1) catalyzes conversion of cholesterol into 7α-hydroxycholesterol. This step is considered to be rate-controlling in bile acid synthesis. In the acidic pathway, the first step involves 27-hydroxylation of the cholesterol side chain (to yield 27-hydroxycholesterol), catalyzed by the enzyme sterol-27-hydroxylase (CYP27A1). Finally, C27-3β-steroid dehydrogenase converts the 7α-hydroxycholesterol formed via either pathway into the two primary bile acids: cholic acid (CA) and chenodeoxycholic acid (CDCA). After their synthesis, primary bile acids are conjugated with glycine or taurine and secreted via the bile into the intestinal lumen, where they facilitate the uptake of dietary fat

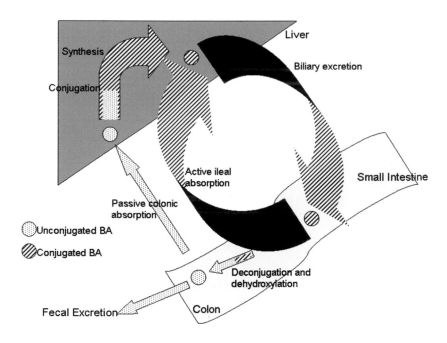

Figure 3. Bile acids are synthesized from cholesterol in the liver. After synthesis, primary bile acids are conjugated with glycine or taurine and secreted into the intestinal lumen. The majority of bile acids is reabsorbed in the ileum and transported back to the liver via the portal system. Some bile acids enter the colon where they are deconjugated and dehydroxylated by the intestinal bacterial flora. These secondary and tertiary bile acids can be passively absorbed from the colon and are transported back to the liver via the enterohepatic circulation. The faecal excretion of bile is a route for removal of excess cholesterol from the body. *Adapted from Volwiler W, Willson RA, Larson AM, et al. The Liver and Biliary System, [Ch 7]. In: The Gut Course; University of Washington, Division of Gastroenterology 2007.*

and other hydrophobic compounds. The majority of bile acids are reabsorbed in the ileum, transported via the portal system back to the liver to complete the enterohepatic circulation. A small fraction of the bile salts escapes ileal reabsorption and enters the colon, where they are deconjugated and subsequently dehydroxylated by intestinal bacteria. These unconjugated bile salts can be passively reabsorbed from the colon, which results in the presence of so-called secondary and tertiary bile acids in the enterohepatic circulation (Figure 3). Bile acids have several important functions in addition to facilitating the absorption of dietary fat and fat-soluble vitamins. The secretion of bile acids from hepatocytes into the biliary system drives bile formation. Bile acids are essential in cholesterol homeostasis; conversion of cholesterol into bile acids and their subsequent faecal loss provides the major route for removal of excess cholesterol from the body.

Inborn errors of cholesterol biosynthesis (Table 1)

Mevalonic aciduria (MA) and hyperIgD and periodic fever syndrome (HIDS)

MA and HIDS are disorders caused by deficiency of mevalonate kinase (MVK). MA is a severe and often fatal disease presenting with a variety of symptoms (dysmorphic features, cataracts, hypotonia, developmental delay, ataxia and cerebellar atrophy, failure to thrive, recurrent febrile illnesses with enteropathy, hepatosplenomegaly, lymphadenopathy, arthralgia, edema and rashes) [2]. HIDS is a less severe condition, characterized by recurrent fever episodes associated with lymphadenopathy, arthralgia, gastrointestinal problems and rash, but without neurological symptoms or dysmorphic features [3]. MA and HIDS are rare diseases with about 30 and 180 patients respectively described worldwide [4]. Since identification of the affected gene in 1992 [5], several disease-causing mutations have been reported. Diagnosis is based on detection of elevated levels of mevalonic acid in urine or plasma. In HIDS, however, this may not always be conclusive. MVK activity is usually below detection levels in MA patients, whereas some residual MVK activity is present in HIDS. Plasma levels of cholesterol are usually in the lower range of normal [6]. In HIDS, serum IgD and IgA are frequently elevated. The diagnosis of MA and HIDS is confirmed by demonstrating mutations in the gene. The pathogenesis of both diseases is still unclear; either accumulation of mevalonic acid or deficiency of cholesterol and intermediates have been postulated to play a role.

Several attempted therapeutic strategies have not been successful in treating MA. Oral cholesterol supplementation worsened diarrhoea [6]. Antioxidant treatment with ubiquinone combined with vitamin C and E to treat a postulated increased sensitivity to reactive oxygen stress, appeared to stabilize clinical symptoms in a few patients [7]. However, a combination of cholesterol, ursodeoxycholic acid (UDCA), ubiquinone and vitamin E did not lead to clinical improvement [6]. Treatment in two patients with lovastatin to block mevalonic acid production resulted in the development of a severe clinical crisis (hyperthermia, vomiting, diarrhoea and marked elevation of serum creatinine kinase levels) [6]. Intervention with prednisone (2mg/kg/d) was effective during a clinical crisis in two patients [6]. One MA patient with associated nephritis was successfully treated with anakinra (an interleukin-I-receptor

Table 1. Features of inborn errors in cholesterol biosynthesis. Reviewed in Porter F, et al. Human malformation syndromes due to inborn errors of cholesterol synthesis. Curr Opin Pediatr 2003; 15(6): 607-13.

	MA	HIDS	SLOS	Desmosterolosis	Conradi-Hunerman (CDPX2)	CHILD	HEM
Deficient enzyme	Mevalonate kinase (EC 2.7.1.36)	Mevalonate kinase (EC 2.7.1.36)	7-dehydrocholesterol Δ^7-reductase (EC 1.3.1.21)	3β-hydroxysterol Δ^{24}-reductase (EC 1.3.1.72)	3β-hydroxysteroid $\Delta^8\Delta^7$-isomerase (EC 5.3.3.5)	3β-hydroxysteroid dehydrogenase (EC 1.1.1.170)	3β-hydroxysterol Δ^{14}-reductase (EC 1.3.1.70)
Gene	MVK	MVK	DHCR7	DHCR24	EBP	NSDHL	LBR gene
Clinical features	Dysmorphic features; Cataracts; Hypotonia; Developmental delay; Ataxia; Cerebellar atrophy; Failure to thrive. Recurrent febrile episodes with: - lymphadenopathy - enteropathy - hepatosplenomegaly - arthralgia - edema - rashes. Often lethal	Recurrent febrile episodes with: - fever - lymphadenopathy - vomiting - diarrhoea - abdominal pain - rash - arthralgia - splenomegaly	Multiple congenital malformations in various organ systems	Multiple congenital malformations in various organ systems	At birth: - ichthyosiform erythroderma - hyperkeratotic rash resolving after a few months; Ichthyosis; Patchy alopecia; Chondrodysplasia punctata; Asymmetrical rhizomelic limb shortening; Scoliosis; Cataracts	Unilateral ichthyosiform skin lesions; Unilateral limb reduction; No cataracts; Alopecia	In utero lethality; Fetal hydrops; Short-limbed dwarfism; Disorganisation of chondro-osseous calcification
Laboratory features	↑ mevalonic acid in urine; ↑ mevalonic acid in plasma	During attacks: ↑ ESR; ↑ leukocytosis; ↑ urinary concentration mevalonic acid. Constantly present: ↑ serum IgD; ↑ serum IgA	↑ 7-DHC/8-DHC; Low/normal plasma cholesterol	↑ plasma desmosterol; ↑ tissue desmosterol	↑ 8-DHC; ↑ 8(9)-cholestenol in plasma and tissues	↑ C4-methylated and ↑ C4-carboxy sterol intermediates in plasma and tissue	↑ cholesta-8,14-dien-3β-ol and ↑ cholesta-8,14,24-trien-33β-ol in tissue
Inheritence	Autosomal recessive	Autosomal recessive	Autosomal recessive	Suggested autosomal recessive	X-linked dominant	X-linked dominant	Autosomal recessive
Prevalence	± 30 cases	± 180 cases	1:20,000-70,000	2 cases	± 100 cases	± 30 cases	± 10 cases
Animal model	Mvk +/- mouse		Dhcr7 -/- mouse (a)	DHCR24 -/- mouse (a)	Tattered (Td) mouse (a)	Bare patches (Bpa) and striated (Str) mouse (a)	Ichthyosis mouse (a)

antagonist) [8]. Remission (during a 15-month follow-up period) of febrile attacks and inflammation after allogenic bone marrow transplantation was described in a 3-year-old patient [9].

The prognosis of HIDS is benign with complications (amyloidosis) being rare. Various pharmacological agents have been tried in the treatment of febrile episodes and associated symptoms in HIDS. Anti-inflammatory drugs (colchicine, thalidomide, cyclosporine and intravenous immunoglobulin) did not consistently suppress or shorten febrile episodes [3, 10, 11]. Individual patients responded to prednisone [3, 10] or non-steroidal anti-inflammatory drugs (NSAIDs) [12]. A randomized, double-blind, crossover study with simvastatin in six patients, did not significantly affect duration or frequency of febrile illnesses [13]. As plasma levels of TNF-α and interleukin (IL)-1β are elevated during febrile attacks, anticytokine therapy has been attempted. Case reports described a limited effect of antitumor necrosis factor (TNF) treatment with etanercept [14, 15]. Anakinra shortened frequency and duration of febrile attacks in sporadic cases [3, 15]. Studies have been performed in small, heterogeneous groups and so far there is no consensus on the treatment of HIDS.

Concluding, for patients with MA, intervention with prednisone or with anakinra may be successful **(III/B)**. The use of statins is not recommended in MA patients **(III/B)**. In the treatment of HIDS, thalidomide **(IIa/B)**, colchicine **(IIa/B)** and statins **(Ib/A)** are not recommended, whereas symptomatic treatment of fever and pain with prednisone or with NSAIDs may be successful **(III/B)**. Anticytokine therapy with etanercept or anakinra may be successful in HIDS patients **(III/B)**.

Smith-Lemli-Opitz syndrome (SLOS)

SLOS was first described in 1964 as an autosomal recessive malformation syndrome with microcephaly, dysmorphic facial features, genital abnormalities, limb defects and mental retardation [16]. Decades later, the underlying biochemical cause was identified [17]. Deficiency of 7-dehydrocholesterol-Δ [7] reductase (7-DHCR) impairs normal cholesterol synthesis leading to hypocholesterolemia and accumulation of the precursors, 7-dehydrocholesterol (7-DHC) and 8-dehydrocholesterol (8-DHC). The gene *DHCR7*, defective in SLOS, was identified in 1998 [18] and since then over 100 different mutations have been reported. SLOS is characterized by a broad spectrum of malformations in various organ systems (reviewed in [19]). Its incidence is estimated between 1:20,000 - 1:70,000 births [19]. The disruption of normal development and growth is classically attributed to the deficiency of cholesterol or to the accumulation and deposition of the (potentially toxic) precursors. SLOS is diagnosed by the determination of elevated concentrations of 7DHC and 8DHC in plasma. *DHCR7* mutation analysis can be performed to confirm the diagnosis. Cholesterol concentrations in plasma are low or normal [19]. Prenatal diagnosis can be performed by measuring elevated levels of 7-DHC concentrations in amniotic fluid or chorionic villus biopsies [20].

No pharmacological strategy has been proven effective in curing SLOS. Dietary supplementation with cholesterol seems a logical treatment because it could be expected to increase plasma and tissue cholesterol levels and to down-regulate its synthesis and the levels of, potentially toxic, precursors. Unfortunately, because brain cholesterol in mammals is dependent on *de novo* synthesis and plasma cholesterol does not efficiently cross the blood brain barrier, the effect of cholesterol supplementation on brain function is expected to be limited. Furthermore, prior developmental defects cannot be reversed by cholesterol treatment. Cholesterol supplementation (administered as natural products such as egg yolk, meat-based formulas and liver or crystalline cholesterol in oil or aqueous suspension) has been evaluated in several trials. Doses of cholesterol used ranged between about 20-150mg/kg/day [21-23]. Cholesterol supplementation improved the serum ratio of cholesterol to total sterols and decreased the level of 7DHC [24]. Some observational studies show improvement in growth, behavior, gastrointestinal symptoms and photosensitivity [21-23]. However, these studies were conducted in small and heterogeneous patient groups and the described improvements have not been correlated to the biochemical changes. Cholesterol treatment does not influence the developmental progress in children and adults with SLOS [24]. Bile acids including CDCA and UDCA added to cholesterol treatment in some studies did not provide benefit in treatment [22, 23]. Treatment of SLOS with simvastatin, an inhibitor of cholesterol synthesis, resulted in inconclusive effects. Adverse effects in two patients are reported [25], whereas simvastatin treatment in two other patients was well tolerated and lowered plasma 7DHC and 8DHC. In these patients, improvement of anthropometric measurements was suggested [26]. Haas *et al* compared cholesterol monotherapy with cholesterol and simvastatin therapy in a group of 39 SLOS patients. Positive effects of simvastatin on anthropometric measurements could not be confirmed. On the other hand, a negative effect of simvastatin on physical development and behavioral problems could not be excluded [27]. In summary, oral cholesterol supplementation may have a positive effect on photosensitivity, behavior and growth in SLOS patients **(II/B)**.

Desmosterolosis

Desmosterolosis is caused by deficiency of 3β-hydroxysterol Δ^{24}-reductase, which catalyses the reduction of the Δ^{24} double bond of sterol intermediates (such as desmosterol) in the cholesterol synthetic pathway. Two patients have been reported so far. The first was a premature infant with multiple lethal malformations and generalized accumulation of desmosterol. Malformations consisted of macrocephaly, a hypoplastic nasal bridge, cleft palate, total anomalous venous drainage, clitoromegaly, short limbs and generalized osteosclerosis [28]. The second patient showed a less severe phenotype at the age of 4 years. His clinical presentation included microcephaly, agenesis of the corpus callosum, dysmorphic facies, submucous cleft palate, persistent patent ductus arteriosus, limb abnormalities and developmental retardation [29]. Desmosterol was elevated in plasma and in cultured lymphoblasts. Parents of both cases had mildly elevated levels of plasma desmosterol suggesting autosomal recessive inheritance. Homozygous mutations in the *DHCR24* gene were demonstrated in both cases [30]. No treatment is currently available.

X-linked dominant chondrodysplasia punctata (Conradi-Hunermann syndrome or Happle syndrome) and congenital hemidysplasia with ichthyosiform nevus and limb defects (CHILD)

Chondrodysplasia punctata is a term used for a heterogeneous group of genetic disorders characterized by abnormal foci of calcification in the cartilaginous skeleton (epiphysial stippling). X-linked dominant chondrodysplasia punctata (CDPX2) is a rare disorder consisting of skeletal, cutanous and ocular malformations (reviewed in [31]). CDPX2 almost exclusively affects females although a few affected males have been reported [31]. Cutaneous manifestations contain ichtyosis, patchy alopecia and atrophoderma. Skeletal abnormalities include epiphysial stippling, asymmetric rhizomelia and scoliosis. Ocular malformations are cataracts, microphtalmus, nystagmus, glaucoma and optic nerve atrophy. Intelligence is usually normal. Other abnormalities (dysmorphic facies, and renal or cardiac manifestations) have been described. CDPX2 is caused by deficiency of 3β-hydroxysteroid-Δ8-Δ7-isomerase which catalyses a step in the conversion of lanosterol to cholesterol. The enzyme defect leads to accumulation of 8-dehydrocholesterol and 8(9)-cholestenol in plasma and tissues. Mutations in the gene encoding the emopamil-binding protein, which functions as a 3β-hydroxysteroid-Δ8-Δ7-isomerase, have been identified as the underlying genetic defect and to date at least 46 different mutations have been described [32]. The pathogenesis of CDPX2 remains to be investigated.

CHILD syndrome is an X-linked disorder with phenotypical similarities to CDPX2 , but with a remarkable unilateral distribution of anomalies. Unilateral skin lesions, characteristically a large epidermal plaque or nevus, are usually present at birth and persist throughout life. Unilateral hypoplasia of limbs and internal organs located at the same side as the skin lesion can be present. Cataracts are not reported in CHILD syndrome and the skeletal malformations are more severe compared to those in CDPX2 (reviewed in [31, 33]). Approximately 30 patients have been reported, amongst which are two males. The defective gene underlying CHILD syndrome has been identified to be *NSDHL*, encoding the enzyme 3β-hydroxysteroid dehydrogenase [34]. Treatment of CDPX2 and CHILD syndrome is symptomatic.

Hydrops-ectopic calcification-moth-eaten skeletal dysplasia (HEM or Greenberg dysplasia)

HEM is a rare, *in utero* lethal, skeletal dysplasia characterized by polyhydramnios, hydrops, dysmorphic facies and short-limbed dwarfism. About 10 cases have been described in the literature. HEM is caused by a deficiency of the enzyme 3β-hydrosterol Δ^{14}-reductase caused by mutations of the *LBR* gene encoding the lamin B receptor [35].

Inborn errors in bile acid synthesis

The conversion of cholesterol into the primary bile acids, CA and CDCA, is disturbed in a number of inborn bile acid synthesis defects (BASD). BASD are rare, with an estimated

Table 2. Features of inborn errors in bile acid synthesis. Adapted from Sundaram SS, et al [78].

Deficient enzyme	Gene	Clinical features	BA profile (urine)	BA profile (serum)	Prevalence	Animal model
Cholesterol 7α-hydroxylase (EC 1.14.13.17)	CYP7A1	Adult patients: ↑serum LDL levels, resistant to statin therapy; Hypertriglyceridemia; Cholesterol gall stones			<10 cases	Cyp7a1 -/- mouse [71]
Oxysterol 7α-hydroxylase (EC 1.14.13.100)	CYP7B1	Neonatal cholestasis; Rapid progression to cirrhosis	Absent primary BA; ↑sulphate/glycosulphate conjugates of 3β-δ5-monohydroxy BA	↑↑ BA level (3β-δ5-monohydroxy BA)	2 cases	Cyp7b1 -/- mouse [72]
3β-hydroxy-Δ5-C27-steroid dehydrogenase (EC 1.1.1.145)	3β-HSD	Cholestasis in children at any age	↓ primary BA; ↑ dihydroxy and trihydroxy-cholenoic acids	↓ or absent primary BA	±40-50 cases	-
3-oxo-Δ4-steroid 5β-reductase (EC 1.3.1.3)	AKR1D1	Neonatal cholestasis; Rapid progression to cirrhosis; GGT can be elevated	↓ primary BA; ↑ 3-oxo-4 bile acids; ↑ allo BA	↓ primary BA; ↑ 3-oxo-4 bile acids; ↑ allo BA	± 5-10 cases	-
Sterol 27-hydroxylase (EC 1.14.13.15)	CYP27A1	Adults (20-30 years): - neurological dysfunction - dementia - cerebellar ataxia - cataracts - premature atherosclerosis - xanthomas; Infancy - juvenile cataracts - chronic diarrhoea - neonatal cholestasis	↑ bile alcohol glucuronides	↑ bile alcohol glucuronides; ↑ cholestanol/cholesterol ratio	Many cases	CYP27 -/- mouse [73]
Alpha-methylacyl-CoA racemase (EC 5.1.99.4)	AMACR	Adult onset peripheral neuropathy; Neonatal cholestasis	↓ primary BA; ↑ C-27 trihydroxycholestanoic acid; ↑ pristanic acid	↓ primary BA; ↑ C-27 trihydroxycholestanoic acid; ↑ pristanic acid	± 5 cases	AMACR -/- mouse [74]
Zellweger syndrome	PEX(1-12)	Malformations in various organ systems; Frequently lethal within 2 years of age	↓ primary BA (a); Atypical mono-, di-, and tri hydroxy C-27 BA (a)	↓ primary BA (a); ↑ long-chain fatty acids (a); ↑ cholestanoic acid (a); ↑ pipecolic acid (a); ↑ C29 dicarboxylic acid (a)	Many cases	Several PEX knock-out mice [75-77]
Bile acid conjugation defects (EC 2.3.1.65)	BAAT	Fat-soluble vitamin deficiency; (Transient) neonatal or childhood cholestasis	Unconjugated CA	Unconjugated CA and CDCA	± 5 cases	-

incidence of 1-2% of childhood cholestasic diseases [36]. BASD can lead to cholestasis and impaired hepatic function based on accumulation of (toxic) intermediates, unusual bile acids and bile alcohols. The lack of competent bile acids in the intestine will frequently cause malabsorption of dietary fat and fat-soluble vitamins. The recognition of BASD was accelerated after the implementation of an international screening program for genetic causes of cholestatic liver disease at the Cincinnati Children's Hospital Medical Center in 2000 [37]. Identification of BASD relies on fast atom bombardment ionisation-mass spectrometry (FAB-MS) or liquid secondary ion mass spectrometry (LSI-MS) of urine and serum to measure absence or reduction of the normal primary bile acids and accumulation of atypical bile acids or bile alcohols [37]. Sequencing of genomic DNA has led to identification of responsible genes in most of the cases. Three clinical symptoms should lead to suspicion of BASD in patients with cholestatic liver disease. First, most BASD are associated with normal to low serum bile acid concentrations, as determined by the conventional laboratory methodologies based on availability of substrates for 3-alpha steroid dehydrogenase, in contrast to elevated bile salt concentrations in other cholestatic liver diseases. Second, serum γ glutamyl transpeptidase (GGT) is usually normal in BASD compared to most other cholestatic liver diseases (except for progressive familial intrahepatic cholestasis type 1 or type 2). Third, pruritis, which is common in cholestatic liver disease, is usually absent in BASD [38]. The clinical picture of BASD depends on the specific defect. In general, defects in modification of the sterol nucleus frequently present with neonatal progressive cholestatic liver disease whereas defects in modification of the side chain cause more neurological symptoms and less severe liver disease. Early recognition of BASD is essential because several of these conditions are treatable with oral bile acid supplementation. General features of inborn errors in bile acid synthesis are depicted in Table 2. Key points and recommendations in the treatment of inborn errors in bile acid synthesis are displayed in the table at the end of the chapter. Due to their low incidence, there is little evidence for therapeutic interventions for inborn errors in bile acid synthesis.

Defects involving modification of the sterol nucleus

Cholesterol 7α-hydroxylase deficiency (CYP7A1)

The most recently described disorder of modification of the sterol nucleus is cholesterol 7α-hydroxylase deficiency, in which bile acid synthesis via the 'classical pathway' is decreased. A prominent feature in adult homozygous patients is an elevated serum LDL level, resistant to statin therapy, elevated serum triglycerides, and decreased (faecal) bile acid excretion. Patients may present with cholesterol gall stones, but liver disease is not observed. Heterozygous subjects present with milder dyslipidemia [39].

Oxysterol 7α-hydroxylase deficiency (CYP7B1)

Deficiency of oxysterol 7α-hydroxylase results in a defective conversion of 27-hydroxy-cholesterol to 7α, 27-dihydroxy-cholesterol. Only two cases of oxysterol 7α-hydroxylase deficiency have been described so far [40, 41]. The first child presented with cholestasis, elevated transaminases and normal GGT at the age of 6 weeks. Hepatic failure with clotting anomalies was present. The serum concentration of total bile acids was low and gas chromatography-mass spectrometry analysis revealed the presence of 3-β-hydroxy-5-

cholenoic and 3-β-hydroxy-5-cholestenoic acids. Serum analysis showed high levels of 27-hydroxy-cholesterol, while 7α-hydroxylated sterols were absent, suggesting a defect at the level of oxysterol 7α-hydroxylase. Genetic analysis revealed a homozygous mutation of *CYP7B1*. Liver biopsy findings consisted of cholestasis, bridging fibrosis, giant cell transformation and proliferation of bile ductules. Treatment with oral UDCA worsened liver function tests and the child was ineffectively treated with oral CA, after which he was subjected to orthotropic liver transplantation (OLT). The second case, a Taiwanese infant of non-consanguineous parents, presented with progressive jaundice at the age of 5 months. Laboratory investigations showed elevated transaminases, a normal GGT and conjugated hyperbilirubinemia. Mass spectrometry in urine revealed large amounts of sulphate or glycosulphate conjugates of monohydroxycholenoic acids, while 'normal bile' acids were absent. In serum, over 90% of bile acids consisted of 3β-hydroxy-5-cholenoic and 3β-hydroxy-5-cholestanoic acid. Liver biopsy findings were consistent with cirrhosis and bile duct proliferation accompanied by giant cell transformation. Genetic analysis showed a homozygous mutation in *CYP7B1*. Treatment with oral UDCA did not improve liver function or cholestasis. CDCA and CA could not be administered because of non-availability in Taiwan. The patient was referred for OLT, but died of cholestatic liver failure before OLT could be performed.

3β-hydroxy-Δ^5-C27-steroid dehydrogenase deficiency (3β-HSD deficiency)

The second step in the bile acid synthesis is catalyzed by 3β-hydroxy-C27-steroid dehydrogenase. Deficiency of this enzyme leads to accumulation of 7α-hydroxycholesterol in hepatocytes. As side chain oxidation and hydroxylation of 7α-hydroxycholesterol by other enzymes progresses, 3β, 7α-dihydroxy-5-cholenoic acid and 3β, 7α, 12α-trihydroxy-5-cholenoic acid will be formed. These non-functional bile acids undergo sulphation, and are found in high concentrations in urine and plasma [42]. Diagnosis of 3β-HSD deficiency includes demonstration of abnormal bile acids in urine or plasma using mass spectrometry. 3β-HSD expression in fibroblasts is absent in affected subjects [43]. Several disease-causing mutations have been identified [44]. 3β-HSD deficiency is a rare autosomal recessive disease with a broad clinical spectrum. Clinical manifestations in children may begin at any age and include cholestasis with jaundice, fat-soluble vitamin deficiency and steatorrhea. Serum transaminases and serum bilirubin are elevated, but the serum GGT is usually normal [42, 45]. In 1999, Akobeng reported two patients with 3β-HSD deficiency, who presented with rickets at the ages of 7 and 9 months, but did not develop clinical signs of liver disease until the age of 3 years [45]. Cholestasis has been identified in adult patients as well, the oldest case being 26 years at the time of diagnosis [46]. The late onset cholestasis is usually preceded by a transient elevation of serum transaminases in the neonatal period. Histopathological findings in the liver, ranging from giant cell hepatitis to cirrhosis, depend on the age of the patient and on the rate of progression of liver disease. The therapeutic approach includes oral administration of primary bile acids. The rationale behind primary bile acid therapy is that these primary bile acids provide bile acid-dependent bile flow, counteracting cholestasis, as CYP7A1 is suppressed by CA and CDCA, thereby reducing the production of the abnormal bile acids. Treatment with oral CDCA (doses ranging from 9-18mg/kg/d) resulted in marked clinical, biochemical and histological improvement [45, 47]. Kobayashi showed that combined therapy with CDCA and CA was more effective than CDCA alone in the treatment of a 23-year-old woman with 3β HSD deficiency [48]. Treatment with oral ursodeochycholic acid (UDCA) may be of temporary benefit [49] but its long-term effect will be limited, because UDCA is not capable of suppressing bile acid synthesis [42]. Thus, oral supplementation of CDCA results in improvement of clinical, biochemical and histological features **(III/B)**. Oral supplementation of CDCA combined with CA was more effective than CDCA treatment alone in an adult patient **(III/B)**.

3-oxo-Δ^4-steroid 5β-reductase deficiency (5βRD)

3-oxo-Δ^4-steroid 5β-reductase deficiency is an autosomal recessive disease caused by mutations in the gene *AKR1D1* (previously known as *SRD5B1*). 5βRD was first described by Setchell *et al* in identical twins suffering from neonatal hepatitis and progressive cholestasis [50]. Deficiency of 5βRD impairs the reduction of the double bond between C4 and C5 of the sterol nucleus, and the conversion of 3-oxo intermediates to their corresponding 3α-hydroxylated products. Urine and plasma levels of primary bile acids are low and intermediate bile acid synthesis products proximal to the enzyme defect (3-oxo-4 bile acids) accumulate, and are detectable by mass spectrometry [36]. However, hyper-3-oxo-Δ^4 bile aciduria is also seen in children with cholestatic liver disease other than inborn errors in bile acid synthesis (e.g. tyrosinemia, α-1-antitrypsin deficiency), rendering it difficult to distinguish between primary 5βRD deficiency and secondary inhibition of the enzyme by liver damage [51]. As 3-oxo-Δ^4-steroid 5β-reductase is not expressed in fibroblasts or leukocytes, cell-based enzyme activity studies are not available. Definite diagnosis of 3-oxo-Δ^4-steroid 5β-reductase deficiency depends on demonstrating mutations in *AKR1D1* [52, 53]. Approximately 10 patients with 5βRD have been described [41, 54]. The clinical picture resembles that of 3β-hydroxy-Δ^5-C27-steroid dehydrogenase deficiency; neonatal cholestasis with elevated plasma concentrations of aminotransferases and conjugated bilirubin. Yet GGT can be elevated in 5βRD. Malabsorption of the fat-soluble vitamin D may cause rickets. Infants with 5βRD tend to have more severe liver disease at an earlier age compared to 3βHSDH. Hepatic histopathology is typical of neonatal hepatitis, with giant cell hepatitis, pseudoacinar transformation, hepatocellular and canalicular cholestasis and extramedullary hematopoiesis [36]. Liver failure will progress rapidly, and without treatment the mortality rate is about 50% [36].

Oral administration of CDCA and CA (both at a dose of 8mg/kg/d) improved liver disease, both clinically and biochemically [53, 55]. Caution with the use of CDCA in patients with normal/high serum concentrations of CDCA should be urged, because CDCA is potentially hepatotoxic [55]. The choleretic bile acid, UDCA, is frequently used in pediatric cholestatic diseases. In 5βRD, UDCA is insufficient as sole therapy, probably because UDCA does not exert a strong negative feedback on bile acid synthesis via CYP7A1 [55]. Concluding, oral supplementation of CDCA combined with CA improved clinical, biochemical and histological features **(III/B)**.

Defects in side chain modification

Cerebrotendinous xanthomatosis (CTX)

CTX is a rare autosomal recessive lipid storage disease caused by the deficiency of the mitochondrial enzyme, sterol 27-hydroxylase, which results in impaired side chain modification during bile acid synthesis. The intermediates 5β-cholestane-3α,7α,12α-triol and 5β-cholestane-3α,7α-diol are not hydroxylated at the c-27 position and therefore side-chain oxidation to the usual C24-primary bile acids cannot take place. These intermediates are hydroxylated at multiple sites to form bile alcohols which become glucuronidated. The production of primary bile acids, in particular CDCA, is reduced while bile alcohol glucuronides (which are diagnostic) accumulate. Some CA can still be synthesized via an alternative C-25 hydroxylation pathway. The absent negative feedback of primary bile acids on CYP7A1 leads to the accumulation of cholestanol which results in its deposition in various tissues. The molecular defect of CTX was identified to reside in the sterol 27-hydroxylase gene (*CYP27A1*) [56] and over 50 different mutations have been described [57].

Plasma concentrations of cholestanol are increased, whereas cholesterol concentrations are normal. Large amounts of bile alcohol glucuronides are excreted in bile, faeces and urine. Patients usually present in the second or third decade of life with various symptoms, including progressive neurological dysfunction, dementia, cerebellar ataxia, cataracts, premature atherosclerosis and the presence of xanthomas in tendons and the brain [57]. Chronic diarrhoea and juvenile cataracts may precede the onset of neurological symptoms, and a few pediatric cases have also been reported [58]. Although liver disease is not observed in CTX, neonatal cholestasis due to mutations in the *CYP27A* gene has been described [59]. Diagnosis is based on an increased plasma cholestanol/cholesterol ratio and the detection of increased levels of bile alcohol glucuronides in urine. Definitive confirmation of the diagnosis is achieved by analysis of the *CYP27A1* gene. For the treatment of CTX, several approaches have been tried, of which oral administration of CDCA was most effective [60]. Berginer *et al* showed clinical and biochemical improvement in 17 adult CTX patients, upon administration of CDCA (750mg/d) for at least 1 year [61]. Comparable results were found after treatment of pediatric CTX patients with CDCA (15mg/kg) [58]. Clinical improvement was most notable if CDCA treatment was initiated before the onset of significant (neurological) symptoms [62]. UDCA is not effective in the treatment of CTX [60, 63]. Statins have been studied as a treatment regime for CTX. Even though data are limited, there is no evidence supporting statin monotherapy as treatment for CTX [63]. Statins combined with CDCA treatment showed additional reduction of cholestanon in one patient [64]. The addition of simvastatin (10-40mg/d) to CDCA did lower serum levels of cholestanol in seven patients; however, additional clinical improvement was not objectified [65]. In summary, oral supplementation of CDCA (15mg/kg/d in children and 250mg/d in adults) improved clinical and biochemical features in CTX patients **(Ib/A)**. Treatment should be initiated before the onset of neurological symptoms.

Alpha-methylacyl-CoA racemase (AMACR) deficiency

AMACR deficiency is an autosomal recessive defect impairing the side-chain oxidation. AMACR catalyzes the racemation of trihydroxycholestanoic acid and pristanic acid into their stereo-isomers. This conversion is required for the subsequent peroxisomal β-oxidation of the C27 bile acid side chain. AMACR deficiency affects both bile acid and fatty acid synthesis, resulting in elevated levels of pristanic acid and trihydroxycholestanoic acid in urine and plasma. Ferdinandusse described two patients presenting with adult-onset peripheral neuropathy and one with symptoms resembling Niemann-Pick type C in childhood [66]. A 2-week-old infant with fat-soluble vitamin deficiency, cholestasis and hematochezia was described. This infant had a sibling who became a liver transplant donor after death in infancy because of intracranial hemorrhage due to vitamin K deficiency. The transplant recipient was diagnosed with AMACR deficiency. Diagnosis was confirmed with absence of AMACR activity, an abnormal bile acid profile, increased plasma pristanic acid concentrations or mutations in the *AMACR* gene. The 2-week-old infant and her sibling's liver recipient were successfully treated with oral CA and fat-soluble vitamins [67]. For the treatment of AMACR deficiency oral supplementation of CA combined with fat-soluble vitamins may improve clinical, biochemical and histological features (III/B).

Zellweger syndrome (ZS or cerebro-hepato-renal syndrome)

The final steps of bile acid synthesis take place in peroxisomes: beta-oxidation of the side chain of specific bile acid intermediates. ZS is an autosomal recessive disorder in which peroxisomes are absent. Patients have dysmorphic facies, hypotonia, chronic liver disease, psychomotor retardation and renal cystic abnormalities. ZS is frequently lethal within 2 years of age. Mutations in 12 genes, *PEX1* to *PEX12*, have been identified with *PEX1* being the most common affected gene in ZS (reviewed in [68]). Amongst biochemical abnormalities, hyperpipecolic acidemia and increased plasma levels of monohydroxy, di- and trihydroxy bile acids with elongated side chains are found, whereas levels of primary bile acids are reduced [68]. Other, less severe peroxisomal disorders (Refsum disease and neonatal adrenoleukodystrophy) have been associated with abnormal bile acid synthesis. The treatment of these conditions is supportive.

Bile acid conjugation defects

The two enzymes catalysing the final step in bile salt synthesis (conjugation of CA and CDCA to taurine or glycine) are bile acid-CoA ligase enzyme and CoA:amino acid N-acyltransferase (encoded by the genes *BAAT* and *BALT*) [69, 70]. Unconjugated bile acids are more rapidly absorbed in the intestine. Due to the decreased secretion of conjugated bile acids, less mixed micelles can be formed. The main feature in patients with bile acid conjugation defects is severe malabsorption of fat and fat-soluble vitamins in infancy or childhood. Conjugated hyperbilirubinemia, pruritis and liver failure have also been described. Mass spectrometry analysis on urine, bile and serum reveals absence of glycine – and taurine – conjugated bile acids whereas unconjugated CA and glucuronide – and sulphate conjugates are present (reviewed in [38]). Mutations in the gene *BAAT* have been found in several Amish patients with this clinical picture [69]. Supplementation with oral primary conjugated bile acids and fat-soluble vitamins could provide a potential treatment.

Conclusions

The recommendations for the treatment of inborn errors in cholesterol or bile acid synthesis are listed as key points below. There is only limited evidence for the treatment of specific indications, which is due to the relative sporadic prevalence. In general, it can be said that the various inborn errors require different approaches and that the diagnosis at the metabolic and/ or genetic level can help to further determine the diagnostic and therapeutic approach.

Key points	Evidence level

Recommendations for the treatment of inborn errors in cholesterol biosynthesis

- MA:
  - prednisone; — III/B
  - anakinra; — 1 case described
  - bone marrow transplant; — 1 case described
  - statins can be dangerous in MA. — III/B
- HIDS:
  - symptomatic treatment of fever and pain:
  - NSAIDs; — III/B
  - prednisone. — III/B
  - anticytokine therapy:
  - etanercept; — III/B
  - anakinra; — III/B
  - thalidomide and colchicine are not recommended; — IIa/B
  - statins are not recommended. — Ib/A
- SLOS:
  - oral cholesterol supplementation (20-150mg/kg/d) may have a positive effect on photosensitivity, behavior and growth. — II/B
- Desmosterolosis:
  - no treatment available.
- Conradi-Hunerman:
  - symptomatic treatment. — IV/C
- CHILD:
  - symptomatic treatment. — IV/C
- HEM:
  - no treatment available.

Recommendations for the treatment of inborn errors in bile acid biosynthesis

- BASD present most frequently as neonatal cholestasis. Presentation as chronic liver disease in older patients occurs. In contrast to other cholestatic liver diseases, patients with BASD commonly present with:
  - normal serum GGT;
  - low serum bile acid levels;
  - pruritus is usually absent.
  Suspicion of, and early diagnosis of, BASD is important, as subsequent early treatment with oral bile acid therapy can prevent progressive cholestatic liver disease.

Continued overleaf

Key points *continued*	Evidence level

Recommendations for the treatment of inborn errors in bile acid biosynthesis *continued*

- Oxysterol 7α-hydroxylase deficiency:　　　　　　　　　　　　IV/C
  - o　OLT was performed in one case.
- 3β-hydroxy-Δ^5-C_{27}-steroid dehydrogenase deficiency:　　　III/B
  - o　oral CDCA or CA and CDCA combined;
  - o　UDCA may be of temporary benefit.
- 3-oxo-Δ^4-steroid 5β-reductase deficiency:　　　　　　　　III/B
  - o　oral CDCA combined with CA (8mg/kg/d);
  - o　caution is required with the use of CDCA in patients with normal/high serum concentrations of CDCA;
  - o　oral UDCA is insufficient as sole therapy.
- CTX:　　　　　　　　　　　　　　　　　　　　　　　　　　Ib/A
  - o　children: oral CDCA 15mg/kg/d;
  - o　adults: oral CDCA 250mg/d;
  - o　treatment should be started before the onset of neurological symptoms.
- AMACR:　　　　　　　　　　　　　　　　　　　　　　　　III/B
  - o　oral CA and fat-soluble vitamins.
- Zellweger syndrome:　　　　　　　　　　　　　　　　　　　IV/C
  - o　treatment is supportive.
- Bile acid conjugation defects:　　　　　　　　　　　　　　　IV/C
  - o　suggested therapy is oral primary BA and fat-soluble vitamins.

References

1. Porter JA, Young KE, Beachy PA. Cholesterol modification of hedgehog signaling proteins in animal development. *Science* 1996; 274(5285): 255-9.
2. Hoffmann G, Gibson KM, Brandt IK, Bader PI, Wappner RS, Sweetman L. Mevalonic aciduria - an inborn error of cholesterol and nonsterol isoprene biosynthesis. *N Engl J Med* 1986; 314(25): 1610-4.
3. van der Hilst JC, Bodar EJ, Barron KS, Frenkel J, Drenth JP, van der Meer JW, *et al.* Long-term follow-up, clinical features, and quality of life in a series of 103 patients with hyperimmunoglobulinemia D syndrome. *Medicine* (Baltimore) 2008; 87(6): 301-10.
4. Haas D, Hoffmann GF. Mevalonate kinase deficiencies: from mevalonic aciduria to hyperimmunoglobulinemia D syndrome. *Orphanet J Rare Dis* 2006; 1: 13.
5. Schafer BL, Bishop RW, Kratunis VJ, Kalinowski SS, Mosley ST, Gibson KM, *et al.* Molecular cloning of human mevalonate kinase and identification of a missense mutation in the genetic disease mevalonic aciduria. *J Biol Chem* 1992; 267(19): 13229-38.
6. Hoffmann GF, Charpentier C, Mayatepek E, Mancini J, Leichsenring M, Gibson KM, *et al.* Clinical and biochemical phenotype in 11 patients with mevalonic aciduria. *Pediatrics* 1993; 91(5): 915-21.
7. Prietsch V, Mayatepek E, Krastel H, Haas D, Zundel D, Waterham HR, *et al.* Mevalonate kinase deficiency: enlarging the clinical and biochemical spectrum. *Pediatrics* 2003; 111(2): 258-61.
8. Nevyjel M, Pontillo A, Calligaris L, Tommasini A, D'Osualdo A, Waterham HR, *et al.* Diagnostics and therapeutic insights in a severe case of mevalonate kinase deficiency. *Pediatrics* 2007; 119(2): e523-7.

9. Neven B, Valayannopoulos V, Quartier P, Blanche S, Prieur AM, Debre M, *et al.* Allogeneic bone marrow transplantation in mevalonic aciduria. *N Engl J Med* 2007; 356(26): 2700-3.

10. Drenth JP, Haagsma CJ, van der Meer JW. Hyperimmunoglobulinemia D and periodic fever syndrome. The clinical spectrum in a series of 50 patients. International Hyper-IgD Study Group. *Medicine* (Baltimore) 1994; 73(3): 133-44.

11. Drenth JP, Vonk AG, Simon A, Powell R, van der Meer JW. Limited efficacy of thalidomide in the treatment of febrile attacks of the hyper-IgD and periodic fever syndrome: a randomized, double-blind, placebo-controlled trial. *J Pharmacol Exp Ther* 2001; 298(3): 1221-6.

12. Picco P, Gattorno M, Di Rocco M, Buoncompagni A. Non-steroidal anti-inflammatory drugs in the treatment of hyper-IgD syndrome. *Ann Rheum Dis* 2001; 60(9): 904.

13. Simon A, Drewe E, van der Meer JW, Powell RJ, Kelley RI, Stalenhoef AF, *et al.* Simvastatin treatment for inflammatory attacks of the hyperimmunoglobulinemia D and periodic fever syndrome. *Clin Pharmacol Ther* 2004; 75(5): 476-83.

14. Demirkaya E, Caglar MK, Waterham HR, Topaloglu R, Ozen S. A patient with hyper-IgD syndrome responding to anti-TNF treatment. *Clin Rheumatol* 2007; 26(10): 1757-9.

15. Bodar EJ, van der Hilst JC, Drenth JP, van der Meer JW, Simon A. Effect of etanercept and anakinra on inflammatory attacks in the hyper-IgD syndrome: introducing a vaccination provocation model. *Neth J Med* 2005; 63(7): 260-4.

16. Smith DW, Lemli L, Opitz JM. A newly recognized syndrome of multiple congenital anomalies. *J Pediatr* 1964; 64: 210-7.

17. Tint GS, Irons M, Elias ER, Batta AK, Frieden R, Chen TS, *et al.* Defective cholesterol biosynthesis associated with the Smith-Lemli-Opitz syndrome. *N Engl J Med* 1994; 330(2): 107-13.

18. Wassif CA, Maslen C, Kachilele-Linjewile S, Lin D, Linck LM, Connor WE, *et al.* Mutations in the human sterol delta7-reductase gene at 11q12-13 cause Smith-Lemli-Opitz syndrome. *Am J Hum Genet* 1998; 63(1): 55-62.

19. Kelley RI, Hennekam RC. The Smith-Lemli-Opitz syndrome. *J Med Genet* 2000; 37(5): 321-35.

20. Tint GS, Abuelo D, Till M, Cordier MP, Batta AK, Shefer S, *et al.* Fetal Smith-Lemli-Opitz syndrome can be detected accurately and reliably by measuring amniotic fluid dehydrocholesterols. *Prenat Diagn* 1998; 18(7): 651-8.

21. Starck L, Lovgren-Sandblom A, Bjorkhem I. Cholesterol treatment forever? The first Scandinavian trial of cholesterol supplementation in the cholesterol-synthesis defect Smith-Lemli-Opitz syndrome. *J Intern Med* 2002; 252(4): 314-21.

22. Irons M, Elias ER, Abuelo D, Bull MJ, Greene CL, Johnson VP, *et al.* Treatment of Smith-Lemli-Opitz syndrome: results of a multicenter trial. *Am J Med Genet* 1997; 68(3): 311-4.

23. Elias ER, Irons MB, Hurley AD, Tint GS, Salen G. Clinical effects of cholesterol supplementation in six patients with the Smith-Lemli-Opitz syndrome (SLOS). *Am J Med Genet* 1997; 68(3): 305-10.

24. Sikora DM, Ruggiero M, Petit-Kekel K, Merkens LS, Connor WE, Steiner RD. Cholesterol supplementation does not improve developmental progress in Smith-Lemli-Opitz syndrome. *J Pediatr* 2004; 144(6): 783-91.

25. Starck L, Lovgren-Sandblom A, Bjorkhem I. Simvastatin treatment in the SLO syndrome: a safe approach? *Am J Med Genet* 2002; 113(2): 183-9.

26. Jira PE, Wevers RA, de Jong J, Rubio-Gozalbo E, Janssen-Zijlstra FS, van Heyst AF, *et al.* Simvastatin. A new therapeutic approach for Smith-Lemli-Opitz syndrome. *J Lipid Res* 2000; 41(8): 1339-46.

27. Haas D, Garbade SF, Vohwinkel C, Muschol N, Trefz FK, Penzien JM, *et al.* Effects of cholesterol and simvastatin treatment in patients with Smith-Lemli-Opitz syndrome (SLOS). *J Inherit Metab Dis* 2007; 30(3): 375-87.

28. FitzPatrick DR, Keeling JW, Evans MJ, Kan AE, Bell JE, Porteous ME, *et al.* Clinical phenotype of desmosterolosis. *Am J Med Genet* 1998; 75(2): 145-52.

29. Andersson HC, Kratz L, Kelley R. Desmosterolosis presenting with multiple congenital anomalies and profound developmental delay. *Am J Med Genet* 2002; 113(4): 315-9.

30 Waterham HR, Koster J, Romeijn GJ, Hennekam RC, Vreken P, Andersson HC, *et al.* Mutations in the 3beta-hydroxysterol Delta24-reductase gene cause desmosterolosis, an autosomal recessive disorder of cholesterol biosynthesis. *Am J Hum Genet* 2001; 69(4): 685-94.

31. Herman GE. X-Linked dominant disorders of cholesterol biosynthesis in man and mouse. *Biochem Biophys Acta* 2000; 1529(1-3): 357-73.

32. Braverman N, Lin P, Moebius FF, Obie C, Moser A, Glossmann H, *et al.* Mutations in the gene encoding 3 beta-hydroxysteroid-delta 8, delta 7-isomerase cause X-linked dominant Conradi-Hunermann syndrome. *Nat Genet* 1999; 22(3): 291-4.

33. Kelley RI, Herman GE. Inborn errors of sterol biosynthesis. *Annu Rev Genomics Hum Genet* 2001; 2: 299-341.

34. Konig A, Happle R, Bornholdt D, Engel H, Grzeschik KH. Mutations in the NSDHL gene, encoding a 3beta-hydroxysteroid dehydrogenase, cause CHILD syndrome. *Am J Med Genet* 2000; 90(4): 339-46.

35. Waterham HR, Koster J, Mooyer P, Noort Gv G, Kelley RI, Wilcox WR, *et al*. Autosomal recessive HEM/Greenberg skeletal dysplasia is caused by 3 beta-hydroxysterol delta 14-reductase deficiency due to mutations in the lamin B receptor gene. *Am J Hum Genet* 2003; 72(4): 1013-7.

36. Bove KE, Heubi JE, Balistreri WF, Setchell KD. Bile acid synthetic defects and liver disease: a comprehensive review. *Pediatr Dev Pathol* 2004; 7(4): 315-34.

37. Heubi JE, Setchell KD, Bove KE. Inborn errors of bile acid metabolism. *Semin Liver Dis* 2007; 27(3): 282-94.

38. Sundaram SS, Bove KE, Lovell MA, Sokol RJ. Mechanisms of disease: inborn errors of bile acid synthesis. *Nat Clin Pract Gastroenterol Hepatol* 2008; 5(8): 456-68.

39. Pullinger CR, Eng C, Salen G, Shefer S, Batta AK, Erickson SK, *et al*. Human cholesterol 7alpha-hydroxylase (CYP7A1) deficiency has a hypercholesterolemic phenotype. *J Clin Invest* 2002; 110(1): 109-17.

40. Setchell KD, Schwarz M, O'Connell NC, Lund EG, Davis DL, Lathe R, *et al*. Identification of a new inborn error in bile acid synthesis: mutation of the oxysterol 7alpha-hydroxylase gene causes severe neonatal liver disease. *J Clin Invest* 1998; 102(9): 1690-703.

41. Ueki I, Kimura A, Nishiyori A, Chen HL, Takei H, Nittono H, *et al*. Neonatal cholestatic liver disease in an Asian patient with a homozygous mutation in the oxysterol 7alpha-hydroxylase gene. *J Pediatr Gastroenterol Nutr* 2008; 46(4): 465-9.

42. Yamato Y, Kimura A, Murai T, Yoshimura T, Kurosawa T, Terazawa S, *et al*. 3beta-hydroxy-delta5 -C27-steroid dehydrogenase deficiency: diagnosis and treatment. *J Paediatr Child Health* 2001; 37(5): 516-9.

43. Buchmann MS, Kvittingen EA, Nazer H, Gunasekaran T, Clayton PT, Sjovall J, *et al*. Lack of 3 beta-hydroxy-delta 5-C27-steroid dehydrogenase/isomerase in fibroblasts from a child with urinary excretion of 3 beta-hydroxy-delta 5-bile acids. A new inborn error of metabolism. *J Clin Invest* 1990; 86(6): 2034-7.

44. Schwarz M, Wright AC, Davis DL, Nazer H, Bjorkhem I, Russell DW. The bile acid synthetic gene 3beta-hydroxy-delta(5)-C(27)-steroid oxidoreductase is mutated in progressive intrahepatic cholestasis. *J Clin Invest* 2000; 106(9): 1175-84.

45. Akobeng AK, Clayton PT, Miller V, Super M, Thomas AG. An inborn error of bile acid synthesis (3beta-hydroxy-delta5-C27-steroid dehydrogenase deficiency) presenting as malabsorption leading to rickets. *Arch Dis Child* 1999; 80(5): 463-5.

46. Fischler B, Bodin K, Stjernman H, Olin M, Hansson M, Sjovall J, *et al*. Cholestatic liver disease in adults may be due to an inherited defect in bile acid biosynthesis. *J Intern Med* 2007; 262(2): 254-62.

47. Ichimiya H, Egestad B, Nazer H, Baginski ES, Clayton PT, Sjovall J. Bile acids and bile alcohols in a child with hepatic 3 beta-hydroxy-delta 5-C27-steroid dehydrogenase deficiency: effects of chenodeoxycholic acid treatment. *J Lipid Res* 1991; 32(5): 829-41.

48. Kobayashi M, Koike M, Sakiyama M, Okuda S, Okuda M, Tanaka T, *et al*. 3beta-hydroxy-delta5-C27-steroid dehydrogenase/isomerase deficiency in a 23-year-old woman. *Pediatr Int* 2000; 42(6): 685-8.

49. Jacquemin E, Setchell KD, O'Connell NC, Estrada A, Maggiore G, Schmitz J, *et al*. A new cause of progressive intrahepatic cholestasis: 3 beta-hydroxy-C27-steroid dehydrogenase/isomerase deficiency. *J Pediatr* 1994; 125(3): 379-84.

50. Setchell KD, Suchy FJ, Welsh MB, Zimmer-Nechemias L, Heubi J, Balistreri WF. Delta 4-3-oxosteroid 5 beta-reductase deficiency described in identical twins with neonatal hepatitis. A new inborn error in bile acid synthesis. *J Clin Invest* 1988; 82(6): 2148-57.

51. Clayton PT, Patel E, Lawson AM, Carruthers RA, Tanner MS, Strandvik B, *et al*. 3-Oxo-delta 4 bile acids in liver disease. *Lancet* 1988; 1(8597): 1283-4.

52. Kimura A, Suzuki M, Murai T, Kurosawa T, Tohma M, Sata M, *et al*. Urinary 7alpha-hydroxy-3-oxochol-4-en-24-oic and 3-oxochola-4,6-dien-24-oic acids in infants with cholestasis. *J Hepatol* 1998; 28(2): 270-9.

53. Lemonde HA, Custard EJ, Bouquet J, Duran M, Overmars H, Scambler PJ, *et al*. Mutations in *SRD5B1* (*AKR1D1*), the gene encoding delta(4)-3-oxosteroid 5beta-reductase, in hepatitis and liver failure in infancy. *Gut* 2003; 52(10): 1494-9.

54. Bove KE, Daugherty CC, Tyson W, Mierau G, Heubi JE, Balistreri WF, *et al*. Bile acid synthetic defects and liver disease. *Pediatr Dev Pathol* 2000; 3(1): 1-16.

55. Clayton PT, Mills KA, Johnson AW, Barabino A, Marazzi MG. Delta 4-3-oxosteroid 5 beta-reductase deficiency: failure of ursodeoxycholic acid treatment and response to chenodeoxycholic acid plus cholic acid. *Gut* 1996; 38(4): 623-8.

56. Cali JJ, Hsieh CL, Francke U, Russell DW. Mutations in the bile acid biosynthetic enzyme sterol 27-hydroxylase underlie cerebrotendinous xanthomatosis. *J Biol Chem* 1991; 266(12): 7779-83.

57. Gallus GN, Dotti MT, Federico A. Clinical and molecular diagnosis of cerebrotendinous xanthomatosis with a review of the mutations in the *CYP27A1* gene. *Neurol Sci* 2006; 27(2): 143-9.

58. van Heijst AF, Verrips A, Wevers RA, Cruysberg JR, Renier WO, Tolboom JJ. Treatment and follow-up of children with cerebrotendinous xanthomatosis. *Eur J Pediatr* 1998; 157(4): 313-6.

59. Clayton PT, Verrips A, Sistermans E, Mann A, Mieli-Vergani G, Wevers R. Mutations in the sterol 27-hydroxylase gene (*CYP27A*) cause hepatitis of infancy as well as cerebrotendinous xanthomatosis. *J Inherit Metab Dis* 2002; 25(6): 501-13.

60. Koopman BJ, Wolthers BG, van der Molen JC, Waterreus RJ. Bile acid therapies applied to patients suffering from cerebrotendinous xanthomatosis. *Clin Chim Acta* 1985; 152(1-2): 115-22.

61. Berginer VM, Salen G, Shefer S. Long-term treatment of cerebrotendinous xanthomatosis with chenodeoxycholic acid. *N Engl J Med* 1984; 311(26): 1649-52.

62. Berginer VM, Gross B, Morad K, Kfir N, Morkos S, Aaref S, et al. Chronic diarrhea and juvenile cataracts: think cerebrotendinous xanthomatosis and treat. *Pediatrics* 2009; 123(1): 143-7.

63. Batta AK, Salen G, Tint GS. Hydrophilic 7 beta-hydroxy bile acids, lovastatin, and cholestyramine are ineffective in the treatment of cerebrotendinous xanthomatosis. *Metabolism* 2004; 53(5): 556-62.

64. Nakamura T, Matsuzawa Y, Takemura K, Kubo M, Miki H, Tarui S. Combined treatment with chenodeoxycholic acid and pravastatin improves plasma cholestanol levels associated with marked regression of tendon xanthomas in cerebrotendinous xanthomatosis. *Metabolism* 1991; 40(7): 741-6.

65. Verrips A, Wevers RA, Van Engelen BG, Keyser A, Wolthers BG, Barkhof F, et al. Effect of simvastatin in addition to chenodeoxycholic acid in patients with cerebrotendinous xanthomatosis. *Metabolism* 1999; 48(2): 233-8.

66. Ferdinandusse S, Denis S, Clayton PT, Graham A, Rees JE, Allen JT, et al. Mutations in the gene encoding peroxisomal alpha-methylacyl-CoA racemase cause adult-onset sensory motor neuropathy. *Nat Genet* 2000; 24(2): 188-91.

67. Setchell KD, Heubi JE, Bove KE, O'Connell NC, Brewsaugh T, Steinberg SJ, et al. Liver disease caused by failure to racemize trihydroxycholestanoic acid: gene mutation and effect of bile acid therapy. *Gastroenterology* 2003; 124(1): 217-32.

68. Steinberg SJ, Dodt G, Raymond GV, Braverman NE, Moser AB, Moser HW. Peroxisome biogenesis disorders. *Biochim Biophys Acta* 2006; 1763(12): 1733-48.

69. Carlton VE, Harris BZ, Puffenberger EG, Batta AK, Knisely AS, Robinson DL, et al. Complex inheritance of familial hypercholanemia with associated mutations in *TJP2* and *BAAT*. *Nat Genet* 2003; 34(1): 91-6.

70. Falany CN, Johnson MR, Barnes S, Diasio RB. Glycine and taurine conjugation of bile acids by a single enzyme. Molecular cloning and expression of human liver bile acid CoA:amino acid N-acyltransferase. *J Biol Chem* 1994; 269(30): 19375-9.

71. Ishibashi S, Schwarz M, Frykman PK, Herz J, Russell DW. Disruption of cholesterol 7alpha-hydroxylase gene in mice. I. Postnatal lethality reversed by bile acid and vitamin supplementation. *J Biol Chem* 1996; 271(30): 18017-23.

72. Li-Hawkins J, Lund EG, Turley SD, Russell DW. Disruption of the oxysterol 7alpha-hydroxylase gene in mice. *J Biol Chem* 2000; 275(22): 16536-42.

73. Rosen H, Reshef A, Maeda N, Lippoldt A, Shpizen S, Triger L, et al. Markedly reduced bile acid synthesis but maintained levels of cholesterol and vitamin D metabolites in mice with disrupted sterol 27-hydroxylase gene. *J Biol Chem* 1998; 273(24): 14805-12.

74. Savolainen K, Kotti TJ, Schmitz W, Savolainen TI, Sormunen RT, Ilves M, et al. A mouse model for alpha-methylacyl-CoA racemase deficiency: adjustment of bile acid synthesis and intolerance to dietary methyl-branched lipids. *Hum Mol Genet* 2004; 13(9): 955-65.

75. Baes M, Gressens P, Baumgart E, Carmeliet P, Casteels M, Fransen M, et al. A mouse model for Zellweger syndrome. *Nat Genet* 1997; 17(1): 49-57.

76. Baumgart E, Vanhorebeek I, Grabenbauer M, Borgers M, Declercq PE, Fahimi HD, et al. Mitochondrial alterations caused by defective peroxisomal biogenesis in a mouse model for Zellweger syndrome (PEX5 knockout mouse). *Am J Pathol* 2001; 159(4): 1477-94.

77. Faust PL, Hatten ME. Targeted deletion of the PEX2 peroxisome assembly gene in mice provides a model for Zellweger syndrome, a human neuronal migration disorder. *J Cell Biol* 1997; 139(5): 1293-305.

78. Sundaram SS, Bove KE, Lovell MA, Sokol RJ. Mechanisms of disease: inborn errors of bile acid synthesis. *Nat Clin Pract Gastroenterol Hepatol* 2008; 5(8): 456-68.

Chapter 16

Differential diagnosis of patients with xanthomas and xanthelasmata

Peter J. Lansberg MD PhD
Co-ordinator, Durrer Center for Cardiogenetic Research
Department of Vascular Medicine, Academic Medical Center
Amsterdam, The Netherlands

Introduction

Dermatological manifestations of lipid accumulations are referred to as xanthomas (Figure 1). Skin, tendon and even osseous manifestations are possible. Case reports have described less common locations such as the gastric lining or even the osseous structures of the cranium. In general they consist of accumulated foam cell-like depositions including histiocytes, fibroblasts, macrophages filled with lipids giving them a characteristic yellowish color. They can be found on any part of the body although certain types of dyslipidemias have characteristic or even pathognomonic locations such as the Achilles tendons in familial hypercholesterolemia. Finding xanthomas is a clear indication to explore possible primary or secondary dyslipidemias, although this is not a 'conditio sine qua non'. A thorough physical examination and complete blood analysis is always necessary for a complete diagnostic evaluation. Rare diseases can manifest with cutaneous xanthoma-like features where histopathological and ultrastructural studies of skin biopsy specimens are necessary to confirm diagnosis. The classification of xanthomas is based on their location and physical characteristics **(IV/C)** (Figure 2).

Xanthoma types

Xanthoma types are as follows:

- palpebral xanthelasma;
- eruptive xanthomas;
- tendon xanthomas;
- tuberous and tuberous-eruptive xanthomas;

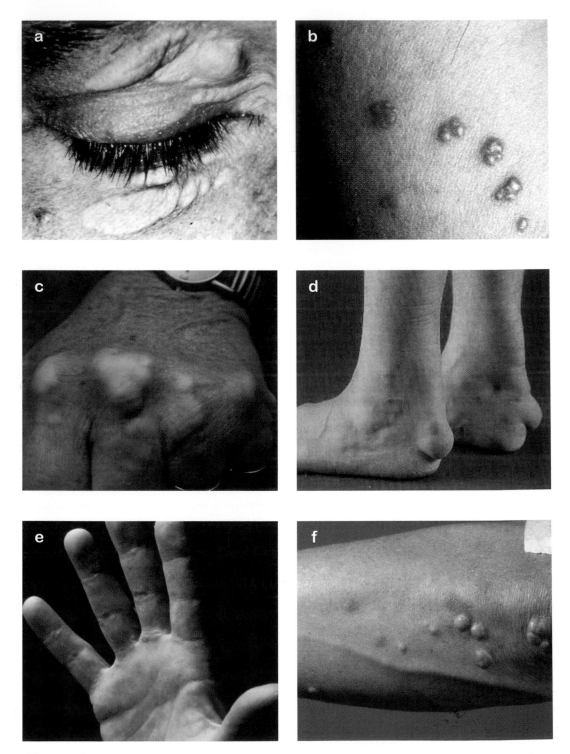

Figure 1. Xanthomas: a) palpebral xanthelasma; b) eruptive xanthomas; c) tendon xanthomas on the hand; d) Achilles tendon xanthomas; e) xanthomas striate palmaris; f) tuberous xanthomas.

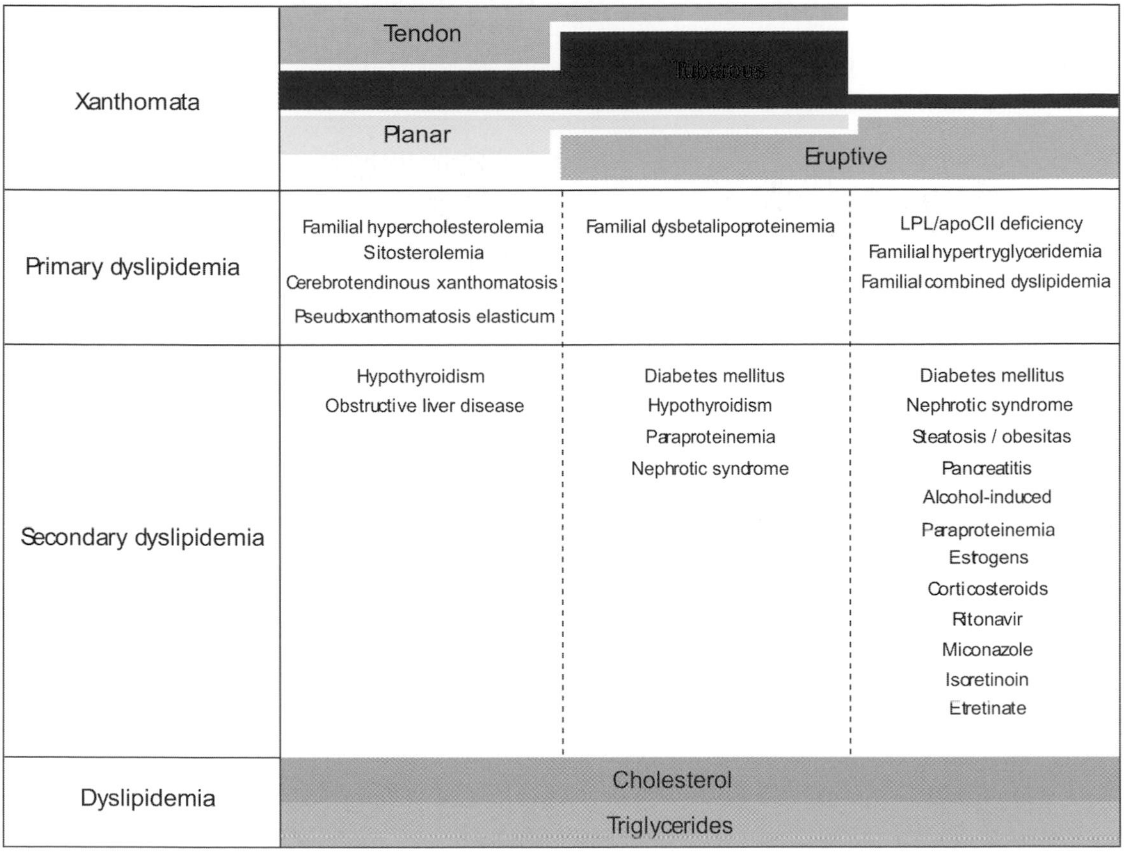

Xanthomata	Tendon		
	Tuberous		
	Planar		
		Eruptive	
Primary dyslipidemia	Familial hypercholesterolemia Sitosterolemia Cerebrotendinous xanthomatosis Pseudoxanthomatosis elasticum	Familial dysbetalipoproteinemia	LPL/apoCII deficiency Familial hypertryglyceridemia Familial combined dyslipidemia
Secondary dyslipidemia	Hypothyroidism Obstructive liver disease	Diabetes mellitus Hypothyroidism Paraproteinemia Nephrotic syndrome	Diabetes mellitus Nephrotic syndrome Steatosis / obesitas Pancreatitis Alcohol-induced Paraproteinemia Estrogens Corticosteroids Ritonavir Miconazole Isoretinoin Etretinate
Dyslipidemia	Cholesterol		
	Triglycerides		

Figure 2. Relationship between dyslipidemic xanthoma type, cause of xanthoma and abnormal plasma lipids [66].

- ◆ xanthomas striate palmaris;
- ◆ rare forms of xanthomas – (normolipidemic):

  - o xanthomata disseminatum - Montgomery;
  - o juvenile granulo-xanthomata;
  - o necrobiotic xanthogranuloma;
  - o verruciform xanthomas;
  - o normolipidemic diffuse plane xanthoma.

Palpebral xanthelasma

The most frequently observed form of xanthomas are the palpebral xanthelasma. They appear as soft yellow plaques, on the medial aspects of the eyelids, that can evolve to a more orange, red-brownish color. They are often bilateral and symmetrical, with the lower eyelids less frequently affected than the upper eyelid. Xanthelasmas are more common in middle-aged and older persons, and is less frequently seen in men (0.3%) than in women (1.1%) [1]. Untreated xanthomas can form larger plaques and sometimes completely circle the eyes.

Dyslipidemia is found in approximately 50% of affected individuals [2]. The most common lipid abnormality is an elevated LDL-cholesterol such as observed in familial hypercholesterolemia (FH), a diagnosis that is more likely when these skin abnormalities are seen before the age of 40. Elevations of total cholesterol as well as triglycerides can be observed in occasional cases as well. For instance, dysbètalipoproteinemia, also referred to as the Fredrickson's type III classification, is a lipid disorder that leads to increased remnant particles that can manifest with xanthelasma [3-5] **(IV/C)**.

Histology

Xanthelasmas contain foamy lipid-laden histiocytes found in the more superficial layers of the skin. Signs of fibrosis and inflammation are observed as well, although this is less common as in tendon or fibrous xanthomas. Cholesterol is the predominant lipid of which the esterified form is most abundant [6]. No ultra-structural differences were observed between normolipidemic and hyperlipidemic patients [7].

Atherosclerosis

The risk of cardiovascular disease is increased, not only in patients with xanthelasma and associated lipid abnormalities, but also in the group of normolipidemic patients where premature atherothrombotic complications have been observed. It remains unclear if this is related to the inherent bias error of observational data or because of metabolic defects that allow for more efficient storage of lipids in the skin as well as in the vasculature [8-9]. A recent small case control study showed no statistical significant difference in the increased carotid intima-media thickness (c-IMT)(1.1mm) of normolipidemic versus hyperlipidemic patients with xanthelasma [10] **(III/B)**.

Differential diagnosis of xanthelasma

Typical lesions:

- primary dyslipidemias:

  o familial hypercholesterolemia (FH);
  o familial combined dyslipidemia (FCH);
  o familial dysbètalipoproteinemia;

- cirrhosis;
- hypothyroidism;
- nephrotic syndrome;
- paraproteinemia;

Atypical lesions:

◆ local trauma and inflammation;
◆ Erdheim Chester disease;
◆ lipoid proteinosis.

Treatment

The most obvious problem with xanthelasma is related to esthetics. There are no other complications other than seldom observed obstruction of vision [11]. In some cases treating the underlying disorder can cause regression. This has been documented in patients with hypothyroidism [12]. The effect of lipid lowering with HMGCoA reductase inhibitors (statins) on xanthelasma seems not to be of great importance. The most effective forms of treatment are:

◆ surgical excision;
◆ laser ablation;
◆ trichloracetic acid.

Regardless of the type of treatment recurrence is likely. In the first year, 25% of patients will need a second procedure and this will increase to 40% in the years to come. After a second procedure 60% of patients will have a recurrence of their xanthelasma [12-14] **(III/B)**.

Eruptive xanthomas

Eruptive xanthomas are generally associated with extremely high plasma triglyceride concentrations. Although eruptive xanthomas are a common characteristic of primary dyslipidemias such as lipoprotein lipase (LPL) deficiency or apoCII deficiency, it is seldom observed in general practice due to the rare occurrence of these primary dyslipidemias. Other more common causes for hypertriglyceridemia and thus eruptive xanthomas are hyperglycemia due to uncontrolled diabetes, and alcoholism (Table 1). Eruptive xanthomas are characterized by small rice-grain-size yellowish cutaneous papules with an erythematous halo. They appear abruptly in clusters and confluence in larger plaques or patches. Preferred locations are the extensor surface of the arms, elbows, buttocks and legs, but a more generalized presence is not uncommon either. They can cause itching, and subsequent scratching can result in bleeding plus scarring.

Diagnosis

The underlying dyslipidemia is hypertriglyceridemia. Lipoproteins that can cause extreme triglyceride concentrations are chylomicrons, very-low-density lipoprotein (VLDL) and remnant particles. Increased synthesis in combination with impaired catabolism of these lipoproteins will thus translate into high plasma levels of triglycerides and the associated eruptive xanthomas. The autosomal recessive LPL and apoCII deficiency are extremely rare

Table 1. Causes of eruptive xanthomas.

Secondary causes

- Uncontrolled diabetes mellitus (type 1 and type 2)
- Excessive alcohol intake
- Chronic renal failure
- Nephrotic syndrome
- Pancreatitis
- Biliary cirrhosis
- Medication:

  o estrogens
  o corticosteroids
  o ritonavir
  o miconazole
  o isoretinoin
  o etretinate

Primary dyslipemias

- LPL-deficiency
- ApoCII deficiency
- Familial hypertriglyceridemia
- Familal combined dyslipidemia
- Familial dysbètalipoproteinemia
- Other metabolic diseases:

  o lysosomal storage disease
  o type I glycogen storage disease von Giercke

Normolipidemic

- Paraproteinemia
- Histiocytosis
- Myeloma
- Trauma or edema
- Pregnancy
- Acquired lipodystrophy

as are some of the metabolic diseases that are associated with triglyceride elevations and eruptive xanthomas, such as von Gierke's glycogen storage disease or lysosomal storage disease [15, 16] **(III/B)**.

Secondary causes

Common diseases and prescription drugs that are associated with eruptive xanthomas share metabolic pathways in which the production or degradation of triglyceride-rich lipoproteins (TRL) are disrupted. Patients with diabetes mellitus, excessive alcohol intake, nephrotic syndrome, chronic renal failure, pancreatitis, biliary cirrhosis, pancreatitis, and obesity have presented with this skin abnormality [17, 18]. Patients with extremely high plasma levels of triglyceride-rich lipoproteins can also manifest lipemia retinalis, abdominal pain, and occasionally acute pancreatitis.

Disorders not associated with hypertriglyceridemia can manifest with eruptive xanthomas as well. Altered lipoprotein content or structure, paraproteinemia, histiocytosis and myelomas are infrequently observed. So called normolipidemic xanthomatosis has been observed during pregnancy, after traumata, edema, or in lipodystrophic patients [19-22]. The mechanism and causes for these local metabolic abnormalities are still obscure and speculative. Increased local uptake, despite normal plasma levels, or *in situ* lipid synthesis of xanthoma tissue have been indicated, the latter as an expression of the biosynthesis of membranous structures in proliferating structures [23] **(IV/C)**.

Histology

In contrast with palpebral xanthoma, eruptive xanthomas contain predominantly triglycerides and less cholesterol. Abundance of lipid-rich vacuoles and foam cells as well as lysosomal organelles has been described. The distribution of cholesterol/triglyceride contents can vary and is dependent on the type of circulating particles as well as dietary content [24].

Atherosclerosis

The risk of cardiovascular disease is associated with the underlying cause of the eruptions. In cases with increased plasma concentrations of chylomicrons, it is not the risk of cardiovascular disease that is a cause for concern, but acute pancreatitis with a very high fatality rate. In patients with familial dysbètalipoproteinemia, the increased remnant particles are associated with accelerated atherosclerosis and subsequent atherothrombotic complications [4]. The risk of atherosclerosis increases with the predominant type of circulating lipids. Cholesterol-containing particles increase this risk while triglyceride-carrying particles are less likely to promote vascular narrowing **(III/B)**.

Treatment

Manifestations of eruptive xanthoma are an expression of underlying pathology in need of proper management. Treatment is important not only because of the disfiguring skin lesions but because of the associated atherosclerosis, hepatosplenomegaly, abdominal pain and pancreatitis. Adequate treatment of the underlying cause will in most cases result in rapid and total disappearance of the disfiguring- and discomfort-causing eruptions. Since an excess of triglyceride-carrying particles are the likely cause in most cases, treatment will focus on trying to reduce these lipoproteins. Apart from the obvious focus on diabetic control, alcohol abstinence or elimination of other secondary causes, a strict dietary approach has proven to be the most promising mode of treatment [25, 26] **(III/B)**. Reducing both caloric and fat intake drastically will show rapid improvements both in plasma lipoproteins as well as the eruptive lesions. Specific treatment such as insulin in patients with insulin deficiency, heparin in extreme hypertriglyceridemic patients to stimulate the degradation of TRL by lipoprotein lipase, or even plasmapheresis can produce dramatic improvements [27] **(III/B)**. For prolonged management of patients with hypertriglyceridemia, lipid-lowering drugs such as fibrates or nicotinic acid (derivatives) as concomitant therapy to diet and lifestyle improvements are indicated. Dietary supplements in the form of omega-3 fatty acids or fish oil have shown triglyceride-lowering properties when used in high dosages of 4-8g/day. In patients at risk for cardiovascular complications, statins would be a first choice as monotherapy or combined with the pharmacological agents mentioned before [28] **(III/B)**.

Tendon xanthomas

Accumulations of cholesterol in tendons, fascia and ligaments are a common feature of FH. Depending on the severity of the underlying LDL-cholesterol elevation clinical expression may vary. Other factors such as mechanical stress caused by enhanced physical activity and/or extreme sports can promote the formation of xanthomas. Homozygous FH children can present prepubertal with extensive xanthomatosis. In heterozygotes, xanthomas manifest in adulthood or could even be absent [4] **(III/B)**.

Tendon xanthomas present as smooth and firm nodules covered by normal skin that is freely moveable over the surface of the lesions and not always easily visible. Careful palpation of extensor tendons of the hands, knees, elbows, feet and the Achilles tendon is necessary to recognize these tissue-specific cholesterol abnormalities. Because of the locations they have been regularly misdiagnosed as rheumatoid nodules or gouty tophy [4].

Diagnosis

Finding tendon xanthomas is an indication of severe lipid abnormalities, in most cases LDL-cholesterol elevations as in FH. Tendon xanthomas are in fact pathognomonic for the diagnosis of FH. Normocholesterolemic xanthomas have been present in patients with pseudo xanthomatosis elasticum, cerebrotendinous xanthomatosis and sitosterolemia, all extremely rare lipid- or sterol-metabolism abnormalities [16] **(IV/C)**. Healed or surgical restored ruptured Achilles tendons might be confused with xanthomas, which is also the case with chronic inflamed tendons because of extreme or prolonged strain. In those instances a proper patient history could eliminate FH as a likely cause for the observed abnormalities. However, one must also realize that a tenosynovitis may develop due to tendon irregularities [29].

Ultrasound

Abnormal Achilles tendons can be missed, even when carefully palpating the tendons. Experienced clinicians have failed to accurately detect the sometimes subtle differences. Using widely available imaging equipment allows for a more accurate measurement of Achilles tendon thickness. This can be crucial for a proper clinical diagnosis and using ultrasound to measure the width of this tendon is considered to be a safe non-invasive imaging tool for more accurate and earlier diagnosis [30] **(IV/C)**. Age-dependent cut-off measurements have been proposed based on C-statistic ROC curves [31] (Table 2).

Table 2. Results of ROC curves and threshold values of sonographic AT thickness for diagnosis of FH. *Reproduced with permission from Junyent M, et al* [31].

Subjects	Area under the curve	95% CI	Tendon thickness threshold (mm)	Sensitivity	Specificity
Men ≤45 years	0.65	0.51-0.78	5.3	49%	91%
Men >45 years	0.84	0.70-0.98	5.7	75%	89%
Women ≤50 years	0.76	0.62-0.89	4.8	50%	88%
Women >50 years	0.79	0.67-0.91	4.9	67%	81%

Atherosclerosis

The clinical significance of tendon xanthomas in patients with FH is still a matter of debate. There are indications that early and extensive xanthomas are associated with higher LDL-cholesterol concentrations and thus result in earlier atherosclerosis. Variability in the phenotypical expression of this disease makes it difficult to draw definite conclusions [32, 33]. It remains confusing that, despite similar plasma LDL-cholesterol levels and sharing the identical mutation, one patient develops distinct xanthomas while the other family member does not [34]. The recently published Spanish FH cohort established a strong and independent association between the presence of tendon xanthomas and premature cardiovascular disease [31] **(IV/C)**.

Treatment

With the introduction of the potent cholesterol-lowering HMG CoA reductase inhibitors or statins, regression of xanthomas has been observed [35], although the response differs between individual patients and depends on the severity of the manifested xanthomas. Combination treatments of statins with cholesterol absorption inhibitors or bile acid binding resins have not been conducted for this specific purpose. Based on their superior LDL-cholesterol-lowering properties one would expect positive results **(III/B)**.

Probucol was one of the first lipid-lowering drugs with additional antioxidant properties that has been used for this particular purpose. In the trials conducted with this compound a marked regression of xanthomas was observed [36, 37]. However, probucol is no longer available in Europe since it was found to cause long QT syndrome in some patients.

Plasmapheresis or LDL-apheresis are treatment modalities commonly reserved for homozygous FH patients. Both tendon and cutaneous xanthomas have regressed and even disappeared following such treatment regimens [38-40]. Liver transplant, a rarely used treatment for homozygous FH patients, has also been shown to markedly reduce xanthomas [41].

A final word of caution should be mentioned with respect to the surgical removal of xanthomas. Although the surgical approach would be an obvious and logical one to eliminate these sometimes disfiguring and disabling anomalies, experience has shown that in the majority of patients xanthomas will reappear and mostly be larger than the ones removed **(IV/C)**.

Tuberous xanthomas

Tuberous xanthomas are characterized by yellow-colored nodules surrounded by a reddish halo. During the early stages they are small and have a soft consistency. They are sometimes mistaken for eruptive xanthomas. During their development the solitary nodules grow and coalesce changing to a darker color and becoming more firm in consistency. They can be found on distinct locations such as knees, elbows, buttocks and knuckles. Their appearance is very noticeable and can be disfiguring. Certain locations such as Achilles tendons can cause disability due to the fact that patients are unable to wear shoes [42] **(IV/C)**.

Diagnosis

The appearance of these distinct and prominent skin anomalies are almost always associated with systemic lipid metabolism disturbances involving cholesterol and/or triglycerides. Primary dyslipidemias that are associated with tuberous xanthomas are (homozygous) FH, familial dysbètalipoproteinemia, cerebrotendinous xanthomatosis and sitosterolemia. Solitary cases of normocholesterolemic xanthomatosis have been described. The etiology is unknown but would point to a distinct and serum lipid-independent metabolic process responsible for the xanthomatosis depositions [42]. Secondary dyslipidemias that can manifest these types of xanthoma are shown in Figure 2 [43-46] **(IV/C)**.

Histology

Tuberous xanthomas contain predominantly cholesterol and cholesterol esters. There is an abundance of diffuse or nodular foamy histiocytes with scanty inflammatory cells as well as lysosomal organelles and fibrous tissue [47].

Treatment

Treatment for tuberous xanthomas is identical as noted in the section on tendon xanthomas.

Xanthomas striate palmaris

Palmar xanthoma are a cutaneous manifestation of lipidosis in which there is an accumulation of lipids in large foam cells within the skin, clinically characterized by flat yellowish to orange plaques that involve the creases of palms and flexural surfaces of the fingers [46, 48]. These typical skin discolorations are pathognomonic for familial dysbètalipoproteinemia. Patients with familial dysbètalipoproteinemia respond very well to dietary restrictions of fats and calories. Combination treatment with a pharmacological regimen of statins or fibrates, depending on their most prominent lipid abnormality, is not uncommon in these types of patients. The characteristic skin discolorations will disappear within days to weeks after initiating treatment **(IV/C)**.

Rare forms of normolipidemic xanthomas

Xanthomata disseminatum – Montgomery

Xanthomata disseminatum (XD) or the Montgomery syndrome is an extremely rare disorder characterized by papulo-nodular red-yellowish lesions that in time change to more distinctive dark brown colored skin papules. The disease is most often discovered at an early age affecting mainly children and adolescents. Unlike eruptive xanthomas their preferable locations are flexural creases, mucous membranes, the central nervous system, cornea, or sclera and, in rare instances, bone. In particular, the mucous membranes of the mouth, tongue, larynx and even the bronchi can be affected. These oral manifestations may cause strictures and subsequent dysphagia, hoarseness and even dyspnea. In 30% of cases, diabetes insipidus develops as a result of lesions in the pituitary gland or the tuber cinereum infundibulum. Plasma lipoproteins are unaffected and therefore the disease is thought to be the result of a local tissue metabolic derangement. It is considered to be part of the spectrum of histiocytosis X, in which a primary proliferation of histiocytotic elements is followed by a reaction of cholesterol deposits in the affected areas. The diagnosis is made on the clinical characteristics in combination with the histological findings. The prognosis is good and treatment is directed at managing the diabetes insipidus or, if the respiratory tree is affected, surgical removal of the oral lesions using a CO_2 laser [49-51] **(IV/C)**.

Juvenile granulo-xanthomata

Juvenile granulo-xanthomata is another form of normolipidemic xanthomatosis where non-Langerhans-cell histiocytosis plays a role. The clinical features consist of a single or sometimes multiple well-delineated solitary papular nodules of firm consistency. They have a yellowish orange color and are mostly found on the upper trunk or head. Microscopically there is a heterogeneous infiltrate of histiocytes with a variable composition of inflammatory cells. Over 80% are found in infants <2 years of age. Ocular manifestations have been described in rare cases (<0.05%). Mucous membrane or visceral involvement is uncommon. Neurofibromatosis (NF) and chronic juvenile myeloid leukemia have been associated with this type of xanthoma, with additional features such as the café au lait skin discoloration in NF. In the majority of cases this is a self-limiting disease that resolves in months to years. Diagnosis is based on clinical features, normal plasma lipid levels and histological characteristics. In the case of ocular involvement, adjuvant therapy with corticosteroids is indicated, which can be administered systemically or locally, by intra-conjunctival injections [52-54] (IV/C).

Necrobiotic xanthogranuloma

Necrobiotic xanthogranuloma (NXG) is a disorder characterized by indurated, yellow-brown nodules or plaques. In time central telangiectasias may form that can eventually ulcerate. It is most commonly found in the face and, less frequently, on the trunk and extremities. In 80% of affected patients a monoclonal IgG paraproteinemia is present combined with leucopenia, anemia, hepatosplenomegaly, reduced plasma complement factors and cryoglobulinemia. Multiple myeloma and hypertension are additional clinical features that have been noted. Visceral involvement is rarely found. Histologically the dermis contains granulomatous infiltrates and bands of hyaline necrobiosis. Foreign body, as well as Touton giant cells, cholesterol clefts, lymphoid nodules and plasma cells are variable but significant features. Plasma lipid levels are normal. Diagnosis is based on clinical features and histological biopsy findings [54-56]. No first-line treatment has been established, although treatments with cyclophosphamide, chlorambucil, plasmapheresis, localized radiation therapy or steroids either local or systemically have been tested, but with mixed results. This is a chronic disease, and a patient's prognosis depends on the degree of extracutaneous involvement [57-59] (IV/C).

Verruciform xanthomas

First described in 1971, this rare form of xanthoma has an unknown etiology. The majority of authors agree about the histiocytic origin of the xanthoma cells [60]. In most cases, the clinical impressions are papilloma or verrucous carcinoma-like. There are some cases reported in conjunction with leukoplakia, carcinoma *in situ*, pemphigus, and discoid lupus erythematosus (DLE), which merits close evaluation of this disease. Localized lesions are mostly found in the mucosal area of the mouth and genitals and occasionally in the inguinal folds. When localized in or around the genital area the similarities with condylomata accuminata make it a difficult diagnosis. Microscopic histological analysis shows a peculiar pattern of a very dense infiltrate of vacuolated foam cells in verruciform xanthomas. Testing for human papillomavirus is the key to making a clear distinction. For the mucosal locations of these lesions a surgical approach seems to be sufficient. The dermal lesions are more difficult to remove. The application of a topical potent antibacterial disinfectant has shown some promising results [61, 62] **(IV/C)**.

Normolipidemic diffuse plane xanthoma

This uncommon form of xanthomatosis is not related to increased plasma lipid levels, is characterized by diffuse yellowish macules or plaques on the neck, axillae, upper trunk, buttocks and inguinal folds and is usually accompanied by persistent itching [63]. Histopathological and ultrastructural studies show foamy histiocytes in the dermis and deposition of neutral fat in the upper papillary dermis. Some authors believe that paraprotein-lipoprotein complexes are deposited in the skin. Others suggest that leukemic cells infiltrate the skin with subsequent xanthomization. Still, others consider this is a form of non-X histiocytosis. Approximately half of all cases are associated with hematological disorders. On rare occasions, they have been described in the context of cutaneous T-cell lymphomas. In patients with limited involvement, the individual lesions can be excised. Other options include chemabrasion, dermabrasion, and ablative laser therapy [64, 65] **(IV/C)**.

Conclusions

Xanthomas are cutaneous lipid accumulations that can give important clues to a variety of internal diseases. In most cases lipoprotein metabolism abnormalities are fuelling the dermatological manifestations and reflect an increased risk for potential life-threatening atherothrombotic complications or pancreatitis. Additional laboratory investigations to determine the underlying lipid abnormalities are always indicated and in certain types of disorder this should be repeated in first-degree family members. Normal plasma lipoprotein concentrations point to rare causes of xanthomas. Specialized dermatological procedures such as skin biopsies are indicated to determine the underlying cause of these types of dermatological manifestations.

Key points	Evidence level
♦ Dermatological manifestations can give important clues for the diagnosis of lipid disorders.	IV/C
♦ Lipid deposits on or around the eyelids (xanthelasma) are an indication for additional diagnostic procedures to rule out primary or secondary dyslipidemias.	IV/C
♦ Approximately half of the patients with lipid deposits on or around the eyelids (xanthelasma) have manifestations of a primary or secondary dyslipidemia.	IV/C
♦ Tendon xanthomas are pathognomonic for the diagnosis of familial hypercholesterolemia.	IV/C
♦ Surgical removal of tendon xanthomas are followed by severe recurrences of these skin manifestations.	IV/C
♦ Tuberous xanthomas are found in patients with severe lipid abnormalities involving cholesterol and triglycerides.	IV/C
♦ Xanthoma striate palmaris is pathognomonic for the diagnosis of familial dysbètalipoproteinemia.	IV/C

References

1.   Jonsson A, Sigfusson N. Significance of xanthelasma palpebrarum in the normal population (Letter). *Lancet* 1976; 1: 372.
2.   Lookingbill DP, Marks JG. *Principles of Dermatology*, 3rd ed. Philadelphia: W.B. Saunders Company, 2000: 119-21.
3.   Polano MK. Xanthomathoses and dyslipoproteinemias. In: *Dermatology in General Medicine*. Fitzpatrick TB, Eisen AZ, Wolff K, Freedberg IM, Austen KF, Eds. New-York: McGraw-Hill, 1993: 1901-15.
4.   Havel RJ, Kane JP. Introduction: Structure and metabolism of plasma lipoproteins. In: *Metabolic Basis of Inherited Disease*. Stanbury JB, Wyngaarden JB, Frederickson DS, Eds. New York: McGraw-Hill, 1989.
5.   Alexander LJ. Ocular signs and symptoms of altered blood lipids. *J Am Optom Assoc* 1983; 54: 123.
6.   Lever WF, Schaumburg-Lever G, Eds. *Histopathology of the Skin*, 6th ed. Philadelphia: JB Lippincott, 1983: 387.
7.   Ferrando J, Bombi JA. Ultrastructural aspects of normolipidemic xanthomatosis. *Arch Dermatol Res* 1979; 266: 143-59.
8.   Douste-Blazy P, Marcel YL, Cohen L, *et al*. Increased frequency of apoE-ND phenotype and hyperapobeta-lipoproteinemia in normolipidemic subjects and xanthelasma of the eyelids. *Ann Intern Med* 1982; 96: 164-9.
9.   Menotti A, Mariotti S, Seccareccia F, *et al*. Determinants of all causes of death in samples of Italian middle-aged men followed up for 25 years. *J Epidemiol Community Health* 1987; 41 : 243-50.
10.   Noel B. Premature atherosclerosis in patients with xanthelasma. *JEADV* 2007; 21: 1244-8.
11.   Pedace FJ, Winkelmann RK. Xanthelasma palpebrarum. *JAMA* 1965; 193: 893.
12.   Kaplan RM, Curtis AC. Xanthoma of the skin. *JAMA* 1961; 176: 859.
13.   Rohrich RJ, Jeffrey E, Janis JE, Pownell PH. Xanthelasma palpebrarum: a review and current management principles. *Plast Reconstr Surg* 2002; 110: 1310-13.
14.   Mendelson BC, Masson JK. Xanthelasma: follow-up on results after surgical excision. *Plast Reconstr Surg* 1976; 58: 535.
15.   Antonio M, Gotto J. Clinical diagnosis of hyperlipoproteinaemia. *Am J Med* 1983; 74: 5-9.

16. Parker F. Xanthomas and hyperlipidaemias. *J Am Acad Dermatol* 1985; 13: 1-30.

17. Ruggero C, Marcello M, Emilio B, Giovanni G. Normolipaemic eruptive cutaneous xanthomatosis. *Arch Dermatol* 1986; 12: 1294-7.

18. Dicken CH, Connolly SM. Eruptive xanthomas associated with isotretinoin (13-cis-retinoic acid). *Arch Dermatol* 1980; 116: 951-2.

19. Parker F. Normocholesterolaemic xanthomatosis. *Arch Dermatol* 1986; 122: 1253-6.

20. Goldstein GD. The Koebner phenomenon with eruptive xanthomas. *J Am Acad Dermatol* 1984; 10: 1064-5.

21. Eeckhout I, Vogelaers D, Gleerts ML, Naeyaert JM. Xanthomas due to generalized edema. *Br J Dermatol* 1997; 136: 601-3.

22. Mahmoud SF Lawrence. Seip syndrome: report of a case from Egypt. *Cutis* 1997; 60: 91-3.

23. Chung-Hong H, Ellefson RD, Winkelmann RK. Lipid synthesis in cutaneous xanthoma. *J Invest Dermatol* 1982; 79: 80-5.

24. Parker F, Odland G. Electron microscopic similarities between experimental xanthomas and human eruptive xanthomas. *J Invest Dermatol* 1969; 52: 136.

25. Archer CB, Macdonald DM. Eruptive xanthoma in type V hyperlipoprotaeinemia associated with diabetes mellitus. *Clin Exp Dermatol* 1984; 9: 312-6.

26. Kuo PI. Hyperlipoproteinemia and atherosclerosis: dietary intervention. Symposium on hyperlipoproteinemia: dietary and pharmacologic intervention. *Am J Med* 1983; 24: 15-8.

27. Tsuang W, Navaneethan U, Ruiz L, Palascak JB, Gelrud A. Hypertriglyceridemic pancreatitis: presentation and management. *Am J Gastroenterol* 2009; 104(4): 984-91.

28. Viljoen A, Wierzbicki AS. Potential options to treat hypertriglyceridaemia. *Curr Drug Targets* 2009; 10(4): 356-62.

29. Beeharry D, Coupe B, Benbow EW, Morgan J, Kwok S, Charlton-Menys V, France M, Durrington PN. Familial hypercholesterolaemia commonly presents with Achilles tenosynovitis. *Ann Rheum Dis* 2006; 65: 312-5.

30. Descamps OS, Leysen X, Van Leuven F, Heller FR. The use of Achilles tendon ultrasonography for the diagnosis of familial hypercholesterolemia. *Atherosclerosis* 2001; 157: 514-8.

31. Junyent M, Gilabert R, Zambon D, Nunez I, Vela M, Civeira F, Pocovi M, Ros E. The use of Achilles tendon sonography to distinguish familial hypercholesterolemia from other genetic dyslipidemias. *Arterioscler Thromb Vasc Biol* 2005; 25: 2203-8.

32. Civeira F. International Panel on Management of Familial Hypercholesterolemia. Guidelines for the diagnosis and management of heterozygous familial hypercholesterolemia. *Atherosclerosis* 2004; 173: 55-68.

33. Kruth HS. Lipid deposition in human tendon xanthoma. *Am J Pathol* 1985; 121: 311-5.

34. Ferrieres J, Lambert J, Lussier-Cacan S, Davignon J. Coronary artery disease in heterozygous familial hypercholesterolemia patients with the same LDL receptor gene mutation. *Circulation* 1995; 92: 290-5.

35. Tsouli SG, Xydis V, Argyropoulou MI, Tselepis AD, Elisaf M, Kiortsis DN. Regression of Achilles tendon thickness after statin treatment in patients with familial hypercholesterolemia: an ultrasonographic study. *Atherosclerosis* 2009; 205(1): 151-5.

36. Kajinami K, Nishitsuji M, Takeda Y, Shimizu M, Koizumi J, Mabuchi H. Long-term probucol treatment results in regression of xanthomas, but in progression of coronary atherosclerosis in a heterozygous patient with familial hypercholesterolemia. *Atherosclerosis* 1996; 120: 181-7.

37. Yamamoto A, Matsuzawa Y, Kishino B. Effects of probucol on homozygous cases of familial hypercholesterolemia. *Atherosclerosis* 1983; 48: 157-66.

38. Scheel AK, Schettler V, Koziolek M, Koelling S, Werner C, Muller GA, *et al*. Impact of chronic LDL-apheresis treatment on Achilles tendon affection in patients with severe familial hypercholesterolemia: a clinical and ultrasonographic 3-year follow-up study. *Atherosclerosis* 2004; 174: 133-9.

39. Mabuchi H, Sakai Y, Watanabe A, Haba T, Koizumi J, Takeda R. Normalization of low-density lipoprotein levels and disappearance of xanthomas during pregnancy in a woman with heterozygous familial hypercholesterolemia. *Metabolism* 1985; 34: 309-15.

40. Mabuchi H, Michishita I, Sakai T, Sakai Y, Watanabe A, Wakasugi T, *et al*. Treatment of homozygous patients with familial hypercholesterolemia by double-filtration plasmapheresis. *Atherosclerosis* 1986; 61: 135-40.

41. Mabuchi H, Koizumi J, Michishita I, Takeda M, Kajinami K, Fujita H, Inazu A, Uno Y, Shimizu M, Takeda R, *et al*. Effects on coronary atherosclerosis of long-term treatment of familial hypercholesterolemia by LDL-apheresis. *Beitr Infusionsther* 1988; 23: 87-96.

42. Fleischmajer R, Tint GS, Bennett HD. Normolipemic tendon and tuberous xanthomas. *J Am Acad Dermatol* 1981; 5(3): 290-6.

43. Roberts WE. Classification and etiology of hyperlipoproteinemia. *Fed Proc* 1971; 30: 829-34.

44. Guirado SS, Conejo-Mir JS, Muñoz MA, Wite JB, Fernandez-Freire LR, Ortíz JV. Sitosterol xanthomatosis. *J Eur Acad Dermatol Venereol* 2007; 21(1): 100-3.

45. Braun-Falco O, Plewig G, Wolff HH, Winkelmann RK. *Dermatology*, 3rd ed. Berlin: Springer Verlag, 1991: 849-60 and 1113-4.

46. Polano MK. Xanthomathoses and dyslipoproteinemias. In: *Dermatology in General Medicine*. Fitzpatrick TB, Eisen AZ, Wolff K, Freedberg IM, Austen KF, Eds. New-York: McGraw-Hill, 1993: 1901-15.

47. Fletcher RF, Gloster J. The lipids in xanthomata. *J Clin Invest* 1964; 43: 2104.

48. Fitzpatrick TB, Johnson RA, Wolff K, Suurmond D. *Color Atlas and Synopsis of Clinical Dermatology*, 4th ed. New-York: McGraw-Hill, 2001: 444-51.

49. Mishkel MA, Cockshott WP, Nazir 01, *et al*. Xanthoma disseminatum. *Arch Dermatol* 1977; 113: 1094-1100.

50. Beylot-Barry M. Histiocytoses non langerhansiennes. In: *Thérapeutique Dermatologique*. Dubertret L, Aractingi S, Bachelez H, Bodemer C, Chosidow O, Cribier B, Joly P, Eds. Paris: Médecine-Sciences Flammarion, 2001: 357.

51. Smoller BR, Horn TD. *Dermatopathology in Systemic Disease*. New York: Oxford University Press, 1993: 197-200.

52. Ferrando J, Campo-Voegeli A, Soler-Carrillo J, *et al*. Systemic xanthohistiocytoma: a variant of xanthoma disseminatum? *Br J Dermatol* 1998; 138: 155-60.

53. Zelger BW, Sidoroff A, Orchard G, Cerio R. Non-Langerhans cell histiocytoses. A new unifying concept. *Am J Dermatopathol* 1996; 18: 490-504.

54. Wolter M, De Prost Y. Xanthogranulome juvénile. In: *Thérapeutique Dermatologique*. Dubertret L, Aractingi S, Bachelez H, Bodemer C, Chosidow O, Cribier B, Joly P, Eds. Paris: Médecine-Sciences Flammarion, 2001: 881-2.

55. Sivak-Callcott JA, Rootman J, Rasmussen SL, Nugent RA, White VA, Paridaens D, Currie Z, Rose G, Clark B, McNab AA, Buffam FV, Neigel JM, Kazim M. Adult xanthogranulomatous disease of the orbit and ocular adnexa: new immunohistochemical findings and clinical review. *Br J Ophthalmol* 2006; 90(5): 602-8.

56. Mehregan DA, Winkelmann RK. Necrobiotic xanthogranuloma. *Arch Dermatol* 1992; 128(1): 94-100.

57. Chave TA, Chowdhury MMU, Holt PJA. Recalcitrant necrobiotic xanthogranuloma responding to pulsed high-dose oral dexamethasone plus maintenance therapy with oral prednisolone. *Br J Dermatol* 2001; 144: 158-61.

58. Venencie PY, Doukan S, Vieillefond A, *et al*. Xanthogranulome nécrobiotique avec paraprotéinémie. *Ann Dermato Venereol* 1992; 119: 825-7.

59. Criado PR, Vasconcellos C, Pegas JR, *et al*. Necrobiotic xanthogranuloma with lambda paraproteinemia: case report of successful treatment with melphalan and prednisone. *J Dermatolog Treat* 2002; 13: 87-9.

60. Gianotti F, Caputo R, Ermacora E. Singuliere histiocytose infantile a cellules avec particules vermiformes intracytoplasmiques. *Bull Soc Fr Dermatol Syphiligr* 1971; 78: 232.

61. Philipsen HP, Reichart PA, Takata T, Ogawa I. Verruciform xanthoma - biological profile of 282 oral lesions based on a literature survey with nine new cases from Japan. *Oral Oncol* 2003; 39(4): 325-36.

62. Connolly SB, Lewis EJ, Lindholm JS, *et al*. Management of cutaneous verruciform xanthoma. *J Am Acad Dermatol* 2000; 42: 343-7.

63. Altman J, *et al*. Diffuse normolipemic plane xanthoma. *Arch Dermatol* 1962; 85: 633.

64. Bragg J. Diffuse plane xanthomata. *Dermatol Online J* 2005; 11(4): 4.

65. Lorenz S, *et al*. Treatment of diffuse plane xanthoma of the face with the Erbium:YAG laser. *Arch Dermatol* 2001; 137: 1413

66. Scoggings RB, Harlan WR. Cutaneous manifestations of hyperlipidemia and uremia. *Postgrad Med* 1967; 41: 537.

Chapter 17

When should we fear statin interactions?

Rob E. Aarnoutse PharmD PhD, Hospital Pharmacist
David M. Burger PharmD PhD, Hospital Pharmacist - Clinical Pharmacologist
Department of Clinical Pharmacy
Radboud University Nijmegen Medical Centre
Nijmegen, The Netherlands

Introduction

The hydroxymethylglutaryl (HMG) CoA reductase inhibitors, or 'statins', are the first-line treatment for dyslipidemia based on several studies that demonstrated a reduction in cardiovascular morbidity and mortality [1]. As a group, the currently used statins (simvastatin, lovastatin, atorvastatin, fluvastatin, pravastatin, rosuvastatin and pitavastatin) are generally well tolerated. Nevertheless, these drugs have an uncommon but serious adverse effect: skeletal muscle abnormalities including myopathy (11 per 100,000 person-years of follow-up) and life-threatening rhabdomyolysis (3-4 per 100,000 person-years) [2].

Over the years, it has become increasingly clear that pharmacokinetic and pharmacodynamic interactions between statins and co-administered agents are the most relevant risk factor for statin-associated muscle toxicity. Consequently, physicians require adequate knowledge of the evidence base of these interactions to prevent morbidity and mortality. Therefore, the objectives of this chapter are:

- to provide a solid background on the risk factors for statin-related myopathy and the role of drug interactions, the general mechanisms of drug interactions, and the pharmacokinetic properties of the statins that determine their interaction profiles;
- to provide an overview and evidence for the most relevant interactions of statins and the circumstances under which they can be expected and should be feared;
- to recognize a set of principles that may be used to prevent relevant drug interactions with statins.

The risk of statin-related myopathy and the role of drug interactions

Aggregate evidence shows that myopathy, the most feared adverse effect of statins, is related to the concentration of statins in blood [3, 4]. This blood concentration is determined by the dose administered, the pharmacokinetics of the statin and by drug interactions (Figure 1). The dose of the statins, an obvious determinant of blood concentration, has been shown to be a risk factor for rhabdomyolysis [5-7] **(III/B)**. Inter-individual variability in pharmacokinetics causes differences between patients in the blood concentrations achieved after the same dose. Genetic polymorphisms in metabolic and transport proteins contribute to this pharmacokinetic variability and some are strongly associated with the risk of myopathy [8-10] **(III/B)**. Finally, interactions may either increase the statin concentrations or potentiate the effect of these concentrations by exerting an additive or synergistic effect.

Apart from the effects of the statin concentration, susceptibility of the patient for myopathy is also relevant (Figure 1). Risk factors include higher age, female sex, renal disease, hepatic disease, existing myopathic conditions, diabetes, hypothyroidism, electrolyte disorders, major trauma, seizures, hypothermia, metabolic acidosis, viral infections and certain drugs of abuse [3, 6, 7, 11, 12] **(III/B)**.

Although the risk of statin-related myopathy is low, this problem is relevant from a societal perspective considering the large numbers of patients who are using statins. Dependent on which guidelines are followed, some 5% to 30% of middle-aged and older patients will

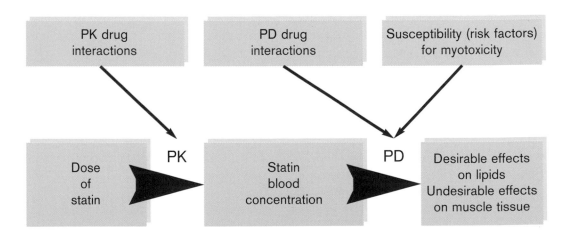

Figure 1. The role of drug interactions in causing statin-related myopathy. PK = pharmacokinetic(s); PD = pharmacodynamic(s).

receive statins, and they will often require life-long therapy [3]. Recent guidelines have even expanded the population of patients that is targeted for cholesterol-lowering therapy and indicated that target cholesterol levels should be lower than recommended previously. The latter change not only further increases the number of individuals prescribed a statin, it also increases the likelihood that statins will be used at higher doses.

Among the many patients who are using these top-selling drugs, the risk of interactions is large. Studies have shown that 6.9% up to 34% of statin prescriptions are issued in combination with drugs that potentially interact with them [13-16] **(III/B)**. This may be related to the type of population in which statins are used. Typically the middle-aged and older population is more exposed to multiple drugs (polypharmacy) with an associated higher risk of interactions with statins [17] **(III/B)**. Of note, some countries have approved over-the-counter or non-prescription access to low-dose statins under certain circumstances [9]. This practice of partly unsupervised therapy may increase the risk of drug interactions.

Drug interactions are not only very prevalent amongst statin users, they have emerged as the most relevant risk factor for myopathy as well. In 2001, cerivastatin was withdrawn from the worldwide market in 2001 because of an unacceptably high incidence of serious myopathy and rhabdomyolysis. It turned out that many of the patients involved were exposed to an interaction between cerivastatin and gemfibrozil [5] **(III/B)**. Furthermore, 50% or more of cases of rhabdomyolysis for any specific statin were associated with a potential drug interaction in the USA [18] **(III/B)**. Likewise, in Australia, interacting drugs featured in 77% of reports for rhabdomyolysis associated with simvastatin, and in 44% of reports associated with atorvastatin [6] **(III/B)**.

General mechanisms of drug interactions

A drug interaction occurs when the response of a patient to a drug is changed by the presence of another substance, which can be a co-administered drug, a food component or an environmental agent. Pharmacokinetic interactions alter the absorption, distribution, metabolism, transport or elimination of a drug, resulting in a change in drug concentrations. Pharmacodynamic interactions involve additive, synergistic or antagonistic effects of drugs acting on the same receptors or physiological systems (Figure 1), yielding altered pharmacological responses to the same drug concentrations.

Most pharmacokinetic interactions are related to changes in the metabolism and transport of drugs. Phase I metabolism mainly involves intestinal and hepatic cytochrome P450 isoenzymes, including the most relevant CYP1, CYP2 and CYP3 families. Phase II metabolism is the coupling of products of phase I metabolism (or the parent drugs) to water-soluble molecules, e.g. glucuronides or sulphates. Drugs interacting with phase I or II enzymes may be characterised as substrates, inhibitors or inducers. Drugs which are substrates for the same enzyme will compete for this system. If the metabolic capacity of the enzyme system is exceeded, the elevated concentrations of substrates may lead to toxicity. Inhibition of enzymes may result in increased concentrations of and exaggerated or prolonged responses to the object drug as well. Furthermore, if the metabolism of a parent drug normally results in the formation of active metabolites, drug response may be diminished when this activation is inhibited. Induction causes an increased synthesis of metabolic enzymes, and a subsequent decrease in drug concentrations. The expression of transporters such as organic anion transporting polypeptide (OATP) 1B1 and p-glycoprotein can also be inhibited or induced.

Pharmacokinetics and pharmacodynamics of statins

Many interactions with statins are based on a pharmacokinetic mechanism, and therefore knowledge of their pharmacokinetic characteristics is essential for understanding, predicting and preventing these interactions. Based on their pharmacokinetic properties (Table 1), the currently available statins can be divided in two groups, with separate risks for drug interactions [3, 4, 8, 12]. One group is often designated as lipophilic statins (based on chemical characteristics, although pitavastatin is also lipophilic) or CYP3A4-dependent statins and comprises simvastatin, lovastatin and atorvastatin. The other group consists of the hydrophilic CYP3A4-independent fluvastatin, pravastatin, rosuvastatin and pivastatin.

The pharmacokinetics of statins can be summarized under the following headings [3, 4, 8, 9, 12].

Absorption

Simvastatin and lovastatin have a low oral bioavailability of 5% or less, which can be explained by their extensive CYP3A4-mediated metabolism on first pass through the liver. In addition, they are substrates for p-glycoprotein (Table 1), a transporter that co-operates with CYP3A4 to reduce their absorption in the intestine. The bioavailability of atorvastatin is somewhat higher, probably because only 20% of this statin is metabolized by CYP3A4. For the other statins, the percent of the dose that reaches the systemic circulation is higher, varying from 18% (pravastatin) to 60% (pitavastatin).

Distribution

All statins are highly bound to plasma proteins, with the exception of pravastatin (50% protein binding). In theory, these highly bound statins could be involved in drug displacement interactions that cause a relatively large increase in unbound (or free, active) statin, but no such interactions have been described so far. For the efficacy of statins such interactions are not expected to be relevant, as statins are relatively insensitive to immediate changes in unbound plasma concentrations due to their slow onset of effect [3]. Temporarily high unbound statin concentrations are not expected to be toxic either, as displaced statin would distribute in the tissues and a larger amount of unbound drug would be available for metabolism and elimination as compensation mechanisms [3].

Table 1. Pharmacokinetic properties of statins [a, b].

	Simvastatin	Lovastatin	Atorvastatin	Fluvastatin	Pravastatin	Rosuvastatin	Pitavastatin
Lipophilicity[c]	++++	++++	+++	+++	+	++	++++
Bioavailability (%)	<5	5	12	30	18	20	60
Protein binding (%)	>95	>98	>98	>98	50	90	96
Hepatic extraction (%)	≥80	≥70	70	≥70	45	63	?
Metabolism[d]	+++	+++	+++	+++	+	+	++
Metabolizing CYP enzymes	3A4, 2C8	3A4, 2C8?	3A4 (2C8)	2C9	(3A4)	2C9 (2C19)	(2C9)
Half-life (h)	2-5	2-5	7-20	1-3	1-3	20	10-13
Urinary excretion (% of dose)	Negl.	10	<2	Negl.	47	<10	2
Substrate of [e]:							
OATP1B1	+	+	+	+	+	+	+
BCRP	?	?	+	+	+	+	+
MDR1 (P-gp)	+	+	+	?	+	-	+
Inhibitor of [e]:							
CYP3A4	+	+	+	+	-	+	-
CYP2C9	-	-	-	+	-	(+)	-
MDR1 (P-gp)	+	+	+	-	-	-	+
BCRP	+	?	+	+	-	+	+

a = adapted from and based on references from Neuvonen *et al*, 2006 [4] and Shitara *et al*, 2008 (urinary excretion data) [8]

b = a question mark indicates 'not known' or 'uncertain', parentheses indicate 'minor significance'

c = five plus signs indicate 'most lipophilic'; one plus sign indicates 'most hydrophilic'

d = three plus signs indicate 'extensively metabolized'; one plus sign indicates 'limited metabolism, eliminated mainly unchanged'

e = a plus sign indicates 'yes'; a minus sign indicates 'no'

Abbreviations: CYP = cytochrome; negl. = neglible; OATP = organic anion transporting polypeptide; BCRP= breast cancer resistance protein; MDR = multi-drug resistance protein; this is p-glycoprotein

Metabolism

CYP3A4 is important to the metabolism of simvastatin, lovastatin and (to a lesser extent) atorvastatin. The metabolism of simvastatin and lovastatin is also mediated by CYP2C8. Fluvastatin is extensively metabolized by CYP2C9. In contrast, pravastatin, rosuvastatin and pitavastatin are excreted largely in their unchanged form. Pravastatin is also partially degraded in the stomach and partially metabolized by non-CYP-enzymes. About 10% of rosuvastatin is metabolized, mainly by CYP2C9.

Transport

For the bioavailability of many statins, p-glycoprotein is important, as mentioned above. As statins are acting inside the hepatocytes, hepatic uptake transporters such as OATP1B1 and OATP2B1, OATP1A2 and sodium-dependent taurocholate cotransporting polypeptide (NTCP) are relevant as well (Table 1). Subsequently, for the transport of statins into the bile, efflux transporters on the hepatocyte are active, including p-glycoprotein, multidrug resistance associated protein (MRP) 2, breast cancer resistance protein (BCRP) and bile salt export pump (BSEP).

Elimination

All statins and their metabolites are mainly excreted through the bile, with pravastatin showing somewhat more renal excretion (Table 1).

The processes of absorption, distribution, metabolism, transport and elimination result in vary large (up to 10-fold [4]) inter-individual variability in the exposure to the same dose of a statin. Genetic polymorphisms in the enzymes and transporters exist and these contribute to this variability as well [4, 8, 9].

From the pharmacokinetic characteristics of individual statins, their interactions can be predicted. Most notably, the CYP3A4-dependent simvastatin, lovastatin and atorvastatin (but not the other statins) are particularly sensitive to interactions with the large group of drugs that inhibit or induce CYP3A4. Atorvastatin is expected to give a less pronounced increase in exposure upon co-administration of strong CYP3A4 inhibitors, as it is less dependent on CYP3A4. Drugs that specifically affect certain transporters will have an interaction with many statins (Table 1).

As to the pharmacodynamics of the statins, it should be noted that their dose-response curve is flat [19]. Approximately two thirds of the maximum response can generally be expected with only one-quarter of the highest dose. This means that relatively small gains in efficacy occur with an increase of the dose, compared to a greater increased risk of adverse effects [20, 21].

Evidence for adverse effects due to drug interactions

Evidence for adverse effects related to drug interactions can not be obtained by controlled clinical trials, as studies with adverse events as a primary outcome are unethical [22]. Instead, identifying specific drugs that cause interaction-related adverse effects relies on sources of evidence that are less definitive [22], including case reports, case series, case-control studies, post-marketing surveillance evaluations, analyses in patient databases, and reports on secondary endpoints in clinical efficacy trials and cohort studies (III/B). Apart from these, pharmacokinetic interaction studies are an important source of evidence for (pharmacokinetic) interactions. These studies, which are often predesigned experiments (trials), could be rated according to the hierarchy of evidence for clinical studies, but it should be recognized that this system is not meant for pharmacokinetic studies. The endpoints in pharmacokinetic studies relate to changes in pharmacokinetic parameters rather than to clinical outcome, and pharmacokinetic data can not always be directly extrapolated to incidence and severity of clinical events [22]. For these reasons only the experimental and non-experimental clinical studies, and not the pharmacokinetic studies, are graded in this chapter.

Pharmacokinetic interactions with statins

Drugs that interact in the intestinal lumen

The most relevant interaction of statins in the intestinal lumen relates to the reduction in statin plasma concentrations by simultaneous ingestion of cholestyramine or colestipol [3]. Therefore, statins should be taken 1 hour before or 4-6 hours after these bile-acid sequestrants. In contrast, colesevelam had no effect on the exposure to lovastatin when the drugs were co-administered with a meal [23]. In addition, the combination of colesevelam with simvastatin or atorvastatin resulted in additive reductions in cholesterol, which indicates that there is no clinically significant interaction between these compounds [24, 25] **(Ia/A)**.

CYP3A4-inhibiting drugs

A large amount of evidence relates to the interactions between individual statins and inhibitors of CYP3A4 [3, 4, 8, 9, 12]. The most relevant interactions are summarized in Table 2 and are mentioned below; these are also the interactions that often present in relation to rhabdomyolysis. Based on the extensive data on individual interactions, general conclusions or guidelines can be drawn. It is important to have these in mind, as many possible interactions between statins and CYP3A4 substrates / inhibitors have not been described yet, but can be anticipated based on these principles.

First, it is clear that concomitant use of any potent inhibitor of CYP3A4 with simvastatin, lovastatin and (to a lesser extent) atorvastatin causes a very strong increase in the exposure to these statins [3, 4, 8, 9, 12]. In turn, this carries a considerable risk of muscle toxicity, particularly if high statin doses are used. For example, pharmacokinetic studies have shown that the strong CYP3A4 inhibitors, ritonavir, itraconazole and ketoconazole, can increase the exposure to simvastatin and lovastatin up to 20-fold, whereas they increase the exposure to atorvastatin by about 3-fold (Table 2 [4]). Other widely used (somewhat less potent) inhibitors of CYP3A4 are the macrolides, clarithromycin and erythromycin, the calcium channel antagonists, verapamil and diltiazem, and grapefruit, all causing strong increases in the exposure to simvastatin and lovastatin (Table 2).

The data from pharmacokinetic studies correspond with information from other sources. Rhabdomyolysis has been described in case reports after the combination of simvastatin, lovastatin or atorvastatin with many CYP3A4 inhibitors, including mibefradil, ritonavir, cyclosporine, itraconazole, fluconazole, clarithromycin, erythromycin, nefazodone, danazol, amiodarone and verapamil [4] **(III/B)**. Epidemiological studies also point to the higher risk

Table 2. Effect of some CYP or transporter inhibitors (fold increase) and inducers (percentage reduction) on exposure to statins (area under the plasma concentration versus time curve) [a, b].

	Simvastatin	Lovastatin	Atorvastatin	Fluvastatin	Pravastatin	Rosuvastatin	Pitavastatin
Inhibitors							
Itraconazole	5-20	5-20	2-4	≈	≈	≈	(≈)
Erythomycin, clarithromycin	4-12	(4-12)	1.5-5	≈	≤2	≈	(≈)
Verapamil, diltiazem	3-8	3-8	?	(≈)	≈	(≈)	(≈)
Grapefruit juice	2-10	2-10	1-4	(≈)	≈	(≈)	≈
Gemfibrozil	2-3	2-3	<1.5	≈	2	2	≤1.5
Cyclosporine	6-8	5-20	6-15	2-4	5-10	5-10	5
Inducers							
Rifampicin, carbamazepine	70-95	(70-95)	60-90	50	30	?	?

a = adapted from and based on references from Neuvonen *et al*, 2006 [4]

b = the doses of inhibitors and inducers, as well as pharmacogenetic factors, can affect the extent of interaction in an individual patient

≈ = practically unchanged

() = estimation based on the pharmacokinetic properties of the statin

? = not known or estimated

associated with the CYP3A4-dependent simvastatin, lovastatin and atorvastatin, due to their interaction profiles. In a systematic review of notifications to national regulatory authorities, cohort studies, randomized trials, and published case reports, the notification rate of rhabdomyolysis to the FDA was about four times higher with simvastatin, lovastatin and atorvastatin compared to fluvastatin and pravastatin [2] (III/B). No cases of rhabdomyolysis occurred in patients on fluvastatin and pravastatin in the cohorts and randomized trials. Data related to the notified cases and case reports showed that 60% of the patients involved used drugs that are known to inhibit CYP3A4 [2]. Another study showed that the proportion of statin users with a potential relevant drug interaction was 12.1% for simvastatin and 10% for atorvastatin compared to 3.8% for fluvastatin and 0.3% for pravastatin [13] (III/B). Finally, in a recent study, the adverse event reporting rate of rhabdomyolysis for simvastatin was strongly dependent on the concurrent administration of a CYP3A4 inhibitor, but this was not observed with pravastatin [26] (III/B).

As a second general conclusion, it can be stated that weak or moderately potent CYP3A4 inhibitors (e.g. verapamil, diltiazem) can be used carefully with simvastatin, lovastatin and atorvastatin as long as these statins are used in low doses [4, 27] (III/B). In such cases, the individual risk factors should be weighed and patients should be monitored, as there is wide variability in susceptibility to the adverse effects of statins.

A third conclusion from available evidence is that selective inhibitors of CYP3A4 do not have a significant pharmacokinetic interaction with the non-CYP3A4-dependent statins, fluvastatin, pravastatin, rosuvastatin and pitavastatin [3, 4, 8, 9, 12]. As an example from Table 2, itraconazole did increase by no more than 1.5-fold the exposure to fluvastatin, pravastatin and rosuvastatin.

HIV-infected patients represent a group of patients who are at risk for dyslipidemia as a result of both HIV infection and certain classes of antiretroviral therapy [28]. A specific guideline has been issued for dyslipidemia in HIV-infected patients [29]. Especially the class of protease inhibitors (PIs) encompasses a risk of increasing the exposure to statins, since they are substrates and inhibitors of CYP3A4. The PI, ritonavir, is a very potent CYP3A4 inhibitor and is frequently used with other PIs to boost their plasma concentrations. Whereas exposure to simvastatin was strongly (32-fold) increased with saquinavir/ritonavir (400mg/400mg), the effect on atorvastatin was less (1.7-fold increase), and pravastatin exposure was actually decreased by 50% [30], possibly due to an effect of ritonavir on glucuronidation or on OATP1B1 [28]. Pravastatin is considered safe for combination with PIs [28]; surprisingly, rosuvastatin exposure was increased moderately (2.1-fold) upon combination with lopinavir/ritonavir [31]. Conversely, the first-choice non-nucleoside reverse transcriptase inhibitor (NNRTI), efavirenz, decreases the exposure to simvastatin, atorvastatin and pravastatin by 35-60% [32]. There are no data on the benefit of increasing the dose of statins under these circumstances.

CYP2C9 inhibitors

Inhibitors of CYP2C9 could increase the plasma concentrations of fluvastatin (Table 1). However, there have only been a few reports of drug interactions with fluvastatin and CYP2C9 inhibitors, including omeprazole and tolbutamide, and multiple cytochrome P450 inhibitors, including cimetidine, fluvoxamine and azole antifungals [8]. Even high doses of fluconazole increased the exposure to fluvastatin by less than 100% [33]. Likewise, the exposure to rosuvastatin (10% metabolized by CYP2C9) was increased by fluconazole to a small extent [34].

CYP2C8 inhibitors

Gemfibrozil and especially its glucuronide inhibit CYP2C8 (but not CYP3A4), which explains the increase in the exposure to simvastatin and lovastatin (both substrates of CYP2C8, see Table 1) with gemfibrozil [35, 36]. This interaction is probably also mediated by inhibition of OATP1B1-mediated hepatic uptake of the statins (see below).

CYP inducers and transporter inducers

Inducers of CYP isoenzymes and transporters (rifampicin, carbamazepine, phenytoin) will not cause any risk of statin-related toxicity, but may cause a very strong decrease in the exposure to statins. Rifampicin strongly decreased the exposure to simvastatin [37] and atorvastatin [36], but shows less effect on fluvastatin [38] and pravastatin [39] (Table 2). Similarly, carbamazepine decreases exposure to simvastatin by 82% [40]. The herbal product, St John's wort (hypericum), a weak inducer of CYP3A4, caused a slight effect on the exposure to simvastatin and had no effect on pravastatin [41]. Such small decreases are of less concern and can be overcome by increasing the dose of the statin.

OATP1B1 inhibitors – gemfibrozil and cyclosporine

Statins are substrates of many transporters in the intestine, liver and kidneys, and many drugs can affect their activity. In fact, many inhibitors of CYP3A4, such as ritonavir and clarithromycin, also inhibit OATP1B1 and p-glycoprotein.

Combination therapy of a statin and a fibrate can be advantageous in the therapy of mixed dyslipidemia. However, it should be recognized that the fibrate, gemfibrozil, and its glucuronide, are not only inhibitors of CYP2C8 (see above), but also of the OATP1B1 transporter that is involved in the hepatic uptake of statins [4, 8, 9]. The extent of this interaction is dependent on the relative role of CYP2C8 and OATP1B1 in the pharmacokinetics of the statin in question (Table 1 [4]). The now withdrawn agent, cerivastatin, showed a strong interaction, whereas only fluvastatin shows no pharmacokinetic interaction with gemfibrozil [42]. The statin-gemfibrozil interaction is probably also pharmacodynamic in nature, as gemfibrozil in monotherapy also shows myotoxicity. Of note, fenofibrate and bezafibrate do not enhance the exposure to simvastatin, lovastatin, pravastatin, rosuvastatin and pitavastatin [4], which means that the pharmacokinetic interaction with statins is not a class effect of fibrates. Other fibrates also show less myotoxicity than gemfibrozil in monotherapy [2, 43].

In agreement with these pharmacokinetic data, the incidence of rhabdomyolysis to statins is about ten times higher upon combination with gemfibrozil [2] (III/B). An analysis of FDA data showed much less cases of rhabdomyolysis per million prescriptions associated with fenofibrate-statin therapy compared with gemfibrozil-statin therapy [44] (III/B). However, physicians should be aware that fenofibrate is an inhibitor of CYP2C9 and should therefore be avoided in combination with fluvastatin. As the fibrates are primarily renally excreted, renal impairment may increase the likelihood of rhabdomyolysis with concurrent use of statins.

Cyclosporine is an immunosuppressant drug that may cause hyperlipidemia. It is an inhibitor of several transporters including OATP1B1 and p-glycoprotein, and it also inhibits CYP3A4 [4, 8, 9]. These properties can explain its strong effects on the pharmacokinetics of the statins (Table 2) and the cases of rhabdomyolysis in patients who were treated for post-transplant hyperlipidemia (III/B). Fluvastatin seems to be least sensitive to the effects of cyclosporine and no report of rhabdomyolysis with this combination has been described [4] (III/B). Although the increased risk of myotoxicity in patients on cyclosporine and statins is acknowledged, its use is considered relatively safe when low doses of statins are used and the patients are monitored [4, 45] (III/B & IV/C).

Pharmacodynamic interactions with statins

Combinations of statins with other lipid-lowering drugs aim to enhance the desirable effect on cholesterol and triglycerides. As mentioned above, statins and gemfibrozil interact in a pharmacokinetic way, but since these drugs are both associated with myopathy, the interaction is probably partly pharmacodynamic in nature.

There are contradictory data on the additional risk of myopathy when combining statins and nicotinic acid (niacin), with most clinical studies showing no additional risk (descriptive analyses on secondary endpoint) **(III/B)**, but with case reports of rhabdomyolysis occurring nevertheless [11, 12] **(III/B)**. Possible interactions between statins and nicotinic acid or ezetimibe are probably of pharmacodynamic origin [4].

Of recent date is the observation that patients with statin-induced myalgias had lower serum vitamin D levels than statin-treated patients without myalgias [46] **(III/B)**. Supplementation of vitamin D during statin use caused an increase in serum vitamin D and a resolution of myalgia in the majority of patients [46] **(III/B)**. These data suggest a pharmacodynamic interaction between vitamin D deficiency and statins on skeletal muscle. However, the interaction may also be pharmacokinetic in nature, as vitamin D is able to induce CYP3A4 *in vitro*, possibly causing a decrease in exposure to statins. In accordance with this, vitamin D supplementation was able to reduce the exposure to atorvastatin in a recent study [47]. This interaction clearly needs further elucidation and may yield a lead for treatment of statin-induced myopathy.

Effect of statins on other drugs

The statins are known to cause an increase in the anticoagulant effect of warfarin and other coumarin anticoagulants, requiring anticoagulant control and a dose reduction of the anticoagulant. The mechanism has been ascribed to inhibition of CYP3A4, CYP2C9 and displacement of the anticoagulant from binding sites, dependent on the statin [4, 48].

Fluvastatin inhibits CYP2C9, which explains the modest increase in the clearance of glibencamide, tolbutamide, diclofenac and phenytoin by this statin [8, 38].

Furthermore, simvastatin, atorvastatin [49] and fluvastatin [50] cause a modest (up to 20%) increase in digoxin concentrations, an interaction which is of minor clinical relevance.

Clopidogrel is a pro-drug that is metabolized in the liver via CYP3A4 to an active compound which inhibits platelet aggregation. It has been suggested that co-administration of clopidogrel with statins that are metabolized by CYP3A4 (simvastatin, lovastatin, atorvastatin) may diminish the conversion of clopidogrel to its active form. However, analyses (mainly post hoc or pharmaco-epidemiologic) **(III/B)** in six out of seven clinical studies or registries revealed no significant influence of different statins on the clinical outcome in patients treated with clopidogrel [51, 52]. Therefore, the interaction between clopidogrel and CYP3A4-dependent statins may occur, but its clinical relevance is doubtful and there is no compelling evidence to prefer CYP3A4-independent statins in patients using clopidogrel at this time. Conversely, it is known that clopidogrel inhibits CYP2C9. However, co-administration of clopidogrel with fluvastatin did not affect the exposure to the statin [53].

Anticipating and preventing relevant drug interactions during statin use

The first step in preventing relevant statin interactions (Table 3) is to recognize the need to evaluate the risk for such an interaction. In practice, this does not appear to be self-evident, but we hope it will be clear from the data provided in this chapter. Next, patient-related risk factors for myopathy should be verified. Co-medication used by the patient represents the other major risk factor for the occurrence of statin-related interactions, and patients should be asked to list or (preferably) bring in all their drugs to their physician.

To evaluate whether an interaction may occur, the physician should have access to reliable and updated sources of information on statin drug interactions, including the information in

Table 3. Anticipating and preventing drug interactions with statins.

- Recognize the need to evaluate the risk for a drug interaction

- Identify possible patient-related risk factors for myopathy

- List currently used drugs by the patient

- Assess the possible occurrence of a relevant interaction based on:

  o   prescribing information
  o   literature
  o   consultation of a pharmacist
  o   pharmacokinetics of the statin and the concomitant drugs

- In the case of a possible relevant interaction consider:

  o   choosing a statin with less interaction potential with the co-administered drugs
  o   choosing co-administered drugs (or change to alternatives) with less interaction potential
  o   withholding either the statin or the co-administered drug for a certain period
  o   using a low dose of an interacting statin
  o   monitoring for signs of statin adverse effects

this chapter, prescribing information and (electronic) access to medical literature. Of note, many possible interactions have not been described; the pharmacokinetic properties of the statins and co-administered drugs may help to predict an interaction. Still the exact probability of an interaction in a given patient is hard to estimate, owing to the inter-individual variability in sensitivity and pharmacokinetics of statins.

From this chapter it is very clear that the choice of a statin may strongly decrease the risk for a relevant drug interaction. The choice for a particular statin can be done individually, based on patient risk profile and concomitant drugs. Of course, apart from the risk of interactions, the availability of clinical event data for a particular statin is an important criterion for the prescribing physician as well.

As to the selection of a statin, it should be noted that switching patients to alternative drugs within a therapeutic class occurs commonly within managed care organizations, based on drug formularies and the availability of cheaper generic equivalents [12]. However, switching statins without regard for the distinct interaction profile of a particular statin in a particular patient may lead to adverse effects. Similar formulary policies may also take place at the national level [54].

Next to the selection of an appropriate statin, it may be considered to withhold the statin for a limited period, or to use another drug that is less likely to interact with statins. When statins have to be prescribed with interactings drugs, the statin dose is an important means to prevent myopathy. Dose limits for statins combined with specific inhibitors are mentioned in statin prescribing information. In this case, it is even more important to inform the patient about signs of myopathy and to monitor the treatment as recommended [55].

Finally, prevention of relevant interactions is a multidisciplinary task. In many countries, community and institutional pharmacists check for drug interactions either manually or by using software. They can fulfill an important role in detecting the majority of relevant interactions, alert prescribing physicians and contribute to minimization of this risk factor for myotoxicity [56] **(III/B)**.

Conclusions

Evidence shows that statin interactions should be feared in patients with risk factors for myopathy, a high dose of a statin, and with co-administration of drugs that inhibit either CYP3A4 or the activity of specific transporters. As a result of differences in pharmacokinetic characteristics, the choice of a statin is a means by which to minimize the risk of relevant interactions.

Key points	Evidence level
◆ A large percent of patients for whom statins are prescribed use concomitant drugs that interact with statins.	III/B
◆ The incidence of rhabdomyolysis, an adverse event to statins, is strongly associated with interactions between statins and concomitant drugs.	III/B
◆ Concomitant use of the CYP3A4-dependent simvastatin, lovastatin and (to a lesser extent) atorvastatin with any potent inhibitor of CYP3A4 causes a strong increase in the exposure to these statins.	PK studies
◆ The CYP3A4-dependent simvastatin, lovastatin and atorvastatin have a higher risk of causing rhabdomyolysis, probably due to their interaction profile.	III/B
◆ Simvastatin, lovastatin and atorvastatin can be used with weak or moderately potent CYP3A4 inhibitors as long as these statins are used in low doses, individual risk factors are weighed and patients are monitored.	III/B
◆ The CYP3A4-independent fluvastatin, pravastatin, rosuvastatin and pitavastatin do not have a relevant pharmacokinetic interaction with selective inhibitors of CYP3A4.	PK studies
◆ Co-administration of gemfibrozil increases the exposure to all statins, apart from fluvastatin.	PK studies
◆ The incidence of rhabdomyolysis to statins is about ten times higher upon combination with gemfibrozil.	III/B
◆ Azole antifungals, ritonavir, clarithromycin, erythromycin, verapamil, diltiazem, gemfibrozil and cyclosporine are most often involved in relevant interactions with statins that may cause statin-related myopathy.	III/B
◆ Rifampicin and carbamazepine strongly decrease the exposure to simvastatin, atorvastatin and probably lovastatin, but have less effect on fluvastatin and pravastatin.	PK studies
◆ The statins cause an increase in the anticoagulant effect of warfarin and other coumarin anticoagulants, requiring anticoagulant control and sometimes a dose reduction of the anticoagulant.	III/B
◆ The effect of statins on clopidogrel is not clinically relevant and does not warrant the preference of some statins over others.	III/B
◆ Myopathy related to interactions of statins can be prevented by evaluating risk factors of individual patients, careful selection of a statin based on interaction profile, using a low dose of the statin and monitoring.	III/B
◆ Pharmacists can fulfil an important role in detecting the majority of relevant statin interactions, alert prescribing physicians and contribute to minimization of this risk factor for myotoxicity.	III/B

PK studies = pharmacokinetic studies

References

1.   Baigent C, Keech A, Kearney PM, *et al.* Efficacy and safety of cholesterol-lowering treatment: prospective meta-analysis of data from 90,056 participants in 14 randomised trials of statins. *Lancet* 2005; 366(9493): 1267-78.

2.   Law M, Rudnicka AR. Statin safety: a systematic review. *Am J Cardiol* 2006; 97(8A): 52C-60.

3.   Williams D, Feely J. Pharmacokinetic-pharmacodynamic drug interactions with HMG-CoA reductase inhibitors. *Clin Pharmacokinet* 2002; 41(5): 343-70.

4.   Neuvonen PJ, Niemi M, Backman JT. Drug interactions with lipid-lowering drugs: mechanisms and clinical relevance. *Clin Pharmacol Ther* 2006; 80(6): 565-81.

5.   Staffa JA, Chang J, Green L. Cerivastatin and reports of fatal rhabdomyolysis. *N Engl J Med* 2002; 346(7): 539-40.

6.   Ronaldson KJ, O'Shea JM, Boyd IW. Risk factors for rhabdomyolysis with simvastatin and atorvastatin. *Drug Saf* 2006; 29(11): 1061-7.

7.   Schech S, Graham D, Staffa J, *et al.* Risk factors for statin-associated rhabdomyolysis. *Pharmacoepidemiol Drug Saf* 2007; 16(3): 352-8.

8.   Shitara Y, Sugiyama Y. Pharmacokinetic and pharmacodynamic alterations of 3-hydroxy-3-methylglutaryl coenzyme A (HMG-CoA) reductase inhibitors: drug-drug interactions and interindividual differences in transporter and metabolic enzyme functions. *Pharmacol Ther* 2006; 112(1): 71-105.

9.   Neuvonen PJ, Backman JT, Niemi M. Pharmacokinetic comparison of the potential over-the-counter statins simvastatin, lovastatin, fluvastatin and pravastatin. *Clin Pharmacokinet* 2008; 47(7): 463-74.

10. Link E, Parish S, Armitage J, *et al.* SLCO1B1 variants and statin-induced myopathy - a genomewide study. *N Engl J Med* 2008; 359(8): 789-99.

11. Ballantyne CM, Corsini A, Davidson MH, *et al.* Risk for myopathy with statin therapy in high-risk patients. *Arch Intern Med* 2003; 163(5): 553-64.

12. Frishman WH, Horn J. Statin-drug interactions: not a class effect. *Cardiol Rev* 2008; 16(4): 205-12.

13. Ratz Bravo AE, Tchambaz L, Krahenbuhl-Melcher A, Hess L, Schlienger RG, Krahenbuhl S. Prevalence of potentially severe drug-drug interactions in ambulatory patients with dyslipidaemia receiving HMG-CoA reductase inhibitor therapy. *Drug Saf* 2005; 28(3): 263-75.

14. Stang P, Morris L, Kempf J, Henderson S, Yood MU, Oliveria S. The coprescription of contraindicated drugs with statins: continuing potential for increased risk of adverse events. *Am J Ther* 2007; 14(1): 30-40.

15. Lafata JE, Schultz L, Simpkins J, *et al.* Potential drug-drug interactions in the outpatient setting. *Med Care* 2006; 44(6): 534-41.

16. Heerey A, Barry M, Ryan M, Kelly A. The potential for drug interactions with statin therapy in Ireland. *Ir J Med Sci* 2000; 169(3): 176-9.

17. Egger SS, Ratz Bravo AE, Hess L, Schlienger RG, Krahenbuhl S. Age-related differences in the prevalence of potential drug-drug interactions in ambulatory dyslipidaemic patients treated with statins. *Drugs Aging* 2007; 24(5): 429-40.

18. Omar MA, Wilson JP, Cox TS. Rhabdomyolysis and HMG-CoA reductase inhibitors. *Ann Pharmacother* 2001; 35(9): 1096-107.

19. Schectman G, Hiatt J. Dose-response characteristics of cholesterol-lowering drug therapies: implications for treatment. *Ann Intern Med* 1996; 125(12): 990-1000.

20. Jones P, Kafonek S, Laurora I, Hunninghake D. Comparative dose efficacy study of atorvastatin versus simvastatin, pravastatin, lovastatin, and fluvastatin in patients with hypercholesterolemia (the CURVES study). *Am J Cardiol* 1998; 81(5): 582-7.

21. Brewer HB, Jr. Benefit-risk assessment of rosuvastatin 10 to 40 milligrams. *Am J Cardiol* 2003; 92(4B): 23K-9.

22. Bottorff MB. Statin safety and drug interactions: clinical implications. *Am J Cardiol* 2006; 97(8A): 27C-31.

23. Donovan JM, Kisicki JC, Stiles MR, Tracewell WG, Burke SK. Effect of colesevelam on lovastatin pharmacokinetics. *Ann Pharmacother* 2002; 36(3): 392-7.

24. Knapp HH, Schrott H, Ma P, *et al.* Efficacy and safety of combination simvastatin and colesevelam in patients with primary hypercholesterolemia. *Am J Med* 2001; 110(5): 352-60.

25. Hunninghake D, Insull W, Jr., Toth P, Davidson D, Donovan JM, Burke SK. Coadministration of colesevelam hydrochloride with atorvastatin lowers LDL cholesterol additively. *Atherosclerosis* 2001; 158(2): 407-16.

26. Rowan C, Brinker AD, Nourjah P, *et al.* Rhabdomyolysis reports show interaction between simvastatin and CYP3A4 inhibitors. *Pharmacoepidemiol Drug Saf* 2009; 18(4): 301-9.

27. Gruer PJ, Vega JM, Mercuri MF, Dobrinska MR, Tobert JA. Concomitant use of cytochrome P450 3A4 inhibitors and simvastatin. *Am J Cardiol* 1999; 84(7): 811-15.

28. Ray GM. Antiretroviral and statin drug-drug interactions. *Cardiol Rev* 2009; 17(1): 44-7.

29. Dube MP, Stein JH, Aberg JA, *et al.* Guidelines for the evaluation and management of dyslipidemia in human immunodeficiency virus (HIV)-infected adults receiving antiretroviral therapy: recommendations of the HIV Medical Association of the Infectious Disease Society of America and the Adult AIDS Clinical Trials Group. *Clin Infect Dis* 2003; 37(5): 613-27.

30. Fichtenbaum CJ, Gerber JG, Rosenkranz SL, *et al.* Pharmacokinetic interactions between protease inhibitors and statins in HIV seronegative volunteers: ACTG Study A5047. *AIDS* 2002; 16(4): 569-77.

31. Kiser JJ, Gerber JG, Predhomme JA, Wolfe P, Flynn DM, Hoody DW. Drug/Drug interaction between lopinavir/ritonavir and rosuvastatin in healthy volunteers. *J Acquir Immune Defic Syndr* 2008; 47(5): 570-8.

32. Gerber JG, Rosenkranz SL, Fichtenbaum CJ *et al.* Effect of efavirenz on the pharmacokinetics of simvastatin, atorvastatin, and pravastatin: results of AIDS Clinical Trials Group 5108 Study. *J Acquir Immune Defic Syndr* 2005; 39(3): 307-12.

33. Kantola T, Backman JT, Niemi M, Kivisto KT, Neuvonen PJ. Effect of fluconazole on plasma fluvastatin and pravastatin concentrations. *Eur J Clin Pharmacol* 2000; 56(3): 225-9.

34. Cooper KJ, Martin PD, Dane AL, Warwick MJ, Schneck DW, Cantarini MV. The effect of fluconazole on the pharmacokinetics of rosuvastatin. *Eur J Clin Pharmacol* 2002; 58(8): 527-31.

35. Backman JT, Kyrklund C, Kivisto KT, Wang JS, Neuvonen PJ. Plasma concentrations of active simvastatin acid are increased by gemfibrozil. *Clin Pharmacol Ther* 2000; 68(2): 122-9.

36. Kyrklund C, Backman JT, Kivisto KT, Neuvonen M, Laitila J, Neuvonen PJ. Plasma concentrations of active lovastatin acid are markedly increased by gemfibrozil but not by bezafibrate. *Clin Pharmacol Ther* 2001; 69(5): 340-5.

37. Kyrklund C, Backman JT, Kivisto KT, Neuvonen M, Laitila J, Neuvonen PJ. Rifampin greatly reduces plasma simvastatin and simvastatin acid concentrations. *Clin Pharmacol Ther* 2000; 68(6): 592-7.

38. Scripture CD, Pieper JA. Clinical pharmacokinetics of fluvastatin. *Clin Pharmacokinet* 2001; 40(4): 263-81.

39. Kyrklund C, Backman JT, Neuvonen M, Neuvonen PJ. Effect of rifampicin on pravastatin pharmacokinetics in healthy subjects. *Br J Clin Pharmacol* 2004; 57(2): 181-7.

40. Ucar M, Neuvonen M, Luurila H, Dahlqvist R, Neuvonen PJ, Mjorndal T. Carbamazepine markedly reduces serum concentrations of simvastatin and simvastatin acid. *Eur J Clin Pharmacol* 2004; 59(12): 879-82.

41. Sugimoto K, Ohmori M, Tsuruoka S, *et al.* Different effects of St John's wort on the pharmacokinetics of simvastatin and pravastatin. *Clin Pharmacol Ther* 2001; 70(6): 518-24.

42. Spence JD, Munoz CE, Hendricks L, Latchinian L, Khouri HE. Pharmacokinetics of the combination of fluvastatin and gemfibrozil. *Am J Cardiol* 1995; 76(2): 80A-3.

43. Graham DJ, Staffa JA, Shatin D, *et al.* Incidence of hospitalized rhabdomyolysis in patients treated with lipid-lowering drugs. *JAMA* 2004; 292(21): 2585-90.

44. Jones PH, Davidson MH. Reporting rate of rhabdomyolysis with fenofibrate + statin versus gemfibrozil + any statin. *Am J Cardiol* 2005; 95(1): 120-2.

45. Kobashigawa JA, Murphy FL, Stevenson LW, *et al.* Low-dose lovastatin safely lowers cholesterol after cardiac transplantation. *Circulation* 1990; 82(5 Suppl): IV281-3.

46. Ahmed W, Khan N, Glueck CJ, *et al.* Low serum 25 (OH) vitamin D levels (<32ng/mL) are associated with reversible myositis-myalgia in statin-treated patients. *Transl Res* 2009; 153(1): 11-6.

47. Schwartz JB. Effects of vitamin D supplementation in atorvastatin-treated patients: a new drug interaction with an unexpected consequence. *Clin Pharmacol Ther* 2009; 85(2): 198-203.

48. Ahmad S. Lovastatin. Warfarin interaction. *Arch Intern Med* 1990; 150(11): 2407.

49. Boyd RA, Stern RH, Stewart BH, *et al.* Atorvastatin coadministration may increase digoxin concentrations by inhibition of intestinal P-glycoprotein-mediated secretion. *J Clin Pharmacol* 2000; 40(1): 91-8.

50. Garnett WR, Venitz J, Wilkens RC, Dimenna G. Pharmacokinetic effects of fluvastatin in patients chronically receiving digoxin. *Am J Med* 1994; 96(6A): 84S-6.

51. Bhindi R, Ormerod O, Newton J, Banning AP, Testa L. Interaction between statins and clopidogrel: is there anything clinically relevant? *QJM* 2008; 101(12): 915-5.

52. Blagojevic A, Delaney JA, Levesque LE, Dendukuri N, Boivin JF, Brophy JM. Investigation of an interaction between statins and clopidogrel after percutaneous coronary intervention: a cohort study. *Pharmacoepidemiol Drug Saf* 2009; 18(5): 362-9.

53. Ayalasomayajula SP, Vaidyanathan S, Kemp C, Prasad P, Balch A, Dole WP. Effect of clopidogrel on the steady-state pharmacokinetics of fluvastatin. *J Clin Pharmacol* 2007; 47(5): 613-9.

54. Devold HM, Molden E, Skurtveit S, Furu K. Co-medication of statins and CYP3A4 inhibitors before and after introduction of new reimbursement policy. *Br J Clin Pharmacol* 2009; 67(2): 234-41.

55. McKenney JM, Davidson MH, Jacobson TA, Guyton JR. Final conclusions and recommendations of the National Lipid Association Statin Safety Assessment Task Force. *Am J Cardiol* 2006; 97(8A): 89C-94.

56. Molden E, Skovlund E, Braathen P. Risk management of simvastatin or atorvastatin interactions with CYP3A4 inhibitors. *Drug Saf* 2008; 31(7): 587-96.

Chapter 18

What are the considerations in patients who are statin 'intolerant'?

Frans L. Opdam [1] MD, Fellow, Vascular Medicine
Henk-Jan Guchelaar [2] PhD, Professor of Clinical Pharmacy and Hospital Pharmacist
Jouke T. Tamsma [1] MD, PhD, Consultant, Vascular Medicine
1 Section of Vascular Medicine, Department of
Endocrinology and Internal Medicine
2 Department of Clinical Pharmacy & Toxicology
Leiden University Medical Center, Leiden, The Netherlands

Introduction

Since the discovery of statins in the seventies of the 20th century by Endo [1], cardiovascular risk management has changed dramatically. By inhibiting the synthesis of endogenous cholesterol, statins are far more effective in reducing elevated blood cholesterol than dietary regimens. In patients with a history of cardiovascular disease, statins decrease cardiovascular disease morbidity and mortality by about 25%. Beyond this efficacy, statins are relatively safe and almost free of serious side effects. It is therefore not surprising that there seems to be an unlimited growing number of patients using statins for hypercholesterolemia, with more than 13 million patients in the United States alone [2].

The currently used statins are well tolerated by most people and present a good safety profile [3]. Side effects of statins include hepatotoxicity characterized by increased plasma levels of transaminases, which is infrequently reported for all of the statins [4]. Myopathy occurs more often and is the most important clinical problem in statin users [5].

Fortunately, serious side effects such as rhabdomyolysis are rare, but with the increasing number of potential users, a significant number of patients experience myalgias and do not tolerate statins in clinical practice. Unfortunately, these benign side effects can adversely affect both quality of life and adherence to a potentially life-saving treatment.

Therefore, this chapter will focus on the management of the clinical important problem of statin myopathy.

Terminology

Statin myopathy includes the spectrum of the clinical entities myopathy, myalgia, myositis and rhabdomyolysis, on which no consensus exists. Proposed definitions for statin-related myopathy by the American College of Cardiology (ACC), American Heart Association (AHA), National Heart, Lung and Blood Insitute (NHLBI) [6], and the National Lipid Association (NLA) [7] are presented in Table 1.

Table 1. Definitions for statin-related myopathy.

Clinical entity	ACC/AHA/NHLBI [6]	NLA [7]
Myopathy	General term referring to any disease of muscle	Complaints of myalgia (muscle pain or soreness), weakness, and/or cramps, plus elevation in serum K >10x the ULN
Myalgia	Muscle ache or weakness without creatine kinase (CK) elevation	N.A.
Myositis	Muscle symptoms with increased CK levels	N.A.
Rhabdomyolysis	Muscle symptoms with marked CK elevation (typically substantially greater than 10 times the upper limit of normal [ULN] and with creatinine elevation (usually with brown urine and urinary myoglobin)	CK elevation >10,000 IU/L or CK >10x the ULN plus an elevation in serum creatinine or medical intervention with intravenous hydration therapy

CK = creatine kinase; ULN = upper limit of normal

Epidemiology

Because high-risk patients are often excluded from clinical trials, the incidence of statin myopathy is artificially reduced in patients participating in trials compared to patients more representative in clinical practice. Therefore, data obtained from observational studies often differ from those obtained from clinical trials. As definitions for myopathy are inconsistent (Table 1), the incidence varies among different studies.

In clinical trials the incidence of statin myopathy is low, ranging from 0.1 to 5% per year [3, 8]. In four randomized trials, the incidence of muscle pain was similar in the treated groups compared to the placebo group [8]. A meta-analysis of 35 double-blind randomized controlled trials (n=48,138) also revealed a non-significant increase in the risk of myalgia incidence among participants who received statins compared to those who received placebo (risk difference/1000 patients [RD], 2,7; 95% CI, -3.2 to 8.7) [9].

In another review of 30 randomized controlled trials (n=83,858), the incidence of myositis (defined by study investigators as a CK elevation of greater than 10 times the upper limit of normal) was only 49 cases in the statin versus 44 cases in the placebo group [10].

In contrast to the low incidence of myalgia reported in clinical trials, higher rates ranging from 5% to 10% are documented in observational studies [11, 12]. The risk of developing statin myopathy was found to be dose-dependent in a large observational study [12], as well as in a meta-analysis of four randomized controlled trials (n=27,545) comparing intensive and moderate dose-statin therapy [13].

Rhabdomyolysis is a rare event in patients taking statins. The incidence of this serious and potential adverse event in a meta-analysis of 20 clinical trials [8], was 1.6 cases per 100,000 patients per year. Based on a review of two cohort studies, the incidence of rhabdomyolysis was 3.4 cases per 100,000 patient years, with a mortality rate of 0.3 per 100,000 patient years [14, 15]. Post-marketing surveillance is probably a better tool to monitor the incidence of rhabdomyolysis. The FDA Adverse Event Reporting System (AERDS) indicates a rhabdomyolysis incidence of 0.70 per 100,000 patient years [16]. Interestingly, the rhabdomyolyis incidence was statin-specific and was lowest for pravastatin (1.63 cases per 1 million prescriptions) and was highest for rosuvastatin (13.54 cases per 1 million prescriptions) [17].

Thus, although rates of myalgia are higher in observational studies than in clinical trials, the incidence rates of rhabdomyolysis fortunately seem to be as rare in adverse events reporting systems as in clinical trials.

Pathophysiology

Various hypotheses have been proposed to explain statin-induced muscle injury. Statin myotoxicity [18] is dose-dependent [19], but seems to appear independent of LDL reduction [19, 20]. However, statin myopathy dose dependency is substance-specific, reporting highest incidences for cerivastatin and lowest for rosuvastatin [19].

Recently, a common DNA polymorphism (rs4149056) in the *SLCO1B1* gene encoding organic anion-transporting polypeptide was strongly associated with simvastatin-induced myopathy [21, 22]. SLCO1B1 encodes the organic anion-transporting polypeptide OATP1B1, which mediates the hepatic uptake of various drugs, including most statins and statin acids [23]. Collective evidence indicates that carriers with the C allele of this polymorphism have higher statin concentrations and a high risk of statin myopathy [21].

Proposed mechanisms for statin-induced myopathy include decreased cholesterol content of skeletal myocyte membranes, modifying muscle membrane excitability. Different ion channels like sodium, potassium and chloride seem to be involved [24]. Furthermore, there are direct myotoxic effects on muscle, including impaired mitochondrial function and impaired calcium signalling.

Ubiquinone (co-enzyme Q10) is an essential electron transporter of the mitochondrial respiratory chain. The role of reduced levels of ubiquinone in statin-induced myotoxicity is highly controversial [24].

Impaired mitochondrial function induced by statins might initiate a cascade of intracellular calcium release, resulting in sarcoplasmatic reticulum calcium overload and calcium waves. In calcium overload, the sarcoplasmatic reticulum may spontaneously release calcium by the ryanodine receptor, although a direct effect of statins on this receptor can not be excluded (Figure 1) [24].

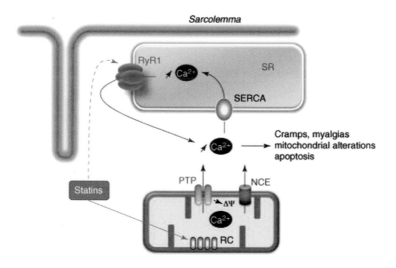

Figure 1. A possible direct physiopathological effect of statins. Although statin myotoxycity may occur through the reduction of cholesterol synthesis, a direct effect of statins has been reported *in vitro* and *in vivo* in muscle fibers from both animal and human models. This diagram summarizes some of the most recent data suggesting a physiopathological mechanism. Statins diffuse into muscle fibers and inhibit complex I of the mitochondrial respiratory chain (RC). This depolarizes the inner membrane (Δψ) triggering a calcium release through the permeability transient pore (PTP) and sodium calcium exchanger (NCE). This results in an elevation of cytoplasmic calcium that will be partially taken up by the sarcoendoplasmic reticulum calcium pump (SERCA) to the sarcoplasmic reticulum (SR). When overloaded, the SR may spontaneously release calcium through the ryanodine receptor (RyR1) to generate a calcium wave. A direct effect of statins on RyR1 may not be excluded (dotted line). Impaired mitochondrial function and consequently calcium signalling may account for muscle symptoms. *Reproduced with permission from Sirvent P, et al* [24].

Clinical presentation and risk factors of statin intolerance

In a large observational study of 7924 hyperlipidemic patients using high-dose statins, muscular symptoms were most commonly manifested as heaviness, stiffness or cramps, with many patients also reporting weakness or loss of strength during exertion. The predominant site of pains was the calves and thighs. Almost 25% of the affected patients experienced general myalgia **(III/B)** (Table 2). Twenty-five percent of patients reported tendon-associated pain, mostly involving several tendons **(III/B)** [12]. In another study of statin-induced rhabdomyolysis, fatigue (74%) was almost as common as muscle pain as the main complaint **(III/B)** [25]. Intriguingly, most of the affected patients experienced an intermittent pain from several minutes to hours **(III/B)** [12].

The time before onset of symptoms after initiation of therapy differed from a mean of 1 month to a mean of 6.3, but could actually occur at any time **(III/B)** [12, 26]. Median duration of myalgia after cessation of statin therapy was 2.3 months with a range of 1 week to 4 months **(III/B)** [26].

Table 2. Muscular symptoms and site of pain in all and affected patients using high-dose statins [12].

Type of pain	% of affected patients	% of all patients
Heaviness/stiffness/cramps	57.9	6.1
Weakness and/or loss of strength during exertion, with or without other symptoms	26.6	2.8
Stiffness/cramps	13.1	1.4
Weakness/heaviness/loss of strength during exertion/stiffness/cramps	1.0	0.1
Unknown	1.4	0.15
Predominant site of pain		
Thighs/calves	25.9	2.7
All over	24.2	2.5
Calves	16.6	1.7
Thighs	9.6	1.0
Trunk	8.2	0.85
Arm/forearm	7.9	0.83
No predominant site	5.7	0.59
Unknown	2.0	0.21

Risk factors for statin myopathy include several patient characteristics, such as for instance female gender, and low BMI. In addition, statin dose and concurrent use of other medications increase the blood level of statins (Table 3) [27, 28]. Gemfibrozil, a fibric acid derivate, has demonstrated one of the highest rates of rhabdomyolysis when combined with most statins [29].

Table 3. Risk factors for statin myopathy [27].

Patient characteristics	Statin-related
Advanced age	High-dose statin therapy
Female sex	Interaction with statin metabolism
Low body mass index	• Grapefruit juice
Renal disease	Drug interactions
Kidney disease	• Fibrates
Hypothyroidism	• Cyclosporine
McArdle disease	• Azole antifungals
Metabolic muscle disease	• Macrolide antibiotics
Genetic polymorphisms	• HIV protease inhibitors
Major surgery or peri-operative period	• Nefazodone
Excessive physical activity	• Amiodarone
History of myopathy while receiving	• Verapamil
another lipid-lowering drug	• Warfarin
History of creatine kinase elevation	
Family history of myopathy	
Unexplained cramps	

In the large observational PRIMO study, patients receiving fluvastatin experienced fewer muscle symptoms than did patients receiving lovastatin, simvastatin or atorvastatin [12].

The clinical importance and the effect of quality of life in patients with statin myopathy was illustrated by the fact that 38% had symptoms that prevented moderate exertion during daily activity. In almost 4% of the affected patients, muscle symptoms were that severe to warrant confinement to bed or to stop working. Almost 40% of patients discontinued their statin or the statin dose was reduced [12].

Management of statin-related myopathy

Two guidelines exist considering screening, monitoring and management of statin-related myopathy [6, 7]. They share similarities but diverge in many aspects.

The ACC/AHA/NHLB1 guideline recommends measurement of creatine kinase prior to the initiation of statin therapy in all patients **(Ib-IV/A-C)** [6], based on clinical trials and safety data from the FDA, whereas the NLA Muscle Expert Panel does not consider a baseline creatine kinase necessary **(Ib-IV/A-C)** [7]. However, it might be useful to assess baseline creatine kinase in patients who are regarded sensitive to the myopathic side effects of statins including those with renal dysfunction, liver disease or on polypharmacy.

Neither guideline recommends routine creatine kinase measurement in asymptomatic patients who are receiving statin therapy [6, 7]. However, when the levels exceed 10 times the upper limit of normal in asymptomatic patients, the ACC/AHA/NHLB advises to discontinue the statin. Intermediate levels of 3 to 10 times the upper limit of normal should be monitored [6]. In asymptomatic hyperlipidemic patients with a high pretreatment creatine kinase, starting statin therapy did not increase these levels. Therefore, high pretreatment creatine kinase levels should not be an impediment to starting or continuing statins for reaching LDL goals **(IIa/B)** [30].

When myalgia develops in a patient, both guidelines advise to measure creatine kinase levels and compare them to baseline levels [6, 7]. The evaluation of a symptomatic patient should include measuring thyroid-stimulating hormone levels and a careful review of concomitant medications and assessment of recent physical activity **(IV/C)** [7]. When symptoms are intolerable or rhabdomyolysis develops, statins should be discontinued, regardless of creatine kinase levels. Where symptoms have disappeared, using a lower dose is an option. When muscle complaints are tolerable and creatine kinase levels are mildly elevated, statins can be continued at the current or lower dose **(IV/C)** [7]. Specific regimens are currently being investigated either using lower dosages or extended-release formulations, increased dose intervals or drug combinations including non-statins.

A flowchart considering the management of statin myopathy is depicted in Figure 2. Details of LDL reduction and the level of evidence of different strategies are illustrated in Table 4.

Low-dose regimens and extended-release formulations

Rosuvastatin in a relative low dose of 5 or 10mg daily was effective and safe in patients with a history of statin myopathy **(IIb/B)** [31]. In our own experience, and based upon earlier observations by Saku *et al* [32], regarding the efficacy of 2.5mg simvastatin daily, we frequently used very low-dose simvastatin treatment. Treatment is initiated as 2.5mg every other day or every third day and titrated upward to a tolerable dose. Approximately 60% of patients tolerate treatment and reach a mean 25% decrease in LDL-C levels at a mean daily dose of 4mg [33]. Extended-release fluvastatin 80mg was well tolerated and gave a 33% LDL-C reduction in patients with a history of muscle-related side effects with other statins **(Ib/A)** [34].

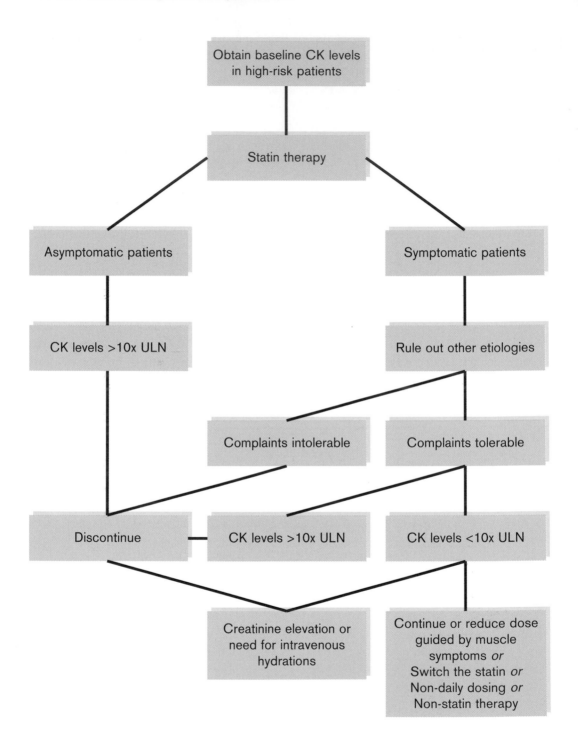

Figure 2. Flow-chart considering recommendations for monitoring statin therapy.

Table 4. Strategy for the treatment of patients intolerant of statins.

Strategy	Study	Design (level of evidence)	Investigated treatment	Number of patients	Duration	LDL reduction	Tolerability
Low-dose rosuvastatin (5-10mg/d)	Glueck et al, 2006 [31]	Prospective, open-label (IIa/B)	Rosuvastatin (5-10mg/d)	61	5mg (16 wk); 10mg (44 wk)	18% (5mg); 24% (10mg)	2%
Extended release fluvastatin	Stein et al, 2008 [34]	RCT (double blind, double dummy)(Ib/A)	Fluvastatin XL (80mg/d) vs. ezetimibe (10mg/d) vs. combination	69 (fluvastatin XL) 66 (ezetimibe) 64 (fluvastatin XL plus ezetimibe)	12 wk	33% (fluvastatin XL) 16% (ezetimibe) 46% (fluvastatin XL plus ezetimibe)	4% (fluvastatin XL) 8% (ezetimibe) 3% (fluvastatin XL plus ezetimibe)
Rosuvastatin (every 2 d)	Backes et al, 2008 [35]	Retrospective (IIb/B)	Rosuvastatin (mean dose 5.6mg)	51	4.6 mo	34.5%	20%
Rosuvastatin (3 times weekly)	Mackie et al, 2007 [36]	Case report (III/B)	Rosuvastatin (2.5mg or 5mg)	2	6 wk	20% (2.5mg); 38% (5mg)	0%
Rosuvastatin (twice weekly)	Gadarla et al, 2008 [37]	Retrospective (IIb/B)	Rosuvastatin (5 or 10mg)	30 (rosuvastatin 5mg) 10 (rosuvastatin 10mg)	3 mo	26%	20%
Rosuvastatin (once weekly)	Backes et al, 2007 [38]	Case report (III/B)	Rosuvastatin (5-20mg)	8	4 mo	29%	20%*
Ezetimibe alone or combination therapy	Gazi et al, 2007 [39]	Retrospective (IIB/B)	Ezetimibe monotherapy (10mg/d); ezetimibe add-on therapy (10mg/d)	25;12	2-3 mo; 2-3 mo	26%; 20%	0%; 17%
Ezetimibe alone or combination therapy	Stein et al, 2008 [34]	RCT (double blind, double dummy) (Ib/A)	Fluvastatin XL (80mg/d) vs. ezetimibe (10mg/d) vs. combination	69 (fluvastatin XL) 66 (ezetimibe) 64 (fluvastatin XL plus ezetimibe)	12 wk	33% (fluvastatin XL) 16% (ezetimibe) 46% (fluvastatin XL plus ezetimibe)	4% (fluvastatin XL) 8% (ezetimibe) 3% (fluvastatin XL lus ezetimibe)
Ezetimibe alone or combination therapy	Rivers et al, 2007 [40]	Retrospective (IIb/B)	Ezetimibe (10mg/d) and colesevalam (3.75g/d)	16	>3 mo	42.2%	0%
Ezetimibe alone or combination therapy	Florentin et al, 2009 [41]	Prospective, randomized, open label study (Ib/A)	Ezetimibe (10mg/d) plus orlistat (120mg 3 dd) vs ezetimibe (10mg/d) plus rimonabant (20mg/d)	15 vs. 15 (non-diabetic overweight/obese)	3 mo	28.4% vs. 15.3%	-
Red yeast rice	Becker et al, 2009 [42]	RCT (Ib/A)	Red yeast rice 1800mg vs. placebo	31 (red yeast rice) 31 placebo	24 wk	12 wk: red yeast rice: 27.3%; placebo: 5.7% 24 wk: red yeast rice: 21.3%; placebo: 8.7%	7% (red yeast rice) vs. 3.5% (placebo)

RCT = randomized controlled trial; tolerability defined as the percentage of patients who discontinued therapy because of recurrent myopathic symptoms; * whether myopathy was the cause of discontinuation is not clear.

Non-daily dosing

In a study by Backes *et al*, patients who previously experienced statin myopathy were treated with rosuvastatin 5 or 10mg on alternate days for a mean of 4.6 months. In this study, 80% experienced no recurrence of muscle symptoms on this treatment. LDL reduction was 34.5% [35]. Comparable results were found for once, twice, and three times weekly dosing [36-38].

Ezetimibe and bile acid-binding resins

Ezetimibe decreases LDL cholesterol levels by inhibiting intestinal cholesterol absorption. Bile-acid resins, such as colesevalam and cholestyramine, interrupt the enterohepatic cycle of bile acids in the terminal ileum. Although there is a lack of evidence in cardiovascular risk endpoints, the combination of ezetimibe and atorvastatin was found to reduce LDL cholesterol and was as effective as high-dose atorvastin alone [43]. In patients with statin intolerance, an LDL reduction of 20% was achieved, with good tolerability [39]. Combination therapy of ezetimibe with colesevalam in diabetic statin-intolerant patients showed a LDL reduction of 42%, without any patient discontinuing therapy because of myopathy [40]. Smaller LDL reductions were found in non-diabetic obese patients with a history of statin myopathy, treated with the combination of ezetimibe and orlistat [41]. Thus, awaiting the data from outcome trials with ezetimibe, ezetimibe alone or in combination with a resin, is an option in statin-intolerant patients.

Red yeast rice

In hyperlipidemic patiens intolerant for statins, a diet with red yeast rice was shown to be an effective therapy in managing LDL levels. However, the treatment group was small and no comparative data exist [30].

Antisense apolipoprotein B

Antisense oligonucleotides to lipoprotein B-100 are a new lipid-lowering strategy in dyslipidemic patients. Besides the effect of reducing apolipoprotein B-100 and LDL cholesterol, this compound also significantly lowers triglycerides. Although of high potential, clinical trials of longer duration are required to demonstrate further safety [44].

Coenzyme Q10 supplementation

Because there may be a depletion of coenzyme Q in statin myopathy, several studies on supplementation of this enzyme in statin-intolerant patients were performed, with alternate success in decreasing muscle pains [45, 46]. A systematic review [47] did not recommend use of coenzyme Q10 in statin myopathy, because of the lack of evidence (Ia/A).

Conclusions

The broad spectrum of statin myopathy is an important problem in daily clinical cardiovascular practice. Although major adverse events such as rhabdomyolysis are extremely rare, myalgias are encountered as frequently as 5-10% in patients receiving statins. Therefore, knowledge and management of this clinical problem is highly recommended, because withdrawing patients from statins could potentially increase cardiovascular morbidity and mortality. Management of statin intolerance includes the combination of identifying risk factors for myopathy, implementing dose and dose-schedule adjustments and switching therapy.

Key points	Evidence level
◆ Myopathy is the most important clinical problem in statin users.	
◆ Although major adverse events, such as rhabdomyolysis, are extremely rare, myalgias are encountered as frequently as in 5% to 10% of patients receiving statins.	III/B
◆ There are several risk factors for statin myopathy, being patient-related as well as statin-related.	
◆ Extended-release fluvastatin 80mg was well-tolerated and gave a 33% LDL cholesterol reduction in patients with a history of muscle-related side effects with other statins.	Ib/A
◆ Rosuvastatin in a relative low dose of 5 or 10mg daily was effective and safe in patients with a history of statin myopathy.	IIb/B
◆ Non-daily low-dose rosuvastatin is an option for intolerant patients, as is very low-dose simvastatin every other day (authors' experience).	IIb/B

References

1. Steinberg D. The statins in preventive cardiology. *N Engl J Med* 2008; 359: 1426.
2. Mitka M. Expanding statin use to help more at-risk patients is causing financial heartburn. *JAMA* 2003; 290: 2243-5.
3. Bays H. Statin safety: an overview and assesement of the data - 2005. *Am J Cardiology* 2006, 97: 6C-26.
4. Cohen DE, Anania FA, Chalasani N. An assessment of statin safety by hepatologists. *Am J Cardiol* 2006; 97 (suppl 8A): 77C-81.
5. Kordas KC, Philips PS, Golomb BA, *et al*. Clinical characteristics of 1053 patients with statin-associated muscle complaints. *Arterioscler Thromb Vasc Biol* 2004; 24: e51-136.
6. Pasternak, RC, Smith SC Jr, Bairy-Merz CN, Grundy SM, Cleeman JI, Lenfant C; American College of Cardiology. ACC/AHA/NHLBI clinical advisory on the use and safety of statins. *J Am Coll Cardiol* 2002; 40: 567-72.
7. McKenney JM, Davidson MH, Jacobson TA, Guyton JR; National Lipid Association Statin Safety Assesment Task Force. *Am J Cardiol* 2006; 97 (suppl.); 89C-94.
8. Law M, Rudnicka AR. Statin safety: a systemetic review. *Am J Cardiol* 2006; 97 (suppl): 52C-60.

9. Kashani A, Phillips CO, Foody JM, Wang Y, Mangamurti S, Ko DT, *et al*. Risk associated with statin therapy: a systematic overview of randomized clinical trials. *Circulation* 2006; 114: 2788-97.

10. Thompson PD, Clarkson P, Karas RH. Statin-associated myopathy. *JAMA* 2003; 289 (13): 1681-90.

11. Nichols GA, Koro CE. Does statin therapy initiation increase the risk for myopathy? An observational study of 32,225 diabetic and nondiabetic patients. *Clin Ther* 2007; 29: 1761-70.

12. Bruckert E, Hayem G, Dejager S, Yau C, Begand B. Mild to moderate muscular symptoms with high-dose statin therapy in hyperlipidemic patients - the PRIMO study. *Cardiovasc Drugs Ther* 2005; 19: 403-14.

13. Silva M, Matthews ML, Jarvis C, Nolan NM, Belliveau P, Malloy M, *et al*. Meta-analysis of drug-induced adverse events associated with intensive-dose statin therapy. *Clin Ther* 2007; 29: 253-60.

14. Gaist D, Rodriquez G, Huerta C *et al*. Lipid-lowering drugs and risk of myopathy - a population-based follow-up study. *Epidemiology* 2001; 12: 565-9.

15. Shanahan RL, Kerzee JA, Sandhoff BG, *et al*. Clinical Pharmacy Cardiac Risk Sevice (CPCRS) Study Group. Low myopathy rates associated with statins as monotherapy or combination therapy with interacting drugs in a group model health maintenance organization. *Pharmacotherapy* 2005; 19: 403-14.

16. Evans M, Rees A. Effects of HMG-CoA reductase inhibitors on skeletal muscle. *Drug Saf* 2002; 25: 649-63.

17. Davidson MH, Clark JA, Glass LM, Kanumalla A. Statin safety: an appraisal from the adverse event reporting system. *Am J Cardiol* 2006; 97: 32C-43.

18. Davidson MH, Stein EA, Dujovne CA, Hunninhake DB, Weiss SR, Knopp RH, Illingworth DR, Mitchel YB, Melino MR, Zupkis RV, *et al*. The efficacy and six-week tolerability of simvastatin 80 and 160mg/day. *Am J Cardiol* 1997; 79: 38-42.

19. Brewer HB. Benefit risk-assessment of rosuvastatin 10 and 40mg. *Am J Cardiol* 2003; 92: 23K-9.

20. Scandinavian Simvastatin Survival Study Group. Randomised trial of cholesterol lowering in 4444 patients with coronary heart disease: the Scandinavian Simvastatin Survival Study. *Lancet* 1994; 344: 1383-9.

21. Link E, Parish S, Armitage J, Bowman L, Heath S, Matsuda F, *et al*. SEARCH Collaborative Group. CO1B1 variants and statin-induced myopathy - a genomewide study. *N Engl J Med* 2008; 359: 789-99.

22. Voora D, Shah SH, Spasojevic I, Ali S, Reed CR, Salisbury BA, Ginsburg GS. The SLCO1B1*5 genetic variant is associated with statin-induced side effects. *J Am Coll Cardiol* 2009; 54(17): 1609-16.

23. König J, Seithel A, Gradhand U, Fromm MF. Pharmacogenomics of human OATP transporters. *Naunyn Schmiedebergs Arch Pharmacol* 2006; 372: 432-43.

24. Sirvent P, Mercier J, Lacampagne A. New insights into the mechanisms of statin-associated myotoxicity. *Curr Opin Pharmacol* 2008; 8: 333-8.

25. Kordas KC, Phillips PS, Golomb BA, *et al*. Clinical characteristics of 1053 patients with statin-associated muscle complaints. *Arterioscler Thromb Vasc Biol* 2004; 24: e51-136.

26. Hansen KE, Hildebrand JP, Ferguson EE, *et al*. Outcomes in 45 patients with statin-induced myopathy. *Arch Intern Med* 2005; 165: 2671-6.

27. Joy TR, Hegele RA. Narrative review: statin-related myopathy. *Ann Intern Med* 2009; 150: 858-68.

28. Harper CR, Jacobson TA. The broad sectrum of statin myopathy: from myalgia to rhabdomyolysis. *Curr Opin Lipidol* 2007; 18: 401-8.

29. Wu J, Song Y, Li H, Chen J. Rhabdomyolysis associated with fibrate therapy: review of 76 published cases and a new case report. *Eur J Clin Pharmacol* 2009; (65)12: 1169-74.

30. Glueck CJ, Rawal B, Khan NA, Yeramaneni S, Goldenberg N, Wang P. Should high creatine kinase discourage the initiation or continuance of statins for the treatment of hypercholesterolemia? *Metabolism* 2009; 58(2): 233-8.

31. Glueck CJ, Aregawi D, Agloria M, Khalil Q, Winiarska M, Munjal J, *et al*. Rosuvastatin 5 and 10mg/d: a pilot study of the effects in hypercholesterolemic adults unable to tolerate other statins and reach LDL cholesterol goals wih non-statin lipid-lowering therapies. *Clin Ther* 2006; 28: 933-42.

32. Saku K, Sasaki J, Arakawa K. Low-dose effect of simvastatin (MK-733) on serum lipids, lipoproteins, and apolipoproteins, in patients with hypercholesterolemia. *Clin Ther* 1989; 11(2): 247-57.

33. De Greef LE, Opdam FL, Teepe-Twiss I, Jukema JW, Guchelaar HJ, Tamsma JT. The tolerability and efficacy of low-dose simvastatin in statin-intolerant patients. *Eur J Intern Med* 2010; in press.

34. Stein EA, Ballantyne CM, Windler E, Sirnes PA, Sussekov A, Yigit Z, *et al*. Efficacy and tolerability of fluvastatin XL 80mg alone, ezetimibe alone, and the comination of fluvastatin XL 80mg with ezetimibe in patients with a history of muscle-related side effects with other statins. *Am J Cardiol* 2008; 101: 490-6.

35. Backes JM, Venero CV, Gibson CA, Ruisinger JF, Howard PA, Thompson PD, *et al*. Effectiveness and tolerability of every-other-day rosuvastatin dosing in patients with prior statin intolerance. *Ann Pharmacother* 2008; 42: 341-6.

36. Mackie BD, Satija S, Nell C, Miller J 3rd, Sperling LS. Monday, Wednesday, and Friday dosing of rosuvastatin in patients previously intolerant to statin therapy. *Am J Cardiol* 2007; 99: 291.

37. Gadarla M, Kearns AK, Thompson PD. Efficacy of rosuvastatin (5mg and 10mg) twice a week in patients intolerant to daily statins. *Am J Cardiol* 2008; 101(12): 1747-8.

38. Backes JM, Moriarty PM, Ruisinger JF, Gibson CA. Effects of once-weekly rosuvastatin among patients with prior statin intolerance. *Am J Cardiol* 2007; 100: 554-5.

39. Gazi IF, Daskalopoulou SS, Nair DS, Mikhailidis DP. Effect of ezetimibe in patients who cannot tolerate statins or cannot get to the low density lipoprotein cholesterol target despite taking a statin. *Curr Med Res Opin* 2007; 23: 2183-92.

40. Rivers SM, Kane MP, Busch RS, Bakst G, Hamilton RA. Colesevalam hydrochloride-ezetimibe combination lipid-lowering therapy in patients with diabetes or metabolic syndrome and a history of statin intolerance. *Endocr Pract* 2007; 13: 11-16.

41. Florentin M, Kostapanos MS, Nakou ES, Elisaf M, Liberopoulos EM. Efficacy and safety of ezetimibe plus orlistat or rimonabant in statin-intolerant nondiabetic overweight/obese patients with dyslipidemia. *J Cardiovasc Ther* 2009; 14(4): 274-82.

42. Becker DJ, Gordon RY, Halbert SC, French B, Morris PB, Rader DJ. Red yeast rice for dyslipidemia in statin-intolerant patients: a randomized trial. *Ann Intern Med* 2009; (150) 12: 830-9, W147-9.

43. Ballantyne CM, Houri J, Notarbartalo A, Melani L, Lipka LJ, Suresh R, *et al*. Ezetimibe study group. Effect of ezetimibe coadministerd with atorvastatin in 628 patients with primary hypercholeaterolemia: a prospective, randomized, double-blind trial. *Circulation* 2003; 107: 2409-15.

44. Akdim F, Stroes ES, Kastelein JJ. Antisense apolipoprotein B therapy: where do we stand? *Curr Opin Lipidol* 2007; 18(4): 397-400.

45. Caso G, Kelly P, McNurlan MA, Lawson WE. Effect of coenzyme Q10 on myopathic symptoms in patients treated with statins. *Am J Cardiol* 2007; 99: 1409-12.

46. Young JM, Florkowski CM, Molyneux SL, McEwan RG, Frampton CM, George PM, *et al*. Effect of coenzyme Q10 supplementation on simvastatin-induced myalgia. *Am J Cardiol* 2007; 100: 1400-3.

47. Maroff L, Thompson PD The role of coenzyme Q10 in statin-associated myopathy: a systematic review. *J Am Coll Cardiol* 2007; 49: 2231-37.

Index

abetalipoproteinemia (ABL) 52, 60-1, 65
ACCORD trial (Action to Control Cardiovascular Risk in Diabetes) 101, 103, 117, 153
ACE inhibitors 174
acetaminophen 189
Achilles tendon xanthomas 252, 258, 259
adipokines 146-7
adiponectin 147-8
adipose tissue 145-8, 154-5
adolescents 126, 132, 219
ADOPT trial (Diabetes Outcome Progression Trial) 153
AFREGS trial (Armed Forces Regression Study) 80
age
      CHD mortality risk 27
      treatment initiation 5-7, 35
AHA (American Heart Association) pediatric guidelines 126-7
alcohol use 78
ALERT trial (Assessment of Lescol in Renal Transplantation) 173
alpha-methylacyl-CoA racemase (AMACR) deficiency 240, 244-5, 247
AMORIS study (Apolipoprotein Mortality Risk) 31, 33, 35
α-amyrin 41, 43
anacetrapib 63, 86, 209-10
anakinra 235, 237
ankylosing spondylitis 186
anticoagulant drugs 277
antifungal drugs 275
antihypertensive drugs 174, 191
antiretroviral drugs 130, 275
antisense oligonucleotides 57, 102, 209, 294
APCSC meta-analysis (Asia Pacific Cohort Studies Collaboration) 26, 31
apheresis 56-7, 136, 209, 260
apolipoprotein AI (apoAI) 17, 32-5, 75, 185
    deficiency 62
    mimetic peptides 84, 85
apolipoprotein B (apoB)
    apoB100 13, 167
    CVD risk and 32-5, 115, 116, 150, 185
    in FCH 112
    mutations 53, 129